MYASTHENIA GRAVIS

T0271983

H.J.G.H. OOSTERHUIS

Myasthenia Gravis

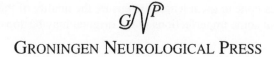

GRONINGEN NEUROLOGICAL PRESS

Transferred to Digital Printing 2010

Groningen Neurological Press
Neurological Department Academic Hospital Groningen
Hanzeplein 1, Postbus 30.001, 9700 RB Groningen
Fax 31.50.3611707

Made in Groningen, the Netherlands
Design: Imelda de Valk, Groningen

ISBN 90-9010600-6
NUGI 742

Publisher's Note
The publisher has gone to great lengths to ensure the quality of this reprint
but points out that some imperfections in the original may be apparent.

PREFACE

The idea to write this book emerged when I was writing a chapter for the *Liber Amicorum* for one of my scientific friends. When it was offered to him, he admitted that he had ambivalent feelings: so many people had been persuaded to do a substantial piece of work that would not be read afterwards except by himself. I shared his feelings.

I therefore decided to write a *Liber Amicis*, as an acknowledgement to so many colleagues who had referred their patients to me, thereby helping me to become an expert.

Most professionals at the end of their carriers are seized by the feeling that their knowledge and experience has suddenly become superfluous and will soon be forgotten. This *'horror vacui'* has been another reason to write down what I learned from a long follow-up of a large number of myasthenic patients. They were my best teachers. I like to thank those who gave me permission to publish their unflattering photographs. I have described the histories of some patients in detail. This will give a better idea of the problems that had to be solved than theoretical considerations only.

Because I have written before on this subject, the text of this book is not entirely new. Chapter 2 and parts of other chapters will remind some readers of my previous book on Myasthenia Gravis (1984) which is out of sale. The illustration 1.6, 1.8-1.10, 2.3-2.6, 2.9-2.12, 2.14, 2.16-2.19, 3.5-3.9 were also used in various chapters of Myasthenia gravis, Ed M. de Baets and H.J.G.H. Oosterhuis, CRC Press Broca Raton U.S.A. 1993; I acknowledge the Publishers for their permission to use them in this book.

Jan Kuks was my reliable and critical companion in the care for myasthenic patients and in the scientific work and contributed largely to the clinical data in the last then years.

I had the invaluable help of Imelda de Valk who made the design and the eventual lay-out of the text.

I owe many thanks to Marc de Baets, clinical immunologist, Han van der Hoeven, clinical neurophysiologist, Chris Höweler, neurologist, Frans Jennekens, neurologist, Jan Kuks, neurologist and Peter Molenaar, neurophysiologist for their comments upon and corrections of the concepts of my text. They also allowed me the use of illustrations of their work.

A also thank Tineke Bysitter for secretarial work, Coen Dobma for making photographs and drawings and Jelly Slager for preparing part of the text.

CONTENTS

PREFACE AND ACKNOWLEDGEMENTS

LIST OF ABBREVIATIONS

1 A SHORT HISTORY OF MYASTHENIA GRAVIS   1
   1.1 The birth of a disease   1
   1.2 Thymus abnormalities and muscle lymphorrhages   4
   1.3 Early aetrological concepts and therapies   5
   1.4 New medical treatments   5
   1.5 Thymectomy   7
   1.6 Pathophysiology   9
   1.7 Autoimmunity   9
       Notes   15

2 CLINICAL ASPECTS AND EPIDEMIOLOGY   17
   2.1 Definition and classification   17
   2.2 Symptoms and signs   18
       2.2.1 Ocular symptoms   18
       2.2.2 Bulbar symptoms   26
       2.2.3 Limb and trunk symptoms   30
       2.2.4 Muscle atrophy   33
   2.3 Clinical scoring and quantified tests   34
   2.4 The course of the disease   35
   2.5 External influences   38
   2.6 Epidemiology   38
       2.6.1 Incidence and prevalence   38
       2.6.2 Age, gender and classification   39
       2.6.3 Death rates   40
       2.6.4 The incidence of thymomas in MG   41
       2.6.5 The incidence of autoimmune diseases in MG   41
       2.6.6 Genetic predisposition   43
   2.7 Myasthenia gravis in childhood   43
       2.7.1 Neonatal MG in children with a myasthenic mother   43
       2.7.2 Congenital myasthenic syndromes   45
       2.7.3 Acquired infantile MG   47
       Notes   48

3 DIAGNOSIS   49
   3.1 Clinical criteria and diagnostic tests   49
   3.2 Clinical assessment   50
   3.3 Diagnostic procedures   53
        3.3.1 Reaction to anticholinesterases   53
        3.3.2 Antibodies to acetylcholine receptor protein (AChR-Ab)   55
        3.3.3 Electromyography   57
        3.3.4 Antimuscle antibodies   60
        3.3.5 Unspecific antibodies   61
   3.4 Human leucocytic antigens (HLA)   62
   3.5 The diagnosis of thymoma and residual thymus   63
   3.6 Summary of diagnostic strategy   65
   Notes   66

4 TREATMENTS   68
   4.1 General remarks   68
   4.2 Anticholinesterases (anti-AChE)   69
   4.3 Drugs to be used with caution   74
   4.4 Thymectomy   75
        4.4.1 Patients without thymoma   75
        4.4.2 Patients with a thymoma   78
   4.5 Immunosuppressive drugs   79
        4.5.1 Corticosteroids and azathioprine   79
        4.5.2 Details of treatment   82
        4.5.3 Management of crisis   86
   4.6 Plasmapheresis and immunoabsorption   88
   4.7 Other immunosuppressive drugs and measures   90
        4.7.1 Cyclosporine (CSA)   90
        4.7.2 Cyclophosphamide, methotrexate, 6-mercaptopurine   90
        4.7.3 Antilymphocyte globulines   91
        4.7.4 Partial or total body irradiation   91
        4.7.5 Intravenous immunoglobulins   91
   4.8 Physical therapy and speech therapy   92
   4.9 Psychological aspects   93
        4.9.1 Reaction to a chronic illness   93
        4.9.2 Uncertain doctors   94
        4.9.3 Communication problems   95
        4.9.4 Central nervous system involvement?   96
        4.9.5 Possible effect of medications   96
        4.9.6 MG is not a lifelong disease   97
   Notes   97

5 EIGHT HUNDRED PATIENTS 1960-1994 · · · 100

5.1 Patients and methods · · · 100
5.2 General features of the 4 subgroups · · · 101
    5.2.1 Epidemiology · · · 101
    5.2.2 Diagnosis · · · 102
    5.2.3 Severity and death · · · 103
    5.2.4 AChR-Ab and AMA · · · 104
    5.2.5 Muscle atrophy · · · 106
    5.2.6 Associated autoimmune diseases · · · 110
    5.2.7 Other associated diseases · · · 110
5.3 Ocular Myasthenia (OMG) · · · 114
    5.3.1 Diagnosis · · · 114
    5.3.2 Epidemiology · · · 115
    5.3.3 Clinical signs · · · 115
    5.3.4 Treatments · · · 118
5.4 Early onset MG · · · 121
    5.4.1 Epidemiology · · · 121
    5.4.2 Thymectomy vs natural course · · · 122
    5.4.3 Pre- and postoperative management · · · 124
    5.4.4 Anti-AChE and IS therapies · · · 127
    5.4.5 Pregnancy and neonatal MG · · · 131
    5.4.6 Infantile MG · · · 131
5.5 Late onset MG · · · 132
    5.5.1 Epidemiology · · · 132
    5.5.2 Therapies · · · 132
    5.5.3 Side effects of immunosuppressive treatment · · · 133
5.6 Patients with a thymoma · · · 137
    5.6.1 Epidemiology · · · 137
    5.6.2 Outcome of treatment · · · 139
5.7 Congenital myasthenic syndromes · · · 143
5.8 Short summary · · · 151
    5.8.1 General features · · · 151
    5.8.2 Ocular MG (OMG) · · · 152
    5.8.3 Early onset MG (EOMG) · · · 152
    5.8.4 Late onset MG (LOMG) · · · 153
    5.8.5 Patients with thymoma (TH) · · · 153
    5.8.6 Congenital myasthenic syndromes (CMS) · · · 153
Notes · · · 154

6 DIFFERENTIAL DIAGNOSIS   157
   6.1 False negative and false positive diagnosis   157
   6.2 Diseases and syndromes with ocular signs and symptoms   158
   6.3 Diseases with bulbar symptoms and signs   165
   6.4 Diseases with weakness of the limb and trunk muscles   165
   6.5 The Lambert-Eaton myasthenic syndrome   166
   6.6 The chronic fatigue syndrome   169
   Notes   171

7 EPILOGUE   172
   7.1 History   172
   7.2 Pathophysiology   173
   7.3 Autoimmunity   175
   7.4 The role of the thymus   177
   7.5 Different types of acquired MG and their treatments   178
       7.5.1 Four different types   178
       7.5.2 Thymectomy   179
       7.5.3 IS therapies   182
   7.6 Becoming an expert   183

REFERENCES   185

LIST OF EUROPEAN PATIENTS ASSOCIATIONS   239

INDEX   243

ABBREVIATIONS

Ab	antibody, antibodies
ACh	acetylcholine
AChR	acetylcholine receptor
AChR-Ab	antibodies to the AChR
A.I.	autoimmune
AMA	anti-muscle antibodies
ANA	anti-nuclear antibodies
anti-AChE	anticholinesterases
AZA	azathioprine
CMAP	compound muscle action potential
CMS	congenital myasthenic syndrome
COPD	chronic obstructive pulmonary disease
CPSC	congenital paucity of synaptic clefts
DS	disability score
EMG	electromyography
EOMG	early onset MG
IS	immunosuppressive
LEMS	Lambert-Eaton myasthenic syndrome
LOMG	late onset MG
M	man
MG	myasthenia gravis, myasthenic
NMT	neuromuscular transmission
OMG	ocular myasthenia gravis
PP	plasmapheresis
PR	prednisone
SFEMG	single fibre EMG
SNMG	seronegative MG (without AChR-Ab)
TH	thymoma
W	woman

N.B.: Notes are indicated in the text with superscript numbers.

1

A Short History of Myasthenia Gravis

1.1 The birth of a disease

On the seventh of January 1895, the German neurologist Friedrich Jolly (1844-1904) proposed a name for a newly emerged disease of which, at that time, 15 cases seemed to be described. He added two cases of his own (1).

The most prominent signs were the inabiltiy to articulate and to swallow, but also drooping of the upper eyelids, eye muscle pareses and weakness of the neck and limb muscles could occur. The disease presented itself in young and middle-aged people, with a sudden onset and progression, although remissions of the symptoms were also reported. More than half of these patients had died in attacks of choking and dyspnoe. **(Fig. 1.1)**

The first patients were reported by Wilhelm Heinrich Erb (1840-1921). He had seen his patients in 1868, '70 and '71. In his paper from 1879 (2) he argues that they seemed to have a bulbar paresis, but their signs and the course of their illness did not fit quite well with the features of the chronic (Amyotrophic lateral sclerosis) or the apoplectic pseudo-bulbar paresis, known at that time. All 3 patients had ptosis of the upper eye lids, weakness of the neck muscles, an inability to chew and a mild or severe weakness of the limb muscles. Although not emphasized in the discussion, it is obvious from the description that the symptoms and signs were fluctuating. One of them, a 30-year-old woman, also had an external ophthalmoplegia and developed difficulties in swallowing and coughing. She suddenly died, but there was no autopsy. One of the male patients recovered during a course of galvano-therapy. The follow-up of these patients was only six months to one year.

In the years between 1877 and 1892 several cases with a similar clinical picture were described (3-11). These patients all had died in a rather short time by sudden respiratory insuffiency. In 6 out of 8 cases there was an autopsy, but no abnormalities in the brain stem or cerebrum were found. Oppenheim (5) referred to his case as "Bulbärparalyse ohne anatomische Befund".

In 1893 Samuel Goldflam (1852-1932), neurologist in Warsaw, reported

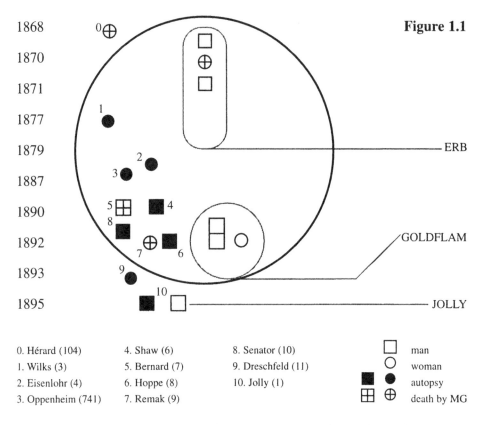

Figure 1.1

1868	0 ⊕
1870	
1871	
1877	1
1879	ERB
1887	2, 3
1890	5, 8, 4
1892	7, 6 · GOLDFLAM
1893	9
1895	10 · JOLLY

0. Hérard (104)	4. Shaw (6)	8. Senator (10)	□	man
1. Wilks (3)	5. Bernard (7)	9. Dreschfeld (11)	○	woman
2. Eisenlohr (4)	6. Hoppe (8)	10. Jolly (1)	■ ●	autopsy
3. Oppenheim (741)	7. Remak (9)		⊞ ⊕	death by MG

Schematic presentation of the cases described between 1877 and 1895 leading, to the concept of myasthenia gravis as a new disease. The large circle comprises the cases that Goldflam included in his analysis. The first clinical description retrospectively recognized as MG was that of Herard in 1868 (case 0).

another 3 patients with the same signs, but with a less progressive course. He also analysed the previous case reports and emphasized the fluctuation of the signs and the spontaneous remissions and exacerbations. He entitled his paper as "Ueber ein scheinbar heilbares bulbärparalytischen Symptomencomplex mit Beteiligung der Extremitäten" (12). It was his merit to recognize the similarity of his cases and the already reported ones. From his later reports (13) the notion "heilbar" (curable) appeared to have been too optimistic: his two male patients died 2 and 9 years after onset from the disease while the woman was suffering from severe dyspnoe attacks. He speculated that the disease was caused by a toxic substance working on the central nervous system.[1]

Jolly had read his paper one month earlier in a meeting of the Berlin medical society. He reported 2 new cases of young men who underwent an extensive examination of their muscles with a faradic electric current. These muscles did not show any signs of denervation, but repeated stimulation diminished the force of muscle contractions, which was restored after a period of rest. **(Fig. 1.2)** Although Jolly was not aware of the cause of the exhaustability, he argued that the disease could best be named according to the asthenia of the muscle, which shoud be called "pseudo-paralytic", since no anatomical lesions were found. Therefore he proposed the name: "<u>Myasthenia gravis pseudo-paralytica"</u> <u>(M.G.)</u>. This name was further supported by Cohn in 1897 (14) and finally accepted after a discussion of the proms - a consensus meeting - of the Berlin Society of Psychiatry and Neurology in 1899 (15).[2]

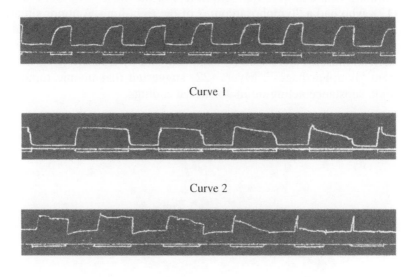

Curve 1

Curve 2

Curve 3

Figure 1.2   Reaction of Jolly from his original paper. (1) Mechanogram during tetanic stimulation of the muscle: 1. tibialis anterior muscle of a healthy man; 2. tibialis anterior muscle of a myasthenic patient; 3. vastus internus muscle of a myasthenic patient

In the next years the disease became more and more recognized. In 1900, Campbell and Bramwell could review 60 cases, 26 of which had proved fatal (16). In 1912 Starr (17) analysed 250 already reported cases, 45% of which were fatal; in 28% an "enlargement" of the thymus was mentioned.
The first Dutch case was described by Van Wayenburg in 1901 (18).[3]

1.2 Thymus abnormalities and muscle lymphorrhages

Although the new disease seemed to lack anatomical abnormalities, at least in the central nervous system, one abnormal finding was noticed: some patients had a tumor of the thymus and if there was no tumor the thymus seemed to be enlarged. Another remarkable finding was the presence of lymphorrhagic infiltrates in the muscles. **(Fig, 1.3)** In 1901 Weigert (19) described a patient who had a thymoma at autopsy. Weigert considered these infiltrates as metastases of the thymoma.

Similar infiltrates were reported in five of the muscles of Goldflam's first case (12), who had a "lymphosarcoma" of the right lung. A tumor situated near the bronchial tree was found by Hoppe (8), and Oppenheim (5) had reported a sarcoma of the thymus. Round cell infiltrations in eye muscles and several skeletal muscles were seen by Link (20) and by Buzzard (21), who coined the term "lymphorrhages". Myers (22) suggested that thymic tumors produce a toxic substance acting on motor-nerve endings.

Figure 1.3

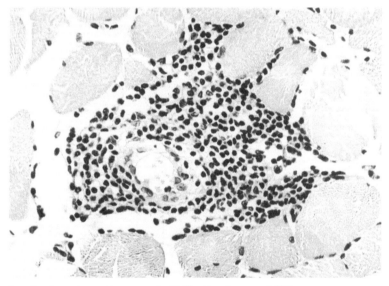

Lymphorrhages in quadriceps muscle. M 60 with a thymoma (x300).

In 1917 Bell (23) reviewed 56 autopsies on MG patients since 1901: in 10 a tumor was found and in another 17 an enlargement of the thymus. At that time the thymus was considered an endocrine gland that activated the thyroid gland. In 1912 Sauerbruch (24) resected the thymus of a young woman with hyperthyroidism and MG. The MG disappeared but the hyperthyroidism persisted and had to be attacked later by a partial thyroidectomy.

1.3 Early aetiological concepts and therapies

The prevailing ideas on the aetiology of MG comprised bacterial toxins, an endocrine disturbance or a substance from the thymus which in the late 1930s and in the 1940s was deemed to be curariform. Neither extracts of thymus tissue from MG patients nor even from foetal whale (25), nor serum of MG patients (26) had convincing and reproducible effects in animals or on neuro-muscular preparations.

Early therapies reflect the general therapeutic endeavours that were undertaken in mental and nervous diseases. A review in 1927 (27) mentioned tonics such as arsenic, phosphorus, quinine and iron, strychnine; or high intake of carbohydrates, albumine or calcium. Also extracts of various endocrine organs including the thymus, the adrenals and the testis were recommended. Electrotherapy (faradism) and the use of hypnotics and anaesthetics were discouraged. In some patients radio-active thorium or irradiation of the mediastinum was tried without systematic evaluation of the outcome.

Beween 1943 and 1960 bilateral sinus caroticus denervation was reported to be useful in young patients, especially by French authors (28), but the results were never convincing (29).

1.4 New medical treatments

The first real therapy was found by chance by a female physician, Harriet Edgeworth, who had a moderate, fluctuating MG herself for years. In 1930 she took ephedrine for relieving her menstrual cramps and noticed an improvement of her ptosis and dysarthria. She subjected herself to a monoblind experiment with a placebo, which confirmed her initial impression (30, 31).

The real therapeutic breakthrough came in 1934, when Mary Walker, a young resident in St Alfege's Hospital near London, tried physostigmine, because the resemblance between MG and curare-intoxication, to which physostigmine was known as an antidote. (Fig. 1.4)[4]

The patient showed a partial but convincing improvement (fig. 1.5), which was specific and could not be produced by the several other substances she tried (32). A year later the same results were achieved with prostigmine (33), which has no effect on the central nervous system and also less peripheral side effects. Besides it could be given orally. This drug brought about a revolution in the treatment of MG, and the neurologist who gives the first neostigmine injection to a newly diagnosed patient will even now be admired as a miracle doctor.

In 1952 a very short-acting anti-cholinesterase, edrophonium-Cl (Tensilon®) was introduced, mainly as a diagnostic test (34). In 1954 pyridostigmine-Br (Mestinon®) (35) and in 1955 ambenomium-Cl (Mytelase®) (36) became available, with a longer action than prostigmin and less parasympathetic side effects.

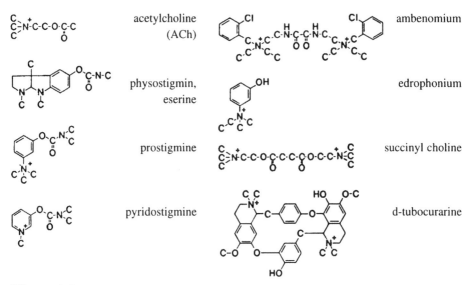

acetylcholine
(ACh)

ambenomium

physostigmin,
eserine

edrophonium

prostigmine

succinyl choline

pyridostigmine

d-tubocurarine

Figure 1.4 Structure of drugs acting on the neuro-muscular transmission. Note the positively charged (N+) quaternary-onium groups, which are partly responsible for the specific action. Only eserine (physostigmine) is a tertiary ammonium base.

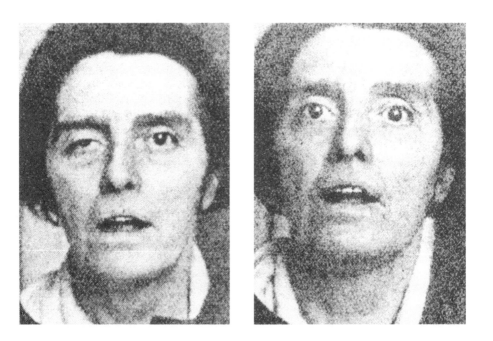

Figure 1.5 Effect of physostigmine on the ptosis in a myasthenic patient. From the original paper of Mary Walker (32).

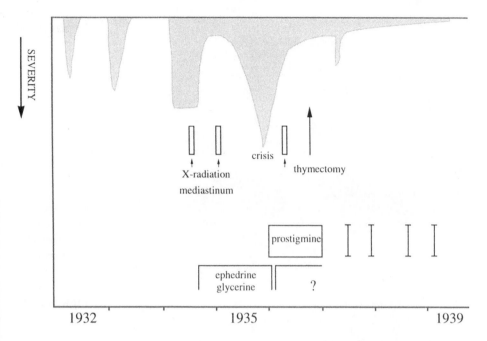

Figure 1.6 Reconstruction of the history of the patient operated on by Blalock (40). Since the age of 16 she suffered from increasingly severe periods of MG. She had received two courses of radiation therapy. In the last period of exacerbation, her life was saved by prostigmine and artificial respiration. The operation took place under intra-tracheal anaesthesia. A 6x5x3 cm cystic and necrotic thymoma was removed, without residual thymus tissue. She recovered without complications from the operation, and the MG improved substantially within a few months. Three years later she was in almost complete remission.

1.5 Thymectomy

The presence of an effective drug, and the improvement of anaesthesia made thymectomy possible. In 1936 Blalock, a surgeon in Baltimore (John Hopkins), operated a young woman with a cystic thymus tumor which had been irradiated previously without effect on the MG. (**Fig. 1.6**) He reported the beneficial effect 3 years later, (37) and decided in 1941 somewhat illogically, to remove also non-tumorous thymuses. However, his decision was later justified by the finding that 7 out of 10 thymuses showed an abnormal histological pattern: the presence of germinal centres (38). (**Fig. 1.7 a and 1.7 b**) The results of his next 20 cases, including 2 thymoma's, were that 3 patients were cured, 5 of them improved considerably, 5 improved moderately, 3 did not respond and 4 died, of whom 3 after the operation (39).

In England the first patient was operated on in 1942 by Sir Geoffrey Keynes, on request of the neurologist Carmichael. Keynes had much experience in thyroid surgery, but had never seen the thymus as he later admitted in his

Figure 1.7a

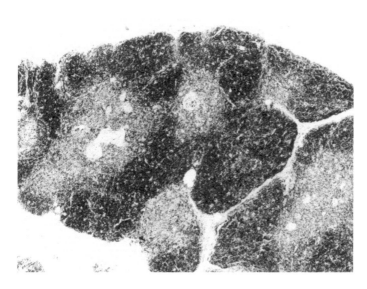

Normal thymus:
(F20):
Cortex : medulla =
1 : 1.
Hassal's corpuscules
in the medulla
(x60).

Figure 1.7b

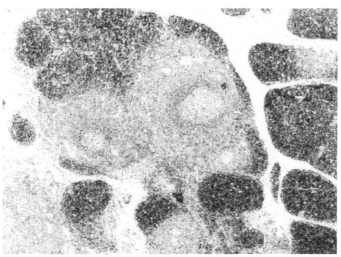

Thymus from MG
patient (F 23):
Cortex : medulla =
1:10.
Large germinal
centres in the
medulla.
About 20% fat
(x56).

memoires (41). The operation on a 37-year-old woman resulted in a complete remission within 7 months. Such a favourable result was of paramount importance to proceed. Between 1942 and 1956 he operated upon 281 patients and he became much involved in the further treatment and follow-up of his patients. However, the results were good in young patients without thymoma's, of whom one third were cured and one third much improved. The results in patients with thymoma's were equivocal. Of his first 21 patients, 8 died, mainly postoperatively, but of the next 30 only 1 died. He emphasized the eminent importance of good postoperative care and a good preparation of the patient before operation, which still holds true (42). Keynes' thymectomy series was compared with non-operated control patients by Simpson (43) who concluded that thymectomy was of substantial benefit, particularly in young patients without thymoma if the MG existed no longer than 5 years.

The effect of thymectomy was initially questioned by American investigators but later confirmed when the less successful thymoma cases were analysed separately. Although no prospective randomised clinical trials have been performed, thymectomy is since the 60s generally considered as the therapy of choice in young onset MG with generalized (i.e. not only ocular) signs. In patients with thymoma's, the operation is indicated because of the potential invasive growth of the tumor (44).

1.6 Pathophysiology

The pathophysiology of MG was since 1934 considered a disturbance of neuro-muscular transmission. This was confirmed by the observation in 1942 that patients with MG are hypersensitive to d-tubocurarine (45). (Curare was since the work of Claude Bernard in 1865 (46) known to be active at this site.) In 1941 Harvey and Masland (47) introduced a refined 'Jolly'-test, showing that the muscle contraction declined by repetitive stimulation of the afferent nerve. The real site of the deficit: presynaptic, synaptic or postsynaptic and the role of a posssible circulating 'curariform' substance was still a matter of conjecture in the 1950s and 1960s. The resistance to intra-arterially administered acetylcholine, although technically difficult, was in favour of a postsynaptic disturbance (48). However, some features comparable with the action of hemicholinium, which impaires the re-uptake of cholinium, were arguments in favour of the presynaptic site (49). This controversy could not be resolved convincingly at the time by histological investigations. in 1962 and 1966 EM pictures of the endplates in intercostal muscles of MG patients and of a myasthenic dog (50, 51) showed postsynaptic changes of the secondary clefts and normal presynaptic nerve endings. These findings were amply confirmed and extended in 1971 (52). In 1973 Fambrough et al (53) demonstrated that the number of acetylcholine receptors at the postsynaptic membrane were considerably reduced, thus combining the morphological and physiological deficits.

1.7 Autoimmunity

In 1959 Smithers in a paper on thyroid tumors suggested that MG might be an autoimmune disease, sometimes associated with neoplasms (57). The suggestion that the pathophysiology of MG could be explained by an autoimmune mechanism, was made in 1960 by the Scottish neurologist

Simpson (58) and independently by Nastuk et al. (59).

Simpson had noticed in a large series of patients the relatively high incidence of concomitant diseases, especially rheumatoid arthritis and disorders of the blood and reticulo-endothelial system. His other arguments were the abnormalities of the thymus, which were at that time discovered of immunological importance (60), the presence of lymphorrhages in muscles, the fluctuating course of the disease, the predominance of women and the occurrence of neonatal MG in children of myasthenic mothers (61). Nastuk and his co-workers (59) had observed that the sera of some MG patients damaged the muscle membrane of the nerve-muscle preparation in their experiments. In search of possible immunological factors they found that serum complement factors were lower during clinical exacerbations than in a clinical remission (62). Simpson expected that an antibody to end-plate protein might be found (58), although the efforts of his own team in this respect were in vain.

A serum globulin fraction that bound to skeletal muscle components and fixed complement was demonstrated by Strauss et al in 1960 (63). Van der Geld (64) demonstrated in a series of my patients that these antibodies also reacted with certain cells in the thymus, which later appeared to be myoid cells (65). (**Fig. 1.8**)

These antibodies were present in 38% of 125 MG patients, compared with 2% in controls and in 100% of the 15 thymoma patients included (66). They were directed against membrane components of striated muscle but obviously not to the end plate zone. Also antinuclear and antithyroid antibodies were increased in the MG patients as compared with matched controls (67), but a firm relation to the pathophysiology of the disease remained enigmatic.

These abnormal immunological findings stimulated the use of immunosuppressive therapies. In the 1950s, the initial exacerbation of myasthenic weakness, following adrenocorticotropic hormone (ACTH) and corticosteroids (68) causing respiratory crises and even death led to the abandonment of these therapies. But in 1965 Von Reis et al (69) reported that ACTH, after an initial deterioration, freed patients from the respirator after 10 days. The beneficial effect of azathioprine in 5 patients was reported by Delwaide et al in 1967 (70) and independently in a large series by Mertens et al in 1969 (71). The usefulness of alternate day prednison was described in 1970 in one patient (72) and soon thereafter confirmed by many clinicians.

The reason why hemodialysis (73, 74) and thoracic lymph drainage (75) caused a transient improvement, was later explained by the discovery of circulating antibodies to acetyl-choline receptor, (AChR), at the postsynaptic membrane in the majority of MG patients (76). The detection of these antibodies became technically possible by the isolation and purification of the AChR protein with the use of snake venoms that have a high and specific affinity for these receptors (77). Serum globulin of MG patients was able to inhibit the binding of alpha-bungarotoxin (alpha-BTX) to the AChR (77a). The reduction of AChR-s in myasthenic muscles could be visualized with [125]I-

Figure 1.8

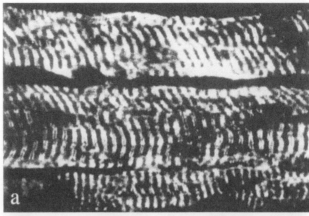

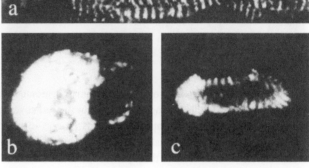

Rat diaphragm incubated
with serum from a MG
patient.
a. Indirect fluorescence
technique. (64)
b, c. Calf thymus incubated
with the same serum:
thymic myoid cell
fluorescence (x 900).

labeled alpha-BTX (78). The IgG of the serum of MG patients enhanced the degradation of AChR's in cultured muscle membranes and further experiments showed that this was caused by cross-linking of two AChR's by one IgG molecule (79). This degradation and final destruction of the AChR's appeared to be medated by complement factors which could be demonstraed by histofluorescence studies. The localization of the membrane attack complex at the postsynaptic membrane involves activation of lytic phase of the complement reaction. The pathogenetic role of these AChR-Ab antibodies was further demonstrated by the passive transfer to recipient mice, which developed muscle weakness and a failure of neuromuscular transmission (81). The simultaneous development of an experimental autoimmune model of MG in animals, following immunization with AChR derived from the electric eel, has given insight into the mechanisms, by which AChR-Ab antibodies cause muscular weakness and into possible new therapies (82). However, in these models thymic abnormalities do not occur, so that they do not mimick an important aspect of the human disease. The role of the thymus in the development of MG is still uncertain, although much more has been discovered about the microenvironment of the thymus and the dynamics of T and B cells. (83). Specific (i.e. AChR-reacting) T-helper cells can be demonstrated in the MG-thymus and in the peripheral blood, which stimulate specific B cells to

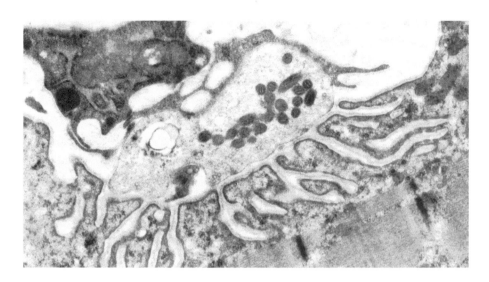

Figure 1.9 a Electronmicrograph of a human neuromuscular junction. The Schwann cell cytoplasm is dense in this micrograph. The Schwann cell covers the nerve terminal. The latter is easily recognizable by its synaptic vesicles. A process of this Schwann cell protrudes in the primary synaptic cleft. The basal membrane in the secondary clefts is split into two layers. The secondary clefts reach close to the myofibrils. Bar = 1 μm.

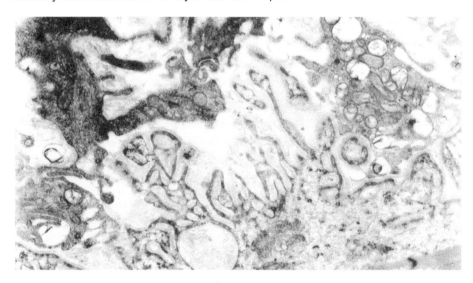

Figure 1.9 b Electronmicrographs of endplate from a patient with myasthenia gravis and circulating antibodies against acetylcholine receptors. The secondary folds are degenerated: they are abnormally irregular, unusually slender, or retracted in comparison to 1.9 a. Bar = 1 μm. (Courtesy of H. Veldman and prof. F.G.I. Jennekens and CRC Press.)

form antibodies against AChR. Myoid cells are found in the thymus which share epitopes with the AChR's are surmised to stimulate AChR-specific T-cells (84). These myoid cells are found in the near vicinity (but never inside) the lymphoid follicles, where immuno-stimulation takes place. Antibody production and the proliferation of specific lymphocytes decline after successful thymectomy, if no thymoma is present (85). Patients with thymomas

Figure 1.10

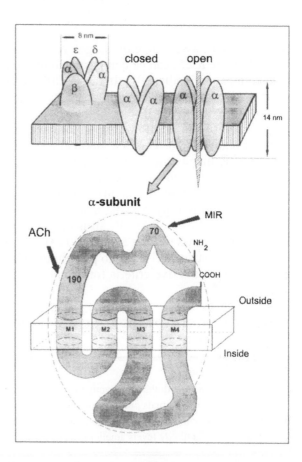

Schematic presentation of the nicotinic acetylcholine receptor (AChR) of the neuromuscular junction. The 5 subunits, protruding from the membrane, form the wall of a funnel shaped space, the ion channel. When both alpha-subunits bind ACh, or another stimulating ligand, the channel opens. The embryonic muscle contains a gamma-subunit which replaces the adult subunit (epsilon), as indicated in the upper figure. The approximate structure of the alpha-unit (lower figure) shows the extramembraneous part with the main immunogenic region (MIR, near position 70) and the ACh-binding site (ACh, near position 190). The numbers indicate the identified aminoacids counted from the terminal NH2 at the hydrophilic side. Courtesy of Dr P.C. Molenaar (88) and CRC Press.

are considered to represent a special category, in which the MG is a paraneoplastic disease (86, 87). The role of the thymus is possibly different in patients with and without thymomas.

The molecular structure of the AChR has become known in detail **(fig. 1.10)** and genes for the 5 subunits have been cloned (88, 89, 89a). The AChR-site, where the acetylcholine binds, is different from the main immunogenic region, where the specific antibody is acting by cross-linking. In most MG patients circulating antibodies reacting with this part of the AChR molecule are found with the immunoprecipitation technique, using denervated human leg muscles from amputees as a source of antigen (90). Still other AChR-Ab, which block the AChR site itself, can be demonstrated in some of the patients, who lack the conventional antibodies (91). In fact AChR-Ab production is heterogenous and every patient might have his own spectrum of AChR-Ab, acting on various parts of the AChR (92). The result however, seems to be the same: accelerated degradation of the AChR which is not counterbalanced by the physiological receptor regeneration. This is accompanied with a structural abnormality of the postsynaptic membrane with loss of membrane folds. **(Fig. 1.9 b)** This process can be demonstrated in all skeletal muscles. The intensity probably varies considerably, although this is difficult to ascertain in living patients. Weakness and exhaustibility only became manifest if at least 50% of the receptors are lost. The causal role of AChR-Ab is demonstrated by the rapid improvement that usually follows plasma-exchange (93). This procedure is especially useful in severe MG-states (crisis) or to prevent these in preparation for thymectomy. MG thus meets the five criteria for an antibody mediated disorder (93a).

Table 1.1 CRITERIA FOR THE PATHOGENESIS OF ANTIBODY MEDIATED DISORDERS

1. antibody is present
2. antibody interacts with the target antigen
3. passive transfer in animals produces disease features
4. immunization with the antigen produces a model disease
5. a reduction of antibody levels ameliorates the disease

From the late 1970's new congenital myasthenic syndromes (CMS) were defined with the use of new neurophysiological, histochemical and electronmicroscopical techniques (94). Although these are rare, the detailed studies have provided more insight into the structure and the (patho)-physiology of the neuromuscular synapse. These studies are still in progress and several entities were newly described (95). These CMS have no immunological origin.

The cause of these disturbances in immunomodulation is not well understood. External causes like viral infections are very unlikely (96), although d-penicillamine may induce MG in patients with rheumatoid arthritis, which is also an autoimmune disease (97). Acquired autoimmune MG occurs in 1-3% in families (98), which is higher than 5 to 7 per 100,000 in the population, but does not follow a known pattern of heredity, as is the case in most congenital (nonimmunogenic) forms. Only the finding that certain human leucocyte antigen (HLA) types are more common in early onset MG without thymoma (99), indicates a genetic propensity. These HLA-types are also more prevalent in patients with other autoimmune diseases and are probably related to the higher incidence of the other autoimmune diseases that occur in MG patients.

NOTES

[1] Physostigmine or eserin was suggested as a possible medicament by Jolly in 1895 (1) and was tried by Murri in 1896 (107), but his patient did not tolerate it. Remen in 1932 described the short-lasting effect of the injection of prostigmine in a study on the effect of glycocoll, but did not mention it in his summary (108). Physiostigmine is a tertiary ammonium-base and is able to pass the blood-brain barrier and to cause central side effects. Prostigmine, pyridostigmine, edrophonium and ambenomium are quaternary ammonium bases which so not pass the blood brain barrier and act only in the peripheral nervous system. Also d-tubocurarine and suxamethonium are quaternary ammonium bases. Long-acting and potent anticholinesterases (such as nerve gases and insecticides) have been tried in patients with MG, but did not prove superior to the other drugs. They were difficult to adjust and exhibited serious side effects, so that they were abandoned by 1958 (109). Anticholinesterases bind to the enzyme acetylcholinesterase situated in the synaptic clefts, and impair the decomposition of acetylcholine in actate and choline thus effecting a longer action of acetylcholine.

[2] Various other names have been proposed: Bulbärparalyse ohne anatomische Befund (5), bulbare Neurose (100), myasthenische Paralyse (100), asthenische Bulbärparalyse (101), asthenische Lähmung (13). The epitheton: pseudoparalytica was soon omitted especially in the English literature. The disease of Erb and Goldflam was an usual eponym until 1950.

[3] The historiography of MG usually starts with Thomas Willis, who had described in 1672 patients with an unusual paralysis under the name: "Paralysia spuria non habitualis". In 1903 Guthrie (102) has drawn attention to this paper in the English translation of Pordage in 1683: "There is another kind of this Disease (i.e. 'the Palsey') depending on the scarcity and fewness of the Spirits, in which tho motion fails wholly in no Part or Member, yet it is performed but weakly only, or depravedly by any: in wit, the affected, tho not become without motion, yet they are not able to move their members, or to sustain any Burthen with strength: moreover in any moving effort they

are troubled with a trembling of the Limbs, which is only the effect of Weakness, or a broken strength in the moving Faculty... they do not dare to set upon any local motion, and if they begin it, they cannot hold it long: nay some, without any considerable sickness, keep their Beds for a long time, as Persons ready to dye: whilst they lye disturbed they discourse with their Friends, and are chearful, but by neither will, nor dare be raised up, or walk about, nay they abhor all motion as some dreadful thing.(...) I have now a prudent and honest Woman in cure, who for many years has been obnoxious to this kind of bastard Palsey not only in the Limbs, but likewise in the Tongue; This person for some time speaks freely and readily enough, but after long, hasty or labourious speaking, presently she becomes as mute as a fish, and cannot bring forth a word, nay, and does not recover the use of her Voice till after an hour or two..." (103).

Although Willis describes the fluctuation of muscle power it is strange for MG to cause weakness of the extremities which confines patients to their beds, but without concomitant bulbar or respiratory symptoms; or in the case of the woman that she becomes "mute as a fish" after speaking which takes two hours to recover.

The first convincing clinical description was that of the French clinician Hérard under the title "De la paralysie glosso-labiolaryngee" in 1868 (104). Although the case was commented upon as uncommon, the French clinicians missed the opportunity to surmise a new disease. Goldflam (13) missed this case in his survey and Charcot quoted it under the title "De l'ophtalmoplégie externe (105). Another typical case was described by Charcot in 1892 (106) under the diagnosis polioencephalitis.

[4] Keynes (41) commented that dr Denny-Brown, visiting neurologist had explained to her the resemblance between MG and curare intoxication, to which physostigmine was known as an antidote. Mary Walker (110) also reported the observation that the ptosis and general muscle weakness in one of her patients increased after ischaemic exercise of both forearm muscles; this effect occurred after a latent period of one minute and a half after the cuff was loosened. This phenomenon which has been known as the Mary Walker effect suggested the accumulation of a curarizing substance produced during ischaemic muscle exercise. Several investigators have tried to reproduce this effect with positive (111-114) or negative (115-116) results. Spontaneous fluctuations of signs and the effect of psychological factors may have influenced the clinical experiments.

2

CLINICAL ASPECTS AND EPIDEMIOLOGY

2.1 Definition and classification

The signs and symptoms of myasthenia gravis (MG) are the result of a fluctuating weakness of the voluntary muscles. The degree of weakness is partly dependent on the exertion of the muscle group concerned, but changes in weakness usually occur spontaneously over shorter or longer periods without apparent cause, and complete remissions may occur (1-4). Apart from a certain degree of local muscle atrophy, no other neurological abnormalities can be expected.

It is usual and relevant to distinguish the following types:
1. Acquired myasthenia, developing at any age after birth, which is by far the most common type;
2. Neonatal myasthenia, occurring in 10-15% of the children of myasthenic mothers;
3. Congenital (hereditary) myasthenia: present at birth or apparent in the first years of life, or rarely later.

The patients with acquired myasthenia (MG) may be distinguished for practical reasons in 4 categories:
A. Purely ocular MG, restricted to the palpebral levator and the eye-moving muscles;
B. Early onset generalized MG, starting before the age of 40 years, without thymoma;
C. Late onset generalized MG, starting from the age of 40 years, without thymoma;
D. Patients with a thymoma, starting at any age.

2.2 Symptoms and signs

2.2.1 Ocular symptoms

2.2.1.1 History

The most frequent single symptom is double vision (diplopia). The patient is immediately aware of it, as it occurs acutely. A common situation is the onset in the evening after a long, busy day, e.g. whilst driving a car or watching television. It may have disappeared the next morning and reappear in the evening, or persist in a variable intensity. No consensus is found in the literature about the ocular sign that most frequently appears first: ptosis or diplopia, or which muscle is involved. In many patients with ocular signs, both are present some time after the onset, when they see a doctor. Double vision is always noticed by the patient, but a mild ptosis may escape his attention. The first sign(s) mentioned by my own patients are given in **table 2.1**.

Some patients notice the fluctuation of the diplopia from onset and are able to analyse the double images themselves. **(Fig. 2.1)** Others only complain of blurred vision, which becomes normal when looking with one eye. Short lasting vertical diplopia after eye opening is mentioned by some patients as the first sign of eye muscle weakness. The diagnosis of MG in that stage is rarely made by the ophthalmologist nor by the neurologist.

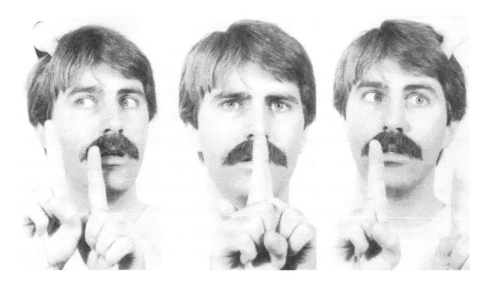

Figure 2.1 M25. MG score $O_2B_1U_0L_0V_0$. Diplopia due to paresis of the external rectus OS, the internal rectus OS, the external rectus OD, and impaired upward and downward movement OD. For interpretation of MG score see table 2.3.

Table 2.1 SYMPTOMS AND SIGNS AT ONSET

	EARLY ONSET 1-39 years	LATE ONSET 40-85 years	THYMOMA	TOTAL
Ocular diplopia	70 (14)	84 (36)	17 (1)	171
ptosis	55 (16)	36 (12)	14	105
ptosis and diplopia	64 (10)	47 (18)	15	126
Bulbar articulation	43	5	6	54
face	20	2		22
chewing	1	6	3	10
swallowing	7	4	1	12
neck muscles	2	5	4	11
combined	23	20	16	59
Oculo-bulbar	25	17	30	72
Limbs: arms	15	3	4	22
hands or fingers	12	1	2	15
legs	45	6	1	52
combined	29	5	5	39
Generalized	4	5	16	25
Respiration	4	2	4	10
Total	419 (40)	248 (66)	138 (1)	805

Very first signs of MG reported by the author's patients. In brackets the patients who remained purely ocular during the follow-up. This was the case in only 1 patient with a thymoma, in 9.5% in the early onset group and 26.6% in the late onset group. The ocular muscles were at onset involved in 59% of all patients, the bulbar muscles in 30%, the ocular and bulbar muscles combined in 80%. Of the 10 patients with respiratory signs, 8 had a prolonged apnoea without previous weakness and 2 were children with high fever. The onset with ocular signs was more frequent in the late onset group than in the early onset group (74% vs 51%). Limb muscle weakness was more frequent in the early onset than in the late onset group (25% vs 8%). Patients with thymomas had the highest incidence of bulbar signs at onset (55% vs 31% in the early onset and 26% in the late onset group).

Diplopia is relatively rare at downward gaze, but may occur in any direction. Particularly at onset, but also in the course of the disease, diplopia may occur without visible squinting or disturbance of movement, if the inspection is done routinely and without provocation.

Drooping of one or both eyelids (ptosis) is the next common sign. It may be present from the onset of the diplopia, or appear any time later. It is not unusual that some degree of ptosis is present but remains unnoticed by the patient, if the upper lid does not cover more than 25% of the cornea. On the other hand, ptosis may be a very prominent sign from onset, so that it obscures the diplopia. If the ptosis is bilateral, it is often asymmetrical and it is very remarkable to see that, even in a short time, the maximal ptosis shifts from one eye to the other. This is certainly not uncommon over longer periods of observation and this ptosis-shift is pathognomonic of MG (5).

The ptosis and the diplopia increase in sunshine or bright light, so many patients prefer to wear sunglasses even at home. Ptosis and diplopia usually increase in the course of the day or are only present in the evening, but about 10% of the patients report that these symptoms are present on awakening in the morning or after a short nap in the afternoon and diminish subsequently in the next 30-60 minutes without medication (3, 6).

2.2.1.2 Examination

Ptosis may be seen in any degree in one or both eyes. If present in both eyes, it is usually asymmetrical and rarely complete in both eyes. Often the ptosis fluctuates rapidly (e.g. 1-5 times per 10 seconds) during the interview, a feature first reported by Oppenheim (7). (**Fig. 2.2**)

This may be falsely interpreted as a sign of nervousness. Patients with an organic ptosis try to compensate this by contraction of their mm frontales or keep their heads in reclination. MG patients usually do so (**fig. 2.3**), except when facial and/or neck muscles are also weak. An easy provocative test is to have the patient look upwards or to one side for at least 30 seconds. In upward gaze this often results in lidtwitching (8) and finally in drooping of the eye lid

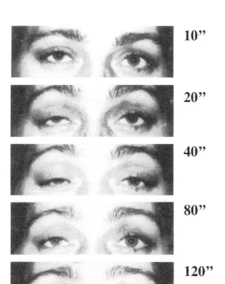

10"

20"

40"

80"

120"

Figure 2.2 W 26. MG score O_2 B_1 L_2 U_1 V_1.
Rapidly fluctuating ptosis during 2 minutes fixed gaze

Figure 2.3

M 60. Ocular MG
Left: Asymmetrical
ptosis relieved by
contraction of the
frontal muscles.
Right: After two
minutes of fixed
gaze, the ptosis OD
has increased.
The patient has to
recline his head in
order to see.

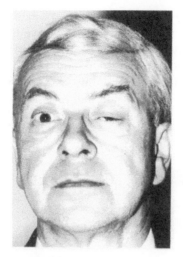
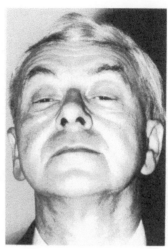

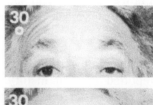
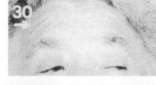
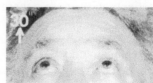

Figure 2.4 (left)
W 26. Ptosis elicited by looking to the side.
Consecutive photographs after 10, 20, 30 etc. seconds.

Figure 2.5
(under) W 80. MG score
$O_1 B_2 U_1 L_0 V_0$. Ptosis is
elicited by looking to the side
and not by looking upwards.

which sign is reversed after eye closing. Usually a more gradual drooping is seen at sidewards-gaze, especially of the abducting eye **(fig. 2.4)**. I found the latter test to be more sensitive. **(Fig. 2.5)** The provocation of the ptosis by repeated eye closure is not recommended. Although some patients will have an increase of their ptosis after this procedure, this test is illogical. Closure of the eye is an activity of the m.orbicularis oculi and rests the m.levator palpebrae. This explains why this test, in my experience, is not sensitive, although proposed by others (4, 9).

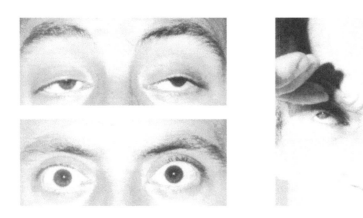

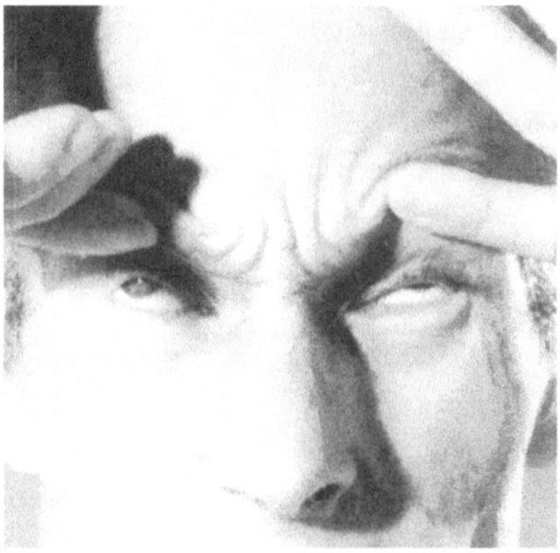

Figure 2.6 (left) M 30. Ocular MG from the age of 7. Drooping eye-lids, lifted by contraction of the frontal muscles (above). After 3 minutes of eye closure the ptosis has disappeared and the palpebral fissure has become wider than normal, due to orbicularis muscle weakness (bottom).

Figure 2.7 (right) M 45. MG score O_1 B_2 U_2 L_1 V_1. Orbicularis weakness. Eyes turn insufficiently upwards due to a superior rectus paresis.

Looking into bright light may induce ptosis, as some patients have already reported in their history. Ptosis may be reduced by eye closure for some minutes. After this, another typical sign may be seen: the palpebral fissure becomes wider than normal **(fig. 2.6)**, which is explained by the weakness of the m.orbicularis oculi, until then obscured by the ptosis. The orbicularis weakness is easily tested and is found to be present in half of the patients with ptosis and/or diplopia (it is in fact the first sign of 'generalization') and in most patients with more generalized weakness. **(Fig. 2.7)** In testing the orbicularis weakness, it may be seen that the eye does not turn upwards as is physiological, due to the paralysis of the superior rectus[1]. The orbicularis 'fatigue' is also the mechanism underlying the 'peek sign': in trying to keep the eyes gently closed, the palpebral fissure widens and the patient seems to 'peek' at the examiner (10). Diplopia may be due to a paresis of just one extrinsic eye muscle, but in most patients more than one muscle of one or both eyes are compromised. Authorities differ in opinion about which muscle is the most often and/or the first to be affected: the superior rectus (11, 12), the medial rectus (9), or the lateral rectus (13). In my experience the medial recti are most commonly affected, followed by the elevators with a preference for the superior recti. In routine testing unconjugated eye movements may be observed. The multiplicity of eye muscle pareses, as well as their fluctuation and ptosis, often make an exact analysis difficult. (**Fig. 2.8**)

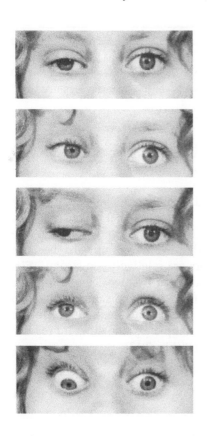

Figure 2.8 Multiple eye muscle pareses in a 15 year old woman with moderate generalized MG.

The red-green glass test (14) and standardized orthoptic procedures may be helpful. In order to get continuous and more or less comparable information, I find it useful to make a rough sketch of the eye movements at every examination. (**Fig. 5.8**) Diplopia may occur without visible squinting. In that case it is likely that a sustained gaze for at least 30 seconds in each of the horizontal and vertical directions will provoke either a visible palsy, or nystagmoid movements, accompanied by an increase of the diplopia. (**Fig. 2.9**) At first, a failure of the adducting eye (medial rectus) may be seen, followed by nystagmoid movements of the abducting eye (lateral rectus), which gradually become coarser and end in a visible paresis of the lateral rectus of the abducting eye. This syndrome is described as pseudo-internuclear ophthalmoplegia (15) and is fairly common in my experience; it may give rise to the erroneous diagnosis of multiple sclerosis.

Another sensitive provocative test is to elicit optokinetic nystagmus during one minute. Diplopia manifesting itself during a drive in a car or by looking out of a moving train may be explained by the same sort of provocation.

External ophthalmoplegia may be nearly complete with some downward movements usually left, and diplopia tends to disappear when the palsies are more symmetrical. In an attempt to move the eyes, tiny isolated high-frequency movements can be observed, which are rapidly exhausted: so called quiver movements (16). Weakness or 'fatigue' of

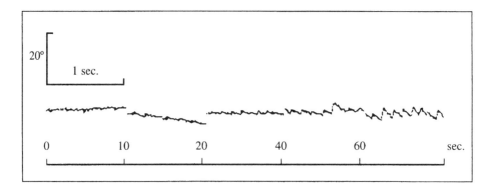

Figure 2.9 Nystagmography (binocular). The patient is looking 30° to one side during 60 seconds. After 20 seconds, nystagmoid movements appeared, which increased in amplitude to 5° after 60 seconds. Courtesy Dr T. Van Weerden

the sphincter pupillae is not detectable with clinical methods, and a narrowing of the pupils still can be observed in an attempt to converge even if the medial rectus is completely paralysed on both sides.[2]

Some curious phenomena may be observed, which may be explained by Hering's law of equal innervation. Hering's law states that yoked muscles receive equal and simultaneous innervation. If the elevators of one eye are paretic and this eye is fixed on a point, the other eye moves upward, because the nerve impulses to the non-paretic elevators are relatively too strong. **(Fig. 2.10)** The same mechanism may widen the palpebral fissure of the non-ptotic eye if the patient tries to open the ptotic eye. **(Fig. 2.11)** The same mechanism explains the observation of the retraction of the eyelid contralateral to the ptosis. If the examiner closes the ptotic eyelid completely, the other lid regains its normal position or even becomes ptotic (17). **(Fig. 2.12)**

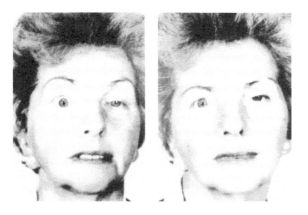

Figure 2.11

Woman (60). Mild ptosis of the right side and annoyingly wide eye at the left side; the eye became normal after suspension of the right eye-lid.

Figure 2.10

M 45. MG score 0_2 B_1 U_0 L_0 V_0.
Multiple eye-muscle pareses,
predominantly of the levators OD and the
depressors OS. When looking with both
eyes the right eye is dominant.
In order to keep the right eye in the
horizontal position, an increased
innervation of the paretic elevator is
needed. The equal innervation of the
elevator of the non-paretic left eye results
in an elevation of the left eye.
When looking with the left eye only, the
patient is easily able to maintain the
horizontal position. This phenomenon
disappeared after a year of prednisone
treatment.

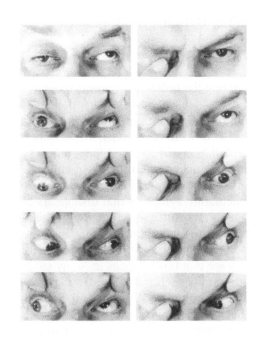

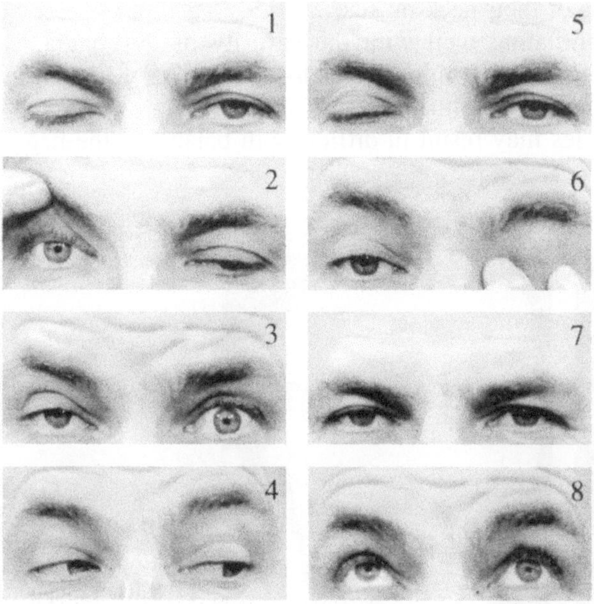

Figure 2.12

Man (37). Ocular MG:
1. Complete ptosis right eye,
slight ptosis left eye.
2. Lifting right eyelid,
enhances the left ptosis.
3. After 30 seconds, with
contraction of mm. frontalis.
4. Ptosis enhanced by looking
to the left side.
5. 30 seconds after figure 4.
6. Right sided ptosis
decreased after passive
closure of left eye.
7. Ptosis disappeared after
neostigmine.
8. Isolate m.rectus sup.paresis
of the left eye.

2.2.2 Bulbar symptoms

2.2.2.1 History

Among the bulbar symptoms, speech difficulties are the most common at onset (in the neurological jargon 'bulbar muscles' are the muscles innervated by motor-neurons originating in the pons and the medulla oblongata - n. V, n. VII, n. IX, n. X, n. Xl, n. Xll). These may be nasality of the voice or a difficulty in articulation. More than any other symptom, dysarthria is likely to occur initially under the influence of emotions. It may be accompanied by difficulties in swallowing and chewing, but at first it is frequently an isolated and very fluctuating symptom that disappears after a 'silent period'. If the dysarthria is due to an insufficient function of the palatum, regurgitation of liquids through the nose is common. A slight insufficiency of the upper pharyngeal muscles will result in the feeling that the food is sticking in the throat, and in fact one can see that this happens in X-ray studies with barium. Patients with dysphagia commonly prefer cold food.

Chewing may be difficult at the end of the meal. Some patients first mention this symptom when chewing bubble-gum or peanuts. If the symptom is more prominent, the jaw sags open and has to be sustained with the hand. A characteristic posture is seen in **figure 2.13**. Most of my patients with chewing problems also had weakness of their neck muscles.

An important symptom correlating well with the severity of dysphagia, is weight loss. Most of my patients with bulbar signs lost 5 - 10 kg of weight in 3 - 6 months, before the diagnosis was made.

Weakness of the neck muscles may result in difficulty in balancing the head,

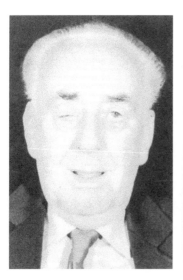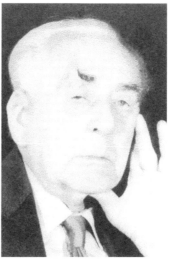

Figure 2.13

M 73.
DS: O_2, B_2, U_1, L_1, V_1.
He had to support his jaw. Adhesive tape is used to relieve the ptosis of his right eye.

which is particularly troublesome if the patient has to perform some work in a forward bent position. Complaints about stiffness, vague pains in the neck and the back of the head, and occasionally paraesthesias are then common, and nearly always set the doctor on the wrong track, unless the strength of the neck muscles is formally tested. Weakness of the facial muscles may occur suddenly - in some patients the initial diagnosis was Bell's palsy (18) (own patients) - but it is more usual for it to occur insidiously. The patient's complaint is often stiffness, the sensation known from dental anaesthesia and sometimes paraesthesias or even hypalgesia (19) are reported. Substantial sensory loss however, is never due to MG. The facial expression may be changed, especially in emotions. Laughing becomes distorted ('we did not know whether she laughed or cried'; **fig. 2.14**) (20). Many patients complain of this change of facial expression and avoid new social contacts (21). People ask them why they always look sad or angry.

Figure 2.14

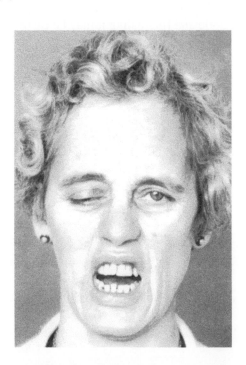

W 45. MG score O_3 B_2 U_2 L_1 V_0.
Myasthenic face with typical vertical laugh
('myasthenic snarl').

Orbicularis oris weakness is first noticed by the inability to whistle or to kiss, in sneezing forcefully, in eating soup with a spoon or by the difficulty in pronouncing certain letters (p, f, s). Some patients complain that their tongues are thick and don't fit in their mouths. The time needed for eating a meal increases, and conversation becomes difficult while eating.
Insufficient strength of the m.orbicularis oculi may cause problems in keeping

the eyes closed while washing the hair. Several of my patients could not close one eye and keep the other open whilst taking photographs. If the eyes are not completely closed whilst sleeping, they may be irritated at awakening.

Some deafness is occasionally reported and is probably due to a disfunction of the Eustachian tube, because of pharyngeal paresis. Hyperacusis is probably caused by a weakness of the stapedius muscle. This may be demonstrated by stapedius reflexometry (22, 23).

As all these symptoms may be minor and fluctuating, they are often detected retrospectively and have not led the patient to consult a doctor in the first stage of the disease.

2.2.2.2 Examination

The most frequent of the bulbar signs in more advanced MG is the facial weakness. In its most prominent form it is easily recognizable **(fig. 2.14)**, but if subtle and fluctuating it may be easily overlooked. In rest, the facial expression may be unremarkable, but any expression of emotion, and particularly laughing, betrays the loss of normal function. A classical feature is the myasthenic snarl (24) or the 'rire verticale'. **(Fig. 2.15)**

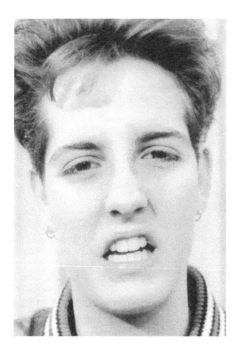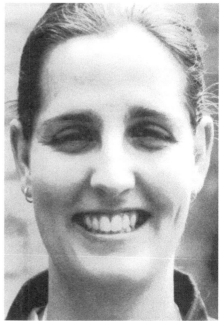

Figure 2.15 W 21. **a.** 'Rire verticale'.
b. Three years after thymectomy.

Since weakness of the upper part of the face is also present, laughing makes the eyelids droop, even if ptosis is not noticeable at rest. An early and sensitive sign of orbicularis oris weakness is the inability to whistle or to kiss (a neglected part of the neurological examination). The patient cannot blow out his cheeks without air escaping, if the cheek is pressed with the finger. The closed eyes can be opened with one finger, or the eyes cannot be closed at all. **(Fig. 2.16)** Facial weakness may be asymmetrical, but this is rarely as pronounced as the ocular signs. The most sensitive function test of the muscles of articulation is speaking aloud without inter-ruption. An easy test is counting (101, 102, etc.) or reading aloud. A certain quantification is pos-sible by annotating, when dys-

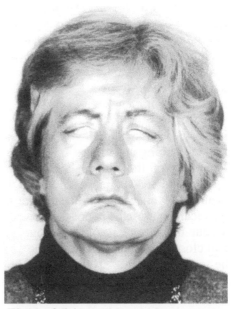

Figure 2.16 W 55. She attempts to close her eyes. Bell's phenomenon.

arthria or nasal twang starts and when the patient becomes unintelligible. **(Fig. 2.17)** In a minority of patients, the voice first becomes weaker and not so much dysarthric, but in general dysarthria and nasality occur whilst the volume is still normal. Seldom some hoarseness occurs but aphonia is not a sign of MG. Slight palatal weakness is demonstrated if peak-flow volume improves as a result of pinching the nose.

Figure 2.17

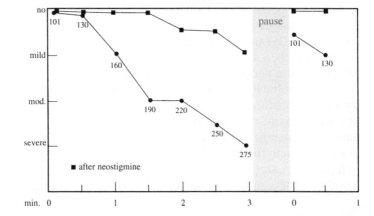

Counting test. Improvement by pausing and by neostigmine.

29

Swallowing difficulties may be due to weakness of the lips, the tongue or pharyngeal muscles and often, although not always, to a combination of these. Few neurologists observe their MG patients during their meals. They might then notice that patients support their jaws, underlips, and the floor of their mouth in order to alleviate gravitation and 'chew with their hands'. Swallowing is in some patients improved if they turn their head, probably thus narrowing their, too wide, atrophic throat. Regurgitation of fluids through the nose is a sign of palatal weakness. Coughing after having finished a glass of water may be another subtle sign of a defective swallowing mechanism. Severe impairment of swallowing is manifested by drooping of saliva, increasing the risk of choking and crisis (4.5.3).

Weakness of the tongue is apparent when the patient cannot protrude his tongue and reach the frenulum of the upperlip. If the tongue is protruded against the inner cheek, the strength can be tested directly. If weakness of the masticatory muscles is not demonstrated on conventional testing (clenching a tongue depressor), it may be provoked by having the patient repeatedly open and close his mouth vigorously, so as to produce an audible click. This should be easily possible 100 times within 30 seconds. The strength of the sternocleidomastoids and of the neck muscles can be felt to be decreased on routine testing. A sensible test is head lifting, in the recumbent position: the patient should be able to look at his toes for 60 seconds.

Muscle atrophy in the face, tongue or throat sometimes occurs and will be discussed later.

2.2.3 Limb and trunk symptoms

2.2.3.1 History

Some 15-20% of the patients complain first of weakness of the arm or hand muscles, or of the legs. In the younger age group (< 30 years) limb muscle weakness, especially of the legs, was the first sign in one third of my patients. This may be explained by situations where these muscles are heavily loaded, e.g. during sports. Inability to keep the arm raised for some time or repeatedly, e.g. when hanging the laundry, hammering a nail or washing hair, are common complaints. Weakness of one or more extensors of the fingers, usually the fourth or fifth, is difficult for the doctor to interpret and sometimes leads to the diagnosis of a peripheral nerve compression.

Weakness of the legs frequently leads to sudden falls and several of my patients had their myasthenia diagnosed after a fall from the stairs. If the first symptoms are weakness of the limbs or of the trunk muscles, most patients complain of undue fatiguability and peculiar feelings of heaviness. If asked about the exact nature of their feelings, they admit that these are different from the normal fatigue after exertion, although some rest is beneficial and restores their normal condition for a shorter or longer time. Most patients have complaints of both arms or legs, but often one of either is more readily exhausted, which may be confirmed by appropriate testing (see **fig. 2.18**).

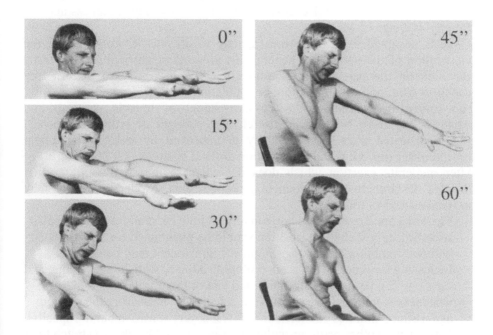

Figure 2.18 Extended arm test (normal 3 minutes).

Pain in the back and girdle muscles occurs in some 10-15% of the patients (1, 18, 24; also reported in older literature) and is readily explained as an insufficiency of the muscles of posture. It usually disappears at rest or after therapy. Chronic pain is not a feature of MG.

Weakness of the respiratory and other trunk muscles is rarely the first single sign of the disease, but it may be the first sign that brings the patient into medical care. I only saw this in rapidly evolving generalized MG during childhood infections, or as an effect of curare during narcosis ('prolonged apnoea'). Some patients report short periods of dyspnoea with inspiratory stridor, which are often the forerunners of longer lasting and life threatening attacks. Rarely, short episodes of unconsciousness occur, which are not always recognized as caused by sudden apnoea and cerebral anoxia. These events should always lead to a rapid hospitalization of the patient.

2.2.3.2 Examination

If a patient is suspected to have myasthenia gravis, it is essential to test the muscle strength after exercise. It should be stated that only weakness and not 'fatigue' is a sign of MG.[3]

All tests designed to measure the capacity to do muscle work require the cooperation of the patient. In general this presents no difficulties, but some suspicion on the part of the examiner may be necessary to discern true weakness from non-organic failure or simulation.

The following procedures in the assessment of muscle strength and exhaustability have been found useful. The strength of individual muscle groups is tested after rest. Accuracy is improved by using a hand-held dynamometer **(fig. 3.1 a)** and the adoption of fixed postures (22, 26). **(Fig. 3.1 b)** After moderate exertion which does not decrease the strength of normal muscles, the strength of the patient is measured again. Moderate exertion may be standardized as follows:

1. The arms are stretched out horizontally and the hand and fingers are also stretched. **(Fig. 2.18)** This position should be maintained for 3 minutes without trembling or shaking. Some encouragement may be necessary. Increasing weakness will produce some shaking or a gradual drooping, and the same can be seen in the hands and one or more fingers. **(Fig. 2.19)** If weakness is minimal, it may only be detected by measuring the strength again after 3 minutes of exertion. This test is very sensitive but not specific. Patients with other neuromuscular diseases may not be able to stretch their arms for more than 1 minute, but the strength before and after this effort remains the same.
2. The grip strength on repeated contraction is to be measured and documented with the hand-held dynamometer. A simple ergometer can be made out of a blood pressure manometer.
3. Kneebending or, in older people, rising from a normal chair without the aid of the hands should be possible 20 times.
4. Walking on the toes and on the heels at least 30 steps.
5. Straight leg rising to 45 degrees during 1 minute in the recumbent position.
6. Vital capacity and peak-flow measurements should give normal values 5 times in a row. A difficulty in these tests may be the weakness of the lips or of the palatum.

In most patients with a generalized MG, but without actual or previous dyspnoea, a decrease of the vital capacity and other respiratory parameters could be found (27-31) and even, in 40% of pure ocular cases, the vital capacity was found to be diminished (29). The most abnormal respiratory parameter was either the maximal expiration pressure (30), or the forced maximal inspiratory flow (28), or the maximal inspiratory pressure (31). Routine lung function tests show that the vital capacity is more decreased than

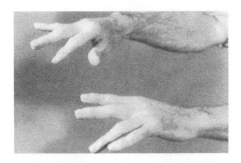

Figure 2.19 Test of the extended hand and fingers. After 30 seconds, extension of the ulnar fingers of the left hand and of the radial fingers of the right hand is affected.

the forced expiratory volume. In most patients, peak-flow or vital capacity measurement is a valuable tool in the follow-up, and can be done easily at any time and in any circumstance.

Most of these tests are quantifiable and some of them can be done by the patient at home, to obtain a reliable picture of the diurnal and periodic fluctuation. According to the complaints of the individual patient, other tests may be appropriate.

The data acquired, may show a convincing difference between the strength at rest and after exertion. They should also serve as a frame of reference in the evaluation of the effect of anticholinesterases and other kinds of treatment.

Some urine incontinence may be a complaint of female patients and is usually paralleled by weakness of the leg and trunk muscles. The most likely interpretation is hypotonia of the muscles of the pelvic floor and the external sphincter of the bladder. This symptom usually disappears if the proximal weakness improves. However, in most older women mild urine incontinence is of the type stress-incontinence, but eventually provoked by the use of anticholinesterases.

2.2.4 Muscle atrophy

The occurrence of local muscle atrophy has caused much confusion in the history of MG. On the one hand, otherwise typical cases with localized atrophy were included in the early series (7, 32), and on the other hand muscle atrophy was used as an argument to place the patient in the category of a myasthenic syndrome, with either a form of myopathy (33, 34), or neuropathy (35), or polymyositis (36), or ophthalmoplegia (37). Others referred to the combination of true MG with myopathy (38-40), with neuropathy (41-43), or with neuromyopathy (44).

Osserman (4) placed his patients with muscular atrophy, comprising 5% of his series, in a separate group. He felt that "the histologic changes in the biopsied muscle are indistinguishable from those seen in polymyositis or muscular dystrophy". From a clinical point of view there is no doubt that localized muscle atrophy is detectable in about 6-10% of the patients (3, 4, 45-47). A still higher percentage is reached if patients with permanent, nearly complete ophthalmoplegia, are included. Remarkably few details about the distribution of the atrophy is found in the literature (45, 46, 48); the atrophy of the tongue however is sometimes mentioned (triple furrowed tongue, first mentioned by Kinnier Wilson; 49). (**Fig. 2.20**) Muscle atrophy in my own patients is further discussed in 5.2.5.

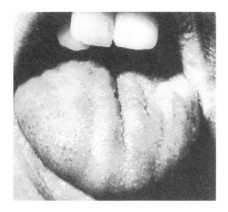

Figure 2.20

W 60. Atrophy of the tongue with two lateral and one medial furrows: 'triple furrowed tongue'. MG existed from early infancy and was diagnosed at age 52.

2.3 Clinical scoring and quantified tests

Several scoring systems of myasthenic signs or of the global state of the patient have been proposed. The classification of Osserman and Genkins (50) is widely used. In fact this is a modification of the initial classification of Osserman (4) in 1958 and altered by Oosterhuis (3) in 1964. In this classification, juvenile patients and patients with muscle atrophy were excluded as separate entities and class 1 was confined to ocular myasthenia. It can be used retrospectively to classify patients to a certain type, but combines localization, severity, and progression and is not well suited to follow individual patients. (**Table 2.2**)

Table 2.2 CLASSIFICATION OF OSSERMAN AND GENKINS (50)

I.	Purely ocular (ptosis, diplopia)
II.A.	Mild generalized (ocular and extemities, no prominent bulbar signs)
II.B.	Moderate generalized (ocular and/or bulbar signs, variable limb muscle involvement, no crises)
III.	Acute fulminating generalized signs with prominent bulbar involvement and crises
IV.	Late severe generalized and prominent bulbar signs and crises

A survey of the maximum clinical severity in several patient populations is given in **table 2.5**.
Various other scoring systems have subscores for ocular, bulbar, limb muscle, and respiratory weakness, either based on description or on quantified tests (51-55). One system gives a detailed scoring for ocular signs (56). They seem to be useful to follow the individual patient by one or a few doctors, accustomed to this particular sysem; in one study the interobservers variation was ≤ 10% (51). Our own global score on a six-point scale is given in **table 2.3**.

2.4 The course of the disease

It should be emphazised that the initial symptoms and signs may have a very variable pattern and evolution in the individual patient. Patients, when treated and relieved of their symptoms, often admit that they have suffered from MG longer than they had reported. Initially Osserman (4) stated: MG does not have a classical clinical course. There is a tendency of spreading to other muscle groups, and only in 10% (57) to 16% (58) of the patients does the MG remain clinically confined to the ocular muscles after 3 years. Spreading beyond ocular muscles occurred in various series after 3 years in 10% (4), 6% (58), or 3% (57).
If the onset is not in the ocular muscles, in most cases spreading of weakness occurs likewise in the first one to three years. It is very rare that weakness remains confined to the bulbar muscles or to the muscles of the extremities.
In most patients the diagnosis is made in the second year after onset, but a much longer delay is not unusual (3, 4). In those patients where the diagnosis is delayed, the natural course may still be observed. In point of fact these patients are often less severely affected. In general, signs and symptoms increase in the first years of the disease, with a tendency to stabilize and to improve or even to subside completely after many years. A typical case history is schematized in **figure 2.21**.
The increase in the first years is reflected in the graphs showing the interval between onset and maximum severity **(fig. 2.22)** and the incidence of crises **(fig. 2.23)**.
Crises rarely occur in the first weeks after onset, except in childhood infections or in patients with rapidly progressive bulbar symptoms who choke and cannot cough vigourously enough. More often crises occur in gradually increasing generalized weakness during respiratory infections, partially induced by aspiration. In patients with thymomas, crises occurred more often than in patients without thymomas (59).
Spontaneous long lasting remissions are rare in the first years, but in the long term they may be expected in 10-20% (2, 58-60). Patients with ocular MG had a higher remission rate than those with the generalized disease (58, 60).

Table 2.3 GLOBAL CLINICAL CLASSIFICATION OF MYASTHENIC SEVERITY

Class 0	No complaints, no signs after exertion or at special testing.
Class 1	No disability. Minor complaints, minor signs. The patient knows that he (still) has MG, but family members or outsiders do not perceive it. The experienced doctor may find minor signs at appropriate testing, e.g. diminished eye closure; some weakness of the foot extensors or triceps muscles; the arms cannot be held extended for 3 minutes; the patient may have complaints such as heavy eyelids or diplopia only when fatigued; inability to perform heavy work.
Class 2	Slight disability, clear signs after exertion. The patient has some restrictions in daily life, e.g. he cannot lift heavy loads, cannot walk for more than half an hour, has intermittent diplopia. Bulbar signs are not pronounced. Family members are aware of the signs, but outsiders (inexperienced doctors included) are not. Weakness is obvious at appropriate testing.
Class 3	Moderate disability, clear signs at rest. The patient is restricted in domestic activities;needs some help in clothing; meals have to be adapted. Bulbar signs are more pronounced. Signs of MG can be observed by any outsider.
Class 4	Severe disability. The patient needs constant support in daily activities. Bulbar signs are pronounced. Respiratory function is decreased.
Class 5	Respiratory support is needed.

Comment
1. The clinical score is made independently from the medication. The qualification 'remission' is to be restricted to class 0, when the patient is not using medication;
2. Patients with purely ocular signs are classified in class 1 or 2;
3. It is sometimes difficult to decide between class 2 and 3. The attitude of the patient and the adaptation to the disease may play a role;
4. The development of respiratory difficulties depends obviously on external factors, such as respiratory infections, inadequate drug regimen or other intercurrent diseases;
5. The function of individual muscle groups may be scored on a 4-point scale:
   •0. normal function (i.e. the specific function tests can be carried out, the patient has no complaints),
   •1. mild or intermittent signs,
   •2. moderate signs,
   •3. severe signs.
   A reasonable use of this semi-quantification can be made by scoring 0(cular), B(ulbar), U(pper extremities), L(ower extremities) and V(entilatory functions) together. For instance a patient with constant diplopia and ptosis, dysarthria after only 3 minutes reading aloud, unable to extend the arms for 1 minute, unable to walk a stairway and with a vital capacity of 75% would be scored as O_3, B_1, U_2, L_2, V_1.

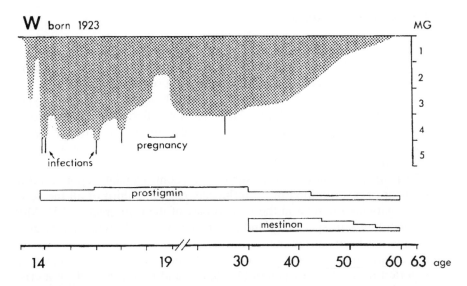

Figure 2.21 Typical case history. Onset of MG with dysarthria, in a stressful situation. Generalization 6 months later. Exacerbations by infections, improvement during pregnancy. During the wartime oral prostigmin was replaced by subcutaneous injections (0.5 mg 6 times a day) because tablets were scarce. She improved very gradually after the age of 30, and after the age of 45 only very slight signs could be found. Several major operations in the last 10 years were performed without any problems concerning her MG. She has been reluctant to omit her medication (prostigmin 7.5 mg and Mestinon 10mg, 3 times a day).

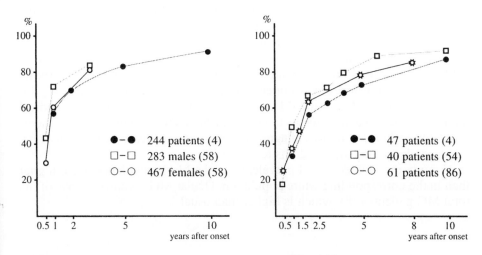

Figure 2.22
Percentage of patients reaching maximum symptoms.

Figure 2.23
Interval between onset and first crisis.

2.5 External influences

Certain events are recognized as influencing the course unfavourably, or at least they are usually followed by an exacerbation or initiate new symptoms. These factors may also preceed the first manifestations of MG.

These are infectious deseases with fever (61), psychological stress (62), hyper- or hypothyroidism, certain drugs, such as antimalaria drugs (quinidine, chloroquine) and d-penicillamine and the puerperium. To a minor degree exacerbations are experienced 3 to 10 days before the menstruation by at least one third of the women exposed (1, 3, 63).

The effect of pregnancy is the subject of controversial reports: either improvement or deterioration or no influence, each one third of all the series (64). Most patients improve in the second part of their pregnancy (65). Most data are acquired retrospectively and no prospective study with standardized examination has been carried out.

Extreme temperatures are not supported well, hot weather in particular has been reported to increase weakness (4, 66, 67) and may even induce a crisis (68). The individual reactivity varies considerably in my experience and several of my patients were considerably better in warm weather.

2.6 Epidemiology

2.6.1 Incidence and prevalence

The annual incidence (newly detected cases) is 3 to 4 per million and the prevalence about 60 per million (69-78), in some surveys even higher. A summary of the more recent epidemiologic studies is given in **table 2.4**.

Since the prevalence rates are based on variable numbers of patients, 95% confidence intervals are given for comparability. In some studies, a striking difference of prevalence was noticed between cities and rural areas (71, 75) which is probably due to the differences in population densities and medical facilities. The prevalence seems to be somewhat increasing in the last decades, problably influenced by new diagnostic tests and a decrease of mortality rate. No dependence on latitude seems to exist (79).

In Virginia the incidence and prevalence in the black population were higher than in the corresponding white population. Ocular MG comprised 25% of the total MG patients (78), which is higher than usual.

Table 2.4 INCIDENCE AND PREVALENCE OF MG PER MILLION INHABITANTS

Country	Period	Incidence	Prevalence	95% CI*	Reference
Norway	1951-81	4.0	90	81-100	69
Finland	1974	--	52	45-59	70
Japan:					
Kumamoto	1982	--	67	52-85	71
Netherlands:					
Amsterdam	1961-65	3.1	53	46-81	72
North Neth.	1982-92	4.6	73	57-92	73
Italy:					
Sardinia	1958-86	2.5	45	--	74
Bologna	1987-88	--	49	36-66	75
Ferrara	1987-88	--	97	64-128	
Denmark:					
(Eastern)	1970-87	4.4	77	67-90	76
Viborg	1973-87	9.8	125	84-180	77
U.S.A.:					
Virginia	1970-84	9.1	142	112-178	78

* confidence intervals

2.6.2 Age, gender and classification

MG may start at any age. In general, women are affected twice as much as men, in the childbearing period even three times as much, while the incidence is about equal before puberty and after the age of 40 (69, 77, 80, 81). The relative incidence is highest in women in the third decade (50, 69, 72), and in some series a late peak is found in older men (50, 69, 58). Ocular MG occurs in about 15% and has a higher prevalence in men, especially over the age of 40 (77, 82). Age at onset, gender, type, and incidence of thymomas in the author's series of 800 patients are given in **fig. 2.24**. A relatively high onset (22%) in the first decade, or 36% before puberty, is reported respectively from Japan (83) and Hong Kong (91). In both series, the signs remained restricted to the ocular muscles in 60% (83) or even 72% (84). However, the incidence of congenital cases is unknown in these series.

The maximum clinical severity scored according to the criteria of Osserman and Genkins (see **table 2.2**) is given in **table 2.5**.

The differences in severity are not readily explained by the periods of observation.

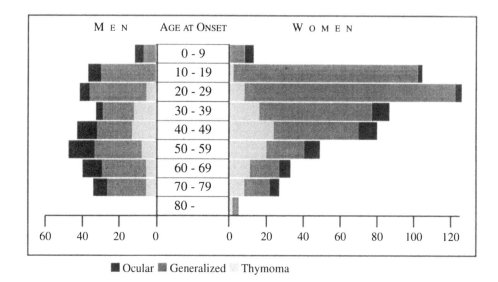

■ Ocular ■ Generalized ▫ Thymoma

Figure 2.24 Myasthenia gravis 1960-1994 - author's series of 805 patients

Table 2.5 MAXIMAL CLINICAL SEVERITY, OSSERMAN AND GENKINS CRITERIA

CLASSIFICATION	PERIOD OF OBSERVATION					
	1926-63	**1950-70**	**±1980-87**	**1984**	**1985-89**	**1985-89**
Ocular I	7	22	8	10	12	15
Mild II A	25	36	24	40	20	30
Moderate II B	45	23	40	38	35	44
Early severe III	9	12	13	4	10	} 11
Late severe IV	14	10	15	8	24	
Number of patients	175	1099[a]	633	48	182	100
Reference	3	50	80	84	76	85

[a] without neonatal and infantile cases

2.6.3 Death rates

Modern treatment modalities have lowered death rates of MG considerably. By comparing several periods, Grob et al (81) found a steady decrease from 40% in 1935 to 1939, 30% in 1940 to 1957, 15% in 1959 to 1965, to 7% in 1965 to 1985. In the last period, thymoma patients still had a death rate of 32%. In another series, mortality declined from 42 to 6% of patients hospitalized in a myasthenic crisis, and from 12 to 3.3% if the total series of the early 1960s and late 1970s were compared (86). In a recent study from six large Italian centers, 3.7% had died (2.6% without, and 8.5% with a thymoma; 80). In the author's series (n = 374) followed from 1965 to 1984, total death rate was 7.8%, of which 1.5% of the patients were under the age of 40 without thymoma, 10% of the patients were over the age of 40 without thymoma (5% by MG and 5% due to complications of medication) and 23% were patients with thymomas (13% by MG, 7% due to thymoma, 3% due to complications of medication) (87). In the Norwegian population, the standardized myasthenia mortality rate was about 150% in the period 1951 to 1981 (69). In Denmark (1970 to 1987), 10% of the patients died from MG, which was about twice the standardized mortality rate (77).

2.6.4 The incidence of thymomas in MG

Thymomas are reported in 9 to 16% of large series of MG patients (50, 77, 91, 92), and in 20 to 34% of series of thymectomies for MG (93-96). The incidence of MG in thymomas was surmised to be 30 to 40% (97), but in two recent series 59 and 61% (95, 96). The incidence of thymomas may have been under-reported in older series collected before CT-scanning of the mediastinum ascertained the detection of small tumors which escape conventional radiography. On the other hand, some selection bias may have occurred in the series of large centers. The incidence of thymomas is lacking in most of the recent epidemiological surveys; in the author's study 19% was found (72). Thymomas in general are very rare under the age of 20 and occur most frequently in the fifth and sixth decade (4, 91, 96, 99, 100). **(Fig. 2.25)**
In the author's series, the relative incidence was the same in men and women (15.8%), but after the age of 40 the incidence in women was twice as much as in men (36 vs 18%). This higher incidence in older women was also found in other series (91), although less prominently. In series of thymectomies, however, thymomas had a higher incidence in men (30 to 46%) than in women (17 to 26%), which may be a selection bias (93-96). In a series reported from Finland, only 4% had a thymoma (70). In general, the myasthenic signs are more severe in patients with a thymoma, and especially this category is liable to develop spontaneous crises (47, 57, 81). In addition, associated autoimmune diseases (57) and extrathymic malignancies (102) are more frequent and contribute to a higher death rate.

2.6.5 The incidence of autoimmune diseases in MG

The hypothesis of the autoimmune (A-I) pathogenesis of MG was partly based on the occurrence of other A-I diseases in a population of MG patients (18). Many associations of MG and other A-I diseases have been reported since then, in case studies and in large series of MG patients (50, 57, 69, 70, 72, 88, 99-

107, 116): the frequencies in these series vary from 2.3 to 24.2%, with a mean of 12.9%. Epidemiologic studies, however, are few (69, 70, 72, 78, 107). In general, A-I diseases have a higher prevalence in women than in men and the same was found in two series of MG patients (16.3 vs 6.4% [57], or 15.3 vs 5.3% [105]). Some occur predominantly in older age, e.g. rheumatoid arthritis and autoimmune gastritis; others are more evenly distributed over a lifetime. It is obvious therefore, that the prevalence in a certain population of patients at a certain moment may vary according to the mean age of that population, to the sex ratio, and to the duration of the follow-up. The prevalence of A-I diseases in the general population is unknown and will depend on inclusion criteria.

The most common association is that with <u>thyroid diseases</u>, usually with hyperthyroidism due to thyroiditis, with frequencies ranging from 2.6 to 16.9% of the reported series. Since the prevalence of hyperthyroidism in population studies was about 1% (108) or 2.5% in adult women (109), the higher prevalence in MG patients is not attributable to chance. In a large series of patients with Graves' disease in Japan (110), MG was present in 0.14%, which is also higher than can be expected (0.005%). Muscle weakness and ophthalmoplegia may also be signs of hyperthyroidism and may obscure the concomitant signs of MG. Signs of MG may be exaggerated by thyroid dysfunction.

<u>Rheumatoid arthritis</u> is the next commonly associated disease, but the prevalence varies from 0 to 10.3% in the reported series. In these series, d-Penicillamin induced MG was not included (111-113); the incidence is probably 1.5% in patients treated for rheumatoid arthritis (114), and should be kept in mind in this category of patients. This complication is not always reversible after omission of the drug. These patients may have true MG.

Less common are systemic lupus erythematosus (50, 58, 70, 91, 99-102, 104, 105, 115), A-I gastritis (pernicious anemia; 57, 70, 88, 99, 101, 102, 116), sarcoidosis (88, 99, 116), Sjögren's disease (70, 99, 100), hemolytic anemia (57, 69, 88), ulcerative colitis (63, 116), Crohn's disease (iliitis terminalis; 117), pemphigus (105, 118), scleroderma (50, 70), polymyositis (50, 57, 70), glomerulonephritis (63, 70, 107, 116), A-I adrenalitis (57, 119, 120), A-I thrombopenia (57, 102, 121, 122), primary ovarian failure (123, 124), Lambert-Eaton myasthenic syndrome (125-129), and pure red cell anemia (72), or pancytopenia (69). The latter two conditions are almost exclusively related to thymoma.

The combination of generalized hair follicle hamartoma (trichoepithelioma), alopecia, and myasthenia gravis has been reported three times in young women (130-132) of whom one is included in the author's series (132). An autoimmune basis for this dermatological disease is not yet established.

The only neurological disease possibly occurring with an increased incidence is multiple sclerosis (MS). Apart from single case reports, in one series from Japan 4 patients were found with both diseases, out of 109 patients with MS and 110 with MG (133), which is an unusually high incidence in both ways. In a Finnish epidemiological survey, 2 patients were found in 94 MG patients (prevalence 6×10^{-5}) and 991 MS patients (prevalence 60×10^{-5}). The expected observed to expected ratio was 40.4 (95% confidence limits 4.9 and 146 [134]). In the author's series of 805 MG patients, 3 patients with MS were diagnosed.

2.6.6 Genetic predisposition

Although MG is not considered as a hereditary disease with a definite mode of genetic transmission, familial cases have been reported in 1 to 4% of several series (4, 82, 88, 135, 136) or even in 7.2% (70). In an analysis of 72 familial cases reported up to 1970, 39% belonged to the congenital type (onset before 2 years of age), 22% had occurred between 3 and 18 years and 39% over the age of 18. In 76% they occurred in one generation, in 24% in two generations and never in three. In 85% of the families, two members had MG, in 10% three and rarely more (135). In twin studies, 6 out of 15 monozygotic twins both were affected and none out of 9 dizygotic twins (137).

In my own series, 7 patients had a near family member with acquired MG (prevalence 1.7%; see Chapter 5).

2.7 Myasthenia in childhood

It is of utmost importance to distinguish between the 3 possible myasthenic syndromes that may occur in childhood: neonatal MG, congenital MG and acquired autoimmune MG (table 2.6).

2.7.1 Neonatal MG in children with a myasthenic mother

In 1942 Strickroot et al. (138) reported the first case of MG in a baby born to a myasthenic woman. Despite treatment with neostigmine, the child died at the 7th day from respiratory insufficiency. Namba et al. (139) gave a review of 82 cases, the incidence being 12% of babies born to myasthenic mothers. About the same figure was found in an epidemiologically defined population, where 2 children out of 11 pregnancies had a transient neonatal MG (72).

The onset was within a few hours after birth in 66%, in 78% in the first day of life and the latest on the third postnatal day. The clinical signs were weak sucking and swallowing, hypotonia and weak movements, feeble crying and respiratory difficulties, while ptosis and squinting and facial weakness were less prominent. The most severe symptoms occurred in the first week, wherein 9 (11%) died of respiratory insufficiency. The mean duration of the symptoms was 18 days and the maximum duration was 47 days, but a prolongation until at least 71 days (140) has been reported. Improvement in strength following an injection of neostigmine (usually 0.1 mg i.m. or subcutaneously) or edrophonium (usually 1.0 mg), occurred in 86%. Management consisted of

Table 2.6 CHILDHOOD MYASTHENIA

	Neonatal	Congenital Myasthenic Syndrome (CMS)	Acquired juvenile
mother with MG	always	not reported	rare, in familial cases
onset	0-72 h after birth	at birth or infancy, rarely later (SCS)[1]	after first year of life (or earlier?)
type	generalized	mostly ocular and limb weakness bulbar signs at infancy, particularly in F.I.M.[1]	any type
course	spontaneous remission in 1-6 weeks	crises may occur in F.I.M. improvement of bulbar signs after infancy stationary or progressive	usually benign, tends to improve after the first years
familial	other sibs occasionally	50% hereditary, or uncertain	±10% familial cases
AChR-Ab	++	–	+/–
reaction to thymectomy	not performed	not performed[2]	no
reaction to prednisone	not given	absent	variable

[1] see text 2.7.2

[2] negative in one of my patients, see 5.7

anticholinesterases and careful nursing (suction of pharyngeal secretions, tube feeding) and artificial respiration, until the signs gradually diminished and disappeared (139). In only one patient out of 39, followed for 1-22 years, a 'recurrence' (?) between the ages of 2 and 3 years was reported (141).

There was no relationship between neonatal MG and the severity of the MG of the mother. Eleven mothers had 2 children with neonatal MG, but had a normal child in between. At least 4 mothers had not had anticholinesterases and 9 were previously thymectomized (139). There was no relation to the presence or absence of anti-muscle antibodies in the mother or child (142. 143), whereas a relation with anti-acetylcholine receptor antibodies (anti-AChR) is certain

(144-148), although these antibodies are usually present in the child without clinical signs (145, 148). It was observed that asymptomatic children and their mothers had relatively low antibody titers (144, 148, 150).

The reason why neonatal MG develops in only 10-15% of the babies is still unclear. The inhibiting effect of alpha-fetoprotein on the interaction between antigen and antibody (149) was not confirmed (150). The class of maternal anti-AChR antibodies might be important: neonatal MG, and especially the severe variety, occurred predominantly in children from mothers with blocking antibodies. The same investigators found that neonatal MG correlated with the presence of antibodies directed against the fetal AChR (containing the gamma instead of the epsilon subunit) extracted from embryonic muscle (151).

2.7.2 Congenital myasthenic syndromes (CMS)

The term congenital myasthenia was first used by Bowman (152) to describe a child with MG from birth, not born from a myasthenic mother. CMS are a conglomerate of uncommon (1-2% of MG) disorders of the neuromuscular transmission, mostly present from birth or infancy (153), although some may develop later in life (154-157). Some patients are born with contractures, so that intra-uterine development may occur (158, 159).

The clinical presentation is variable, but most patients have ptosis **(fig. 2.25)**, ophthalmoparesis, and limb muscle weakness, increased by exercise. The earliest recognized entity was familial infantile myasthenia (FIMG), characterized by bulbar signs (poor sucking, choking, weak crying) in the neonatal period, with life threatening exacerbations also in later childhood, especially during infections (160-163). Other types usually have a smooth course, without remissions and exacerbations, and are usually detected at a later age, sometimes after prolonged apnoea due to the use of muscle relaxant agents. Localized muscle atrophy is reported of the hand muscles in Slow Channel syndrome (SCS) (155) and of the trunk and hand extensors in older patients with acetylcholinesterase deficiency (167). With the use of modern neurophysiological and morphological techniques, the precise localization and the nature of the deficit is recognized; these may be presynaptic, synaptic or postsynaptic (153). **(Table 2.7)**

Presynaptic deficits are related to the release or storage of ACh (154, 161), the synaptic defect is related to absence (167) or reduction (169) of acetylcholinesterase, and the postsynaptic defects are caused by a reduction or abnormal structure of the AChR (155, 156, 171), usually combined with structural abnormalities of the postsynaptic membrane (159, 170) or with a (putative) defect of the interaction of ACh with the AChR (166, 174).

In some types an autosomal recessive heredity is probable, since several cases occurred in only one generation; in the SCS an autosomal dominant heredity exists, with subclinical (electromyographical) expression (156), but of many other types only single cases were studied. It is unclear whether the familial

Table 2.7 CONGENITAL MYASTHENIC SYNDROMES

	HEREDITY	REFERENCES
A Presynaptic defects		
1. Reduced size synaptic vesicles (FIMG)	AR	154, 161
2. Paucity of synaptic vesicles	1 patient	164
3. Congenital Lambert-Eaton syndrome	2 patients	165, 166
B Synaptic defects		
1. Absence ACh-esterase, small nerve terminals	AR (5 patients)	167, 168
2. Deficiency ACh-esterase and of AChR	1 patient	169
C Postsynaptic defects		
1. Slow Channel syndrome (SCS)	AD (12 patients)	155, 157
2. Congenital paucity of synaptic clefts (CPSC)	AR (4 patients)	159, 170
3. Epsilon subunit mutation	2 patients	171
4. AChR deficiency and short channel open time	1 patient	172
5. High conductance fast closure AChR channel	1 patient	173
6. Abnormal interactions ACh to AChR	1 patient	174
7. AChR deficiencies	9 patients	166
D Undefined syndromes		
1. Familial limb girdle MG	2 patients (+2?)	175
2. Benign congenital MG with facial malformations	AR	179

AR = autosomal recessive; AD = autosomal dominant

limb girdle MG (175) belongs to the acquired familial MG or to the congenital entity.

The course in FIMG is rather benign if patients survive the exacerbations in infancy; in the SCS a gradual progression occurred (155, 156), as was the case in 2 patients with the CPSC syndrome (170); some patients with arthrogryposis at birth improved by anticholinesterases (159).

The diagnosis of CMS is confirmed by the absence of AChR-ab and by the decrement of the CMAP at repetitive nerve stimulation, although in FIMG this feature only occurred after exercise or prolonged stimulation (154). A decisive diagnostic EMG feature was a double CMAP at single stimulation in patients with SCS (155, 156) or ACh-esterase deficiency (167). The patient with these types of CMS does not respond to anticholinesterases, or even gets worse. In other types, the reaction to anticholinesterases is moderate, the ptosis and ophthalmoparesis being refractory. In some patients 3,4-diaminopyridine gave a significant improvement (177).

Genetic mutations were demonstrated in SCS patients, concerning the beta-subunit (178) of the AChR; in one other CMS-type the epsilon-subunit was abnormal (171).

The practical importance of distinguishing CMS from acquired MG is the avoidance of thymectomy and immunosuppressive therapies and in genetic counseling. My own experience with 8 CMS patients is reported in Chapter 4.

2.7.3 Acquired infantile MG

Acquired MG may occur at any age. The prevalence of cases with onset in the first decade in European and American series varies from 1.1 to 3.1% (**table 2.8, fig. 2.1**), which is lower than the overall prevalence in the population.

Table 2.8 MYASTHENIA IN CHILDHOOD

	PERIOD	N	CONGENITAL	ACQUIRED			REF.
				0-9	10-12	13-15	
Osserman	1958	319	2.5[1]	3.1		3	4
Millichap	1935-59	437	1.4	1.6		5.2	179
Szobor	1951-87	1050				10.8	180
Batocchi	1971-80	580		2.1		6.0	181
Somnier*	1970-87	182		◀----5.5----▶			76
Giagheddu*	1958-86	110		2			74
Storm*	1912-81	458		1.1			69
Oosterhuis	1960-94	805	1.1	2.8	1.7	4.8	

* Epidemiological investigation; [1] percentages

A relative large prevalence was found in Japanese (82) and Chinese (182) populations, with a peak at the ages of 2-3 years of ocular MG. The relatively high incidence of ocular MG in prepubertal MG was also found in European series (181). **(Table 2.1)**

The prognosis of infantile MG is usually favourable, although exacerbations may occur during fever, requiring hospitalization. In sporadic cases, a fulminating onset with life threatening respiratory insufficiency may occur (183, 184). Thymectomy and immunosuppression were effective in the prepuberal generalized MG, and without severe side effects, e.g. growth retardation accompanying the use of prednisone (181).

In children up to 3-4 years, AChR-ab tests may be negative (own experience; 185), so that these tests cannot be used to decide between congenital and acquired MG.

NOTES

[1] This Bell's phenomenon was present in 23 normal individuals under the age of 40, but after that age a steadily increasing percentage did not show it:
40-49: 11%, 50-59: 22%, 60-70: 35%, 70-79: 44%. In this older group, it could be found in either one or both eyes (186).

[2] I could not confirm the observation of diminished pupillary contractions on repeated exposure to light (187), nor the complete loss of light-reaction after 2-3 minutes of repeated illumination reversed by edrophonium (188). However, with infra-red pupillography about 30% slowing of the pupillary contraction-dilatation cycles was demonstrated (189, 190).

[3] 'Fatigue' denotes a subjective feeling impairing the impulse to move and only in extreme conditions the muscle power. Weakness occurring or increasing after moderate exertion is accompanied by strange, heavy feelings, which may be called 'fatigue', but a better term would be 'exhaustion'. Muscle work during partial curarization was accompanied by the reduction of the normal feeling of fatigue (191) and with a recognition of the limitation of capacity, rather than a feeling of increased effort (192). The isometric maximal voluntary contraction in normals results quickly in a loss of force due to the high metabolic demand in combination with an impeded blood flow. Several parameters measurable with surface EMG change during maximal voluntary contraction: the average muscle fibre velocity, the median frequency of the power spectrum and the amplitude of the integrated EMG all decrease as well as the final power of the contraction (193). In MG patients the muscle force (Newton) measured in the m.biceps was initally much lower, and declined more rapidly and the integrated EMG had a lower amplitude. However the conduction velocity of the muscle fibres did not change and the median frequency much less than in normals. (**Fig. 2.25**)

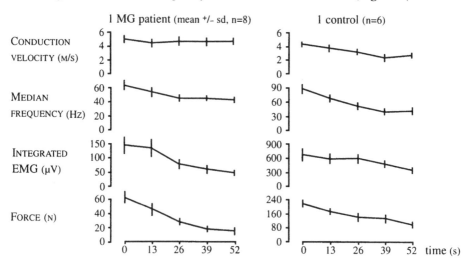

3

DIAGNOSIS

3.1 Clinical criteria and diagnostic tests

MG is not difficult to diagnose if the patient has a typical history of fluctuating weakness and clinical signs. Unfortunately many patients present at onset with vaguely formulated complaints and most doctors do not know the disease from their own medical experience. A doctor's delay of one to two years is not unusual, and in many patients the diagnosis is only made after unnecessary investigations, e.g. CT-scan of the cerebrum, angiography, muscle biopsy to exclude other diseases. On the other hand, a falsely positive diagnosis is sometimes made in patients with ptosis, blepharospasm (1), bulbar syndromes and somatization disorders (2).

Table 3.1 CRITERIA FOR THE DIAGNOSIS OF MG

- •1. Symptoms and signs are explained by muscle weakness of a peripheral type*;
- •2. The weakness is fluctuating, either spontaneous over short (minutes to hours) or longer (days to months) periods or due to exertion and rest;
- •3. A deficit of neuromuscular transmission is confirmed by one of the following tests:
   - a. the specific effect of anticholinesterases: neostigmine, pyridostigmine, edrophonium;
   - b. electromyographic procedures: repetitive nerve stimulation tests or single fibre EMG;
   - c. the presence of antibodies to acetylcholine receptors (AChR-Ab)

* The involvement of ocular or bulbar muscles contributes considerably to the clinical probability of the diagnosis, but weakness confined to the limb muscles is not unusual at onset in young patients (table 2.1), but persistence without involvement of ocular or bulbar muscles is very rare (3,4).

Not all MG patients will meet the criteria sub 2-3c in every stage of their disease: the effect of anti-AChE may be lacking at the first onset, particularly in ocular signs, or in crisis. AChR-Ab are absent in 10-15% of patients with generalized signs and in 50-60% with purely ocular signs. If the criteria sub 1-3 are met, a congenital myasthenic syndrome (2.7.2) and the Lambert-Eaton Myasthenic syndrome (6.5) should also be considered.

The sensitivity and specificity of these diagnostic tests is somewhat different in generalized and ocular MG. (**Table 3.2**)

Table 3.2 SENSITIVITY AND SPECIFICITY OF DIANOSTIC TESTS
IN GENERALIZED AND OCULAR MYASTHENIA[a]

	Generalized Myasthenia		Ocular Myasthenia	
	SENSITIVITY	SPECIFICITY	SENSITIVITY	SPECIFICITY
AChR-ab	0.92 (0.89-0.95)[b]	0.97 (0.94-1.00)	0.36 (0.23-0.49)	0.97 (0.94-1.00)
Edrophonium or Neostigmine test	0.97 (0.94-1.0)	0.90 (0.82-0.98)	0.80 (0.69-0.91)	0.90 (0.82-0.98)
Repetitive nerve stimulation	0.82 (0.72-0.92)	0.92 (0.86-0.98)	0.45 (0.28-0.62)	0.88 (0.79-0.97)

[a] Data from 450 MG patients and 173 patients with "pseudo-myasthenia", referred to the author). Not all tests were performed in each patient (15); [b] 95% confidence interval.

A proper use of these tests depends upon the present probability which must rely on the clinical signs and symptoms, eventually combined with the results of another test.

3.2 Clinical assessment

If MG is surmised, given the history or certain clinical signs (e.g. ptosis, eye muscle pareses, dysarthria, chewing difficulties), it is mandatory to prove that the signs can be influenced by exertion ("fatigue") and rest.

The tests listed in **table 3.3** and described in Chapter 2 have proved to be very useful in search for myasthenic weakness. They are simple, quantifiable and practicable in the consulting room as well as at the bedside. These tests have been used by the author for more than 25 years and the normal values are reliable.

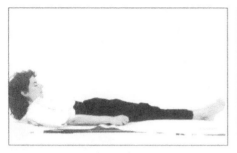

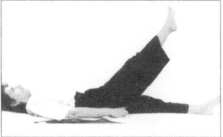

Figure 3.1 "Look at your toes."   **Figure 3.2** Leg raising test.

Table 3.3 QUANTITATIVE TESTS TO ASSESS MYASTHENIC WEAKNESS

1. Looking to one side (30°) during 30 s provokes diplopia and/or ptosis on the side of the abducting eye; nystagmoid movements, usually of the abducting eye may occur.
2. Ptosis decreases after 3 min eye closure or increases after looking into a bright light or at a fixed point.
3. Eye closure is weak and becomes weaker after repeated squeezing of the eyelids.
4. Reading aloud or counting (101, 102 etc.) provokes dysarthria or nasal speech within 3 minutes.
5. Closing of the jaws with an audible click is not possible for at least 100 times.
6. Swallowing (glass of water) is not possible without coughing or regurgitation through the nose.
7. Head raising in recumbent position is not possible during 60". **(Fig. 3.1)**
8. Arms and hands (in pronation) cannot be kept stretched out horizontally for 3 minutes: arms begin to tremble or to shake and one or more fingers may drop (fig. 2.18).
9. Straight leg raising to 45° in recumbent position is not possible for one minute. **(Fig. 3.2)**
10. Deep knee bends are not possible > 20 times; in older patients 20 times rising from a normal table chair is not possible.
11. Vital capacity (VC) or peak flow (maximal expiratory pressure) is diminished, or decreases after repeated testing. The difference in the VC with closed or open nose gives an indication for the palatum closure.

The strength and exhaustability of separate muscle groups can also be tested with a hand-held dynamometer (5, 6, 7) **(fig. 3.3)** and compared with the normal values for age and gender. In this way weakness may be detected which remained unnoticed or at least unreported by the patient. In mild cases, such weakness may only appear after exertion, e.g. a weakness of the deltoid muscle after performing the arm test for 3 minutes.

A typical profile of muscle weakness is given in **figure 3.4**.

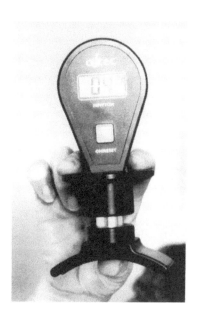

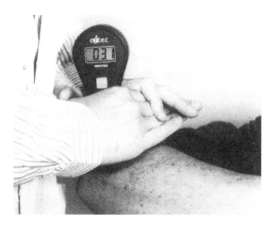

Figure 3.3 (Left) Hand-held dynamometer.[1] The positions for testing the three point grip (left) and the strength of the shoulder abductors muscle (right) are shown.

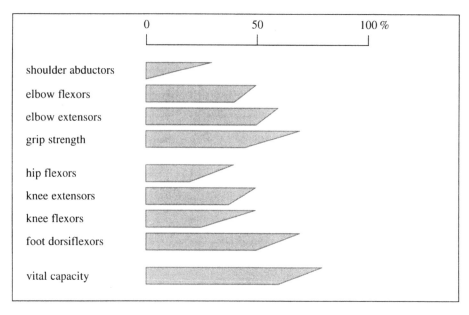

Figure 3.4 Muscle strength in MG. Typical profile of myasthenic weakness. Man 50 years (DS 4: O_2, B_2, U_3, L_3, V_1). Values by measurement with hand-held dynamometer, expressed as percentage of normal reference values (5). Upper part of bar is value of first contraction, lower part is value of fifth contraction. Arm extension test: 10 seconds, leg extension test: 5 seconds, one deep knee bend was possible.

In my experience it is exceptional that the typical complaints cannot be confirmed by one or more of these tests. If this specific examination is negative, the patient should be seen at the end of the afternoon or in a period of complaints.

3.3 Diagnostic procedures

3.3.1 Reaction to anticholinesterases

The specific effect of an anticholinesterase drug (pyridostigmine, prostigmine, ambenomium, edrophonium) is the key-stone for the diagnosis. A placebo-effect may be ruled out by the preceding use of atropine (which also serves as an anticholinergic) or by the immediate effect on oculobulbar functions. The use of atropine is advisable in case of predominant limb muscle weakness or diplopia without visible eye muscle pareses, which may occur in fatigue syndromes.

It is important to choose specific symptoms which can be quantified and compared before and after administration of the medicaments and not to rely upon subjective feelings of the patient. Previous oral anticholinesterases should be stopped for at least 24 hours if the test is equivocal.

For the first diagnostic test, I prefer the atropine-neostigmine test as originally described by Viets and Schwab (8, 9), instead of the edrophonium (Tensilon®) test (10, 11). The main reason is that the effect of neostigmine lasts longer (1 to 2 hours) than the effect of Tensilon (5 minutes, rarely 30 minutes) thus providing enough time for standardized clinical testing. Secondly, neostigmine is given intramuscularly while Tensilon is administered intravenously and may have unpleasant and sometimes alarming cholinergic side effects, such as bradycardia, asystoly, lacrimation, nausea, and glottis spasm, which may also hamper the interpretation of the specific effect. Patients with chronic obstructive pulmonary disease (COPD) may develop bronchoconstriction (12). Although serious side effects at fractionated administration are rare (1-1.5% [11, 13]), atropine should always be at hand.

In the atropine-neostigmine test, the cholinergic side effects may be present, but they rarely impede the assessment of the specific effect.

The technique for each test is given in **table 3.4**.

The sensitivity and specificity of both tests are given in table 3.1 (9, 11, 14-17). False negative tests are sometimes seen in the early stage of the disease, when the signs may be very fluctuating (for example in patients with eye muscle paresis only, in patients with muscle atrophy, or in very weak patients). If the diagnosis is still suspected, the test should be repeated after vigorous muscle exertion or at the end of the day. In patients with ocular signs only, some additional tests may be helpful.

Table 3.4 ATROPINE-NEOSTIGMINE TEST

Prepare the patient by telling her that she will get one or two injections, depending on the effect of the first
- test target signs
- administer 0.5 mg atropine subcutaneously
- test target signs after 10 minutes
- administer 1-2 mg (1 mg/50 kg) neostigmine i.m.
- test target signs after 10, 20, 30 min. and 2 hours

*Maximal effect to be expected 10-30 minutes after the second injection!

*Effect of first injection should be negative!

*Symptoms should reappear 1-2 hours after the second injection.

EDROPHONIUM (TENSILON®) TEST

- patient in half seated position with possibility to lay down
- test target signs
- prepare 1 ml syringe with 1.0 ml Tensilon® (10 mg) and syringe with 0.5 ml atropine (1 mg)
- fix the needle after venapunction so that change of syringe is easy
- administer 0.2 ml (2 mg) Tensilon® i.v.
- test target signs; if unequivocal improvement, stop the test
- if negative: add 0.3 ml (3 mg) Tensilon® i.v. after 1 minute
- test target signs: if improvement, stop the test
- if negative and no side effects: administer 5 mg Tensilon® after 1-2 minutes

*Effect to be expected 30-60 seconds after injection

*Control target symptoms after 5-30 minutes: signs should reappear!

*If not the slightest cholinergic effects are noticed by the patient, nor fasciculations in the face, one can doubt about the proper administration

False positive tests are reported in patients with polymyositis (18), ALS (19), botulism (20), the Guillain-Barré syndrome (21), the Lambert-Eaton myasthenic syndrome (21,22) and in patients with cranial nerve syndromes due to brainstem involvement (18, 23), tumors of the orbital or parasellar region (24), and bilateral intracavernous carotid aneurysm (24, 25). Also in mitochondrial myopathies (26) and nonmyasthenic ocular palsies (27), these tests are occasionally positive.

Apart from the qualitative aspect (the diagnosis), the neostigmine or pyridostigmine test has a quantitative aspect: it sets the limit for the effect of oral administration (see 3.6).

3.3.2 Antibodies to acetylcholine receptorprotein (AChR-ab)

The detection of AChR-ab has greatly facilitated the diagnosis of MG. With the conventional immunoprecipitating test (28), AChR-ab could be demonstrated in 76 to 93% of large series of MG patients (15, 29-34), but in patients with purely ocular MG only in 36 to 54% (15, 17, 31, 32, 35, 36). They are nearly always present in patients with MG and thymomas (30, 37, 38). The AChR-ab concentrations had a log-normal distribution, 95% ranging from 0.2 and 1549 nMol/l, with highest values up to 5000 nMol/l (33). **(Table 5.4)** In general, the concentration is not indicative for the severity of MG, though in most studies ocular patients have lower antibody titers. In the above mentioned study, a positive correlation of severity and AChR-ab levels was found with regression analysis (33). If individual patients are followed during the course of MG, a good correlation between the changes in clinical condition and the changes in AChR concentration is found in about 80% of the cases (38-40). AChR-ab remain demonstrable in most patients with complete clinical remission (30).

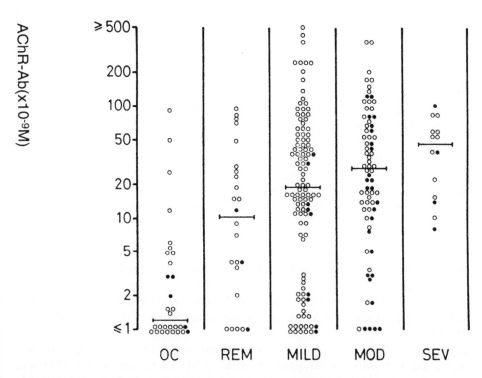

Figure 3.5 Antibodies to acetylcholine receptors in 250 MG patients grouped according to the severity of the disease at the time of serum sampling. Concentrations below 1 nM are negative. Rem(ission), Oc (ular), Mild (stage 1 or 2), Mod(erate) (stage 3 or 4), Sev(ere) (stage 5); closed circles represent patients receiving corticosteroids at the time of serum sampling (30).

Other techniques are used that can demonstrate the presence of blocking (of the ACh-binding site or alpha-Bungarotoxin binding site) or modulating (AChR's in muscle cultures) antibodies (29, 41-43a), which may have a more close relation to the severity of the disease (43). The additional test for blocking antibodies is no routine, since the yield is minimal and the tests are rather complex (43a, 56). Antibodies specific for ocular muscle have been reported, but their specificity is rather low (45). If important for the diagnosis, the help of specialized laboratories can be sought. Women with blocking and modulating antibodies probably have a higher frequency of children with neonatal MG (44). False positive tests, usually with low concentrations, have been described in various other conditions with contradictory results.[2] **(Table 3.5)**

Table 3.5 FALSE POSITIVE ACHR-AB TEST

	References	
• Thymoma without MG: 2/11[a], 5/11		30, 31
• Rheumatoid arthritis treated with d-penicillamine: 3/35, 3/100		30, 46
• Biliary cirrhosis: 16/17, 0/16		47, 48
• Systemic lupus erythematosus: 0/20, 2/70		30, 49
• Hematological diseases: 8/62		50
• Following bone marrow grafting: 21/52		50
• Down's syndrome: 9/38, 0/30		51, 52
• CVA patients older than 60 years: 9/50		51
• Old patients (> 70 y) with anti-thyroid antibodies: 3/40		52
• Amyotrophic lateral sclerosis: 2/22		43
• Tardive dyskinesias: 22/34		53
• Relatives of MG patients: 34/68, 0/48		54, 55
• Pseudo-MG patients: 5/157 (own patients)		15

[a] In 2 out of 11 patients with a thymoma without MG the AChR-ab test was positive, etc.

It should be emphasized that the sensitivity and the specificity of the test depend on the chosen cutoff point (46).[3] Since the predictive value of a positive test is more influenced by the specificity than by the sensitivity, the cutoff point should not be too low. If the conditions listed in table 3.5 are reasonably excluded, the AChR-ab test has a specificity of 0.97 to 0.994% (15, 16, 47).

Seronegative MG patients (i.e., without binding AChR-ab) with generalized signs did not differ from patients with AChR-ab in one series (34) and responded equally well to thymectomy and plasmapheresis. In other series (36, 37), including that of the author, young men with mild and spontaneously remitting disease were over-represented and patients with thymomas were absent (30, 37) or rare.[4]

3.3.3 Electromyography

3.3.3.1 Repetitive nerve stimulation

A prominent feature of myasthenic weakness is the increase during exertion. This phenomenon is the basis of a functional test using slow (2 to 3 Hz) supramaximal stimulation of a peripheral nerve and recording the compound muscle action potential (CMAP) from the muscle with surface electrodes. The typical finding in MG is a decrement in CMAP amplitude below 90% of the first CMAP, with a lowest amplitude at the fifth CMAP (57-60; **fig. 3.5**), although other patterns may occur (58).

Figure 3.6

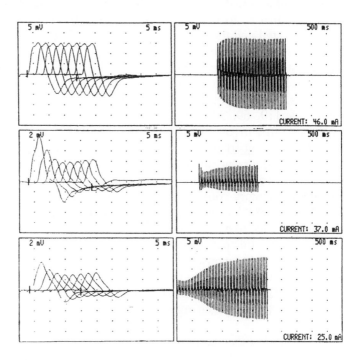

Repetitive nerve stimulation. Supramaximal stimulation of the ulnar nerve at the wrist. Compound muscle action potentials (CMAP) from the hypothenar muscles with surface electrodes. Stimulation rate 3/sec (left) and 20/sec (right). Upper trace: normal man, aged 35; middle trace: woman, aged 68 with myasthenia gravis (MG); lower trace: man aged 45 with Lambert-Eaton myasthenic syndrome (LEMS). Note the differences in calibration (2mV and 5mV). The initial amplitude of the CMAP in MG is within normal limits for age and gender, but too low in LEMS. In MG and LEMS the smallest amplitude of the CMAP is in the 4th and 5th CMAP with a slight increase in the following. At 20/sec stimulation a 25% increase of the CMAP is a normal finding. In LEMS the increase is 500% due to the low initial amplitude; the final value after 3 seconds is the same as in normals. (Courtesy Dr J.H. van der Hoeven.)

The decrement is enhanced by maximum voluntary contraction and by warming up the muscle to 36° (61, 62) or by ischemia (63, 64). This test is routinely done in the small hand muscles, but other muscles such as the m.orbicularis oculi (58, 65), the wrist extensors and deltoid muscle (58), the trapezius muscle (66) and even the diaphragm (67), are accessible and increase the yield of positive tests if the hand muscles are not clinically affected. Precautions should be made to avoid movement artifacts (60). Supramaximal stimuli are necessary and the stimulation rate should not exceed 3/sec. If these tests are negative, short intermittent stimulations may be continued up to 5 minutes to demonstrate post-tetanic exhaustion (57, 60). In some patients with severe initial weakness the response may be only positive after administration of anticholinesterase drugs (68). The sensitivity of this test in generalized MG varied from 0.32 to 0.89 (15, 16, 35, 58, 60), depending on the number of muscles tested and the severity of clinical weakness. In ocular MG, abnormal responses are less common (0.04 to 0.50) (15, 16, 35, 37, 38). The specificity of the test in generalized MG is about 0.90 (15, 16) and 0.90-0.99 in ocular MG (15, 16). False positive responses are reported in various other neuromuscular disorders, e.g. amyotrophic lateral sclerosis (first CMAP usually of low amplitude [19, 69, 70]), myotonic dystrophy (nonspecific steady decrement [71]) and other myopathies (26, 58).

Also in the Lambert-Eaton Myasthenic Syndrome (LEMS, see Chapter 6.5), a decrement occurs at stimulation of 1 to 3 Hz, but in this condition these CMAP's have an unusually low initial amplitude (1 to 3mV). After a brief maximal voluntary contraction or during a short (1 to 2 sec) nerve stimulation of 20 Hz, the CMAP reaches the normal size (72, 73). **(Fig. 3.6)** If other rare presynaptic disorders, e.g. botulism, hypermagnesemia, or hypocalcemia are excluded (60), this pattern is specific for LEMS.

A double muscle reponse to a single nerve stimulus **(fig. 5.16)** is characteristic for the Slow Channel syndrome and for the congenital acetylcholinesterase deficiency (2.7.2). This phenomenon should be tested routinely in seronegative patients with generalized signs.

3.3.3.2 Single Fiber Electromyography (SFEMG)

With SFEMG it is possible to record the action potentials (AP) of single muscle fibers. For this investigation a special needle electrode is used with a recording surface of only 25 μ in diameter, mounted in the side of the needle shaft (74, 75). With this needle, potential pairs from two muscle fibers, belonging to the same motor unit, are searched for (75). The time interval between the two AP's has a certain variability of about 10 to 50 μsec which is called "jitter". If neuromuscular transmission is impaired, the mean jitter is increased and often intermittent failure of transmission occurs ("blocking" [59, 75]). These blockings are the cause of the decrement in the CMAP at repetitive nerve stimulation. Criteria for abnormality are the mean jitter in 20 different fiber pairs (normally about 25 to 35 μsec), the number of fibers that have a jitter exceeding the statistically defined upper limit, and the occurrence of blockings. The m.extensor digitorum communis (EDC) of the forearm and the m.frontalis are commonly examined during voluntary contraction, but more proximal muscles (biceps, deltoid) may be used. In patients with ocular MG, the examination of the facial muscles (orbicularis oculi [76, 80], orbicularis oris [77]) will show more abnormalities.

Drawbacks of the method are the examination time (it takes 30 minutes to examine one muscle and at least 20 fiber pairs should be analyzed) and the dependency on the cooperation of the patient. The latter is not needed if intramuscular stimulation of the axonal nerve twigs is used (75), which is also possible in the examination of the facial muscles (76). This method is less time consuming and is well supported (78). The jitter values at stimulation are lower than those obtained by voluntary contraction (76). (**Fig. 3.7**)

SFEMG has a high sensitivity in patients with MG (59, 76). The mean jitter

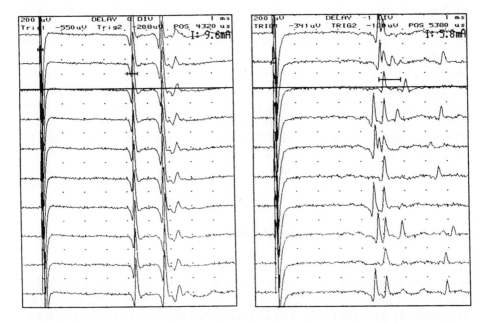

Figure 3.7 Examples of stimulated single fiber EMG. Stimulation of a branch of the facial nerve with a monopolar needle electrode, recording of the orbicularis oculi muscle with a single fiber electrode. Stimulation frequency during recording 10 Hz. On the left side of both figures, stimulation artifact, on the right side, the acquired potentials. Left: normal situation. Note the stable response consisting of three single fiber potentials. Right: myasthenia gravis. Unstable potentials, increased jitters, and frequent blocking. (Courtesy Dr J.H. van der Hoeven.)

values and the percentages of blockings increased according to the severity of the clinical signs, although a large variation was found in individual patients (59, 77). In mild generalized MG where SFEMG will be used preferentially, abnormal findings were reported in 84 to 96% in EDC alone (77), but additional examination of one or more facial muscles increased the yield of abnormal findings to 95% (77). In patients with moderate to severe MG, EDC had abnormal findings in 97 to 100% (35, 77). In ocular MG, abnormal findings in EDC varied from 63% (77) to even 94% (79-80); the used definition of ocular MG may play a role. Also, in clinical remission, SFEMG findings were abnormal in 75% (77). The specificity of SFEMG has not been reported in a large group of "pseudo-myasthenia", but several incidental false positive findings have been reported. This is not unexpected in a very sensitive test. *A priori* they are to be expected in disorders with regeneration of nerve fibers (59), such as motor neuron disease (75), peripheral neuropathies (81-83), but they have also been reported in chronic myopathies (59) and in chronic external ophthalmoplegia (84). Less well explained are abnormal jitter values in 6 of 15 patients with multiple sclerosis (85) and in 30 of 40 patients complaining of abnormal fatigue, following an identified viral infection (86). In the latter group of patients, neurological findings and repetitive nerve stimulation test results were normal but muscle biopsies showed mild abnormalities (86). Since MG is usually not a familial disease, the findings of increased jitter in 27% (87) or 30% (88) of asymptomatic close relatives in Swedish patients are remarkable, especially since 28 close relatives in an American study were completely normal (55).

The very high sensitivity of SFEMG makes it a useful tool to exclude the diagnosis of generalized MG if no abnormal jitter is found in a limb muscle nor in a facial muscle. In the suspicion of ocular MG, a negative finding in the facial muscles leaves some doubt. If SFEMG shows abnormal findings, some other (neuromuscular) diseases should also be considered.[5]

3.3.4 Antimuscle antibodies (AMA)

An early finding in the search for abnormal antibodies in MG patients was the detection of antibodies reacting with components of striated muscle (AMA). The indirect immunofluorescence technique (IIF) with rat diaphragm was and is commonly used (89). **(Fig. 1.8)** The incidence of AMA was 20% in patients without, and 100% in patients with thymomas (TH). The latter also had higher titers. The incidence increased with age (90). AMA were found in 2% of close relatives of MG patients and 0,2% of 441 matched controls (91). In a later study these findings were confirmed, though 16% of myasthenic TH patients had no AMA, probably these patients will develop AMA only after thymectomy (92, 93). AMA were also found in patients with a TH without (yet) MG (94), in patients with acute cardiac conditions (89) and in patients with rheumatoid arthritis treated with d-penicillamin (95).

In TH patients without MG, the presence of AMA predicted the subsequent development of MG (94).

Antibodies to a citric acid extract (CAE) of skeletal muscle were reported to be 100% specific in an indirect hemagglutination test, where the IIF technique had a sensitivity of 80% and a specificity of 60% (96). These findings were not confirmed in another study (97) when an Elisa and Western blot technique using CAE was compared with the conventional IIF. The Elisa and IIF showed the same findings; the Western Blot was superior in the detection of TH in young onset patients, but less useful in the late onset group. With these techniques AMA were found in 19% of MG patients without TH. The incidence increased with age up to 75% in the 60^+ group, which makes the positive predictive value neglegible in older patients (98). AMA-titers fluctuated in 42 patients in relation to their clinical condition and immunosuppressive therapies (IS). In 10 of 12 patients who underwent thymectomy without concomitant IS, AMA appeared de novo after the operation (93). AMA could also be detected in saline soluble components of skeletal muscle with the highest incidence in patients with TH (90%) and in older patients (99). Also IgG antibodies against titin, a large ($\pm$ 2,800 KD) myofibrillar protein have a high sensitivity (29/30) for the detection of TH (100), but their specificity is low since these antibodies were also present in 43% of late onset non-TH MG patients (101).

The high incidence of AMA in patients with MG and TH is only partly explained by common antigens of epithelial and muscle cells (102), because of the high incidence of these various antibodies in older patients without TH.

3.3.5 Disease non-specific antibodies

In 1963 an increased production of auto-antibodies (Ab) was demonstrated in an unselected populaton of MG patients, compared with controls matched for age and sex. Besides AMA these included antinuclear (ANA) and antithyroid Ab. A relatively high incidence of auto-Ab was found in TH-patients, especially of ANA (103). These findings were confirmed by others (104-106). Ab production increased with advancing age, which is a feature in common with other autoimmune diseases and with normal aging. Gross abnormalities in serum globulins are rare (107), but hypergammaglobulinaemia (108-110) was reported.

Other Ab against muscle constituents with a higher incidence in MG than in controls include those against filamin and vinculin (but not against tropomyosin) (111), reticulin (112), myosin, acto-myosin, especially in TH-patients, but not against actin and alpha-actin (113). Anti-neuroblastoma Ab measured with IIF, were found in 40% of MG patients, but also in patients with other autoimmune diseases without MG, and in neurological controls. These Ab were not well correlated with AChR-Ab (114).

An unexpected finding were Ab to muscarine AChR, extracted from rat brain:

IgG from MG patients blocked the specified binding sites, but not the affinity of antagonists to the AChR (115). Anti-presynaptic membrane receptor Ab, tested on an antigen extracted with beta-bungarotoxin were found in the sera of 67% of Chinese MG patients, in 80% overlapping with the postsynaptic AChR-Ab. These presynaptic binding Ab were also found in 6% of neurological controls and had no correlation with the clinical status (116).

These findings suggest a global imbalance of immunomodulation in MG patients, but are of minor clinical importance.

A good routine in the treatment of MG patients seems the search for ANA (anti-DNA), antithyroid and antigastric Ab as well as for rheuma factors, since these Ab have a predicting value for the presence or later appearence of the specific autoimmune diseases that have a higher incidence in MG.

3.4 Human leucocytic antigens (HLA)

Autoimmune (A-I) diseases have an increased familial incidence. In MG familial cases occur in 1-3% of patients (2.6), which is much higher than the incidence in the general population) (2.5), indicating a genetic factor. A possible explanation for genetic influence was found in the increased incidence of HLA-B8 antigens in early onset MG without thymoma (60-80% vs 20-30% in the general population (90, 117-120). The presence of HLA-B8 was related to higher mean AChR-Ab concentrations (105, 121), but not to the severity of the disease. The relative risk for a HLA-B8 positive individual to contract MG is 6, compared to HLA-B8 negativity, and even 28 if the individual is homozygous (122). In patients with thymomas HLA-B8 is relatively absent, but no special HLA group had a higher incidence. HLA-B8 is in linkage disequilibrium with A1 and also with DR3. Later it was found that the HLA-DR3 positive MG patients showed a close association with the presence of a 15 Kb restriction fragment, but this was not the case in DR3-positive patients with other A-I diseases (123). The relative risk for a HLA-DR3 individual expressing the 15 Kb restriction fragment to contract MG is 35 compared to a relative risk factor of 6 for HLA-B8 (123). An increase in DQw2 was found in our early onset group (124). No HLA group was indicative for the effect of thymectomy (124). In young Japanese females, the predominant HLA group was B12 (125); certain DR-subgroups seemed to be related to disease severity or clinical subgroups (126, 127). In young Chinese patients with mainly ocular MG, a strong association with HLA-Bw46 and DRw9 was found (128, 129).

The determination of HLA-antigens in MG patients is mainly of theoretical importance and does not contribute to the management of the individual patient.

3.5 The diagnosis of thymoma and residual thymus

Before the development of the CT-scan (±1975) the diagnosis of a TH relied upon conventional radiography of the thorax. If also 10° oblique lateral views were made, 50-60% of the TH diagnosed by operation or autopsy could be detected (130-133). In about 12 to 25% of these calcification is seen, mainly on the lateral view. The typical aspect is a rounded or lobulated mass in the normally empty space of the anterior mediastinum, but not infrequently they present as a mass overshadowing the hilus of the lung (130, 131). **(Fig. 3.8)**

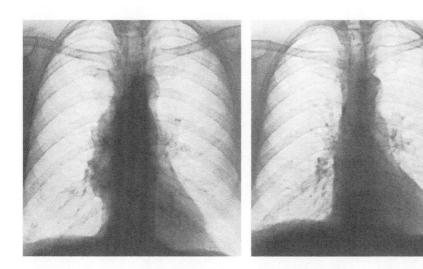

Figure 3.8 Thymoma on X-ray thorax: (left) before, and (right) after treatment of prednisone.

Computer tomography (CT) **(fig. 3.9)** is a more sensitive method of detecting a thymoma and possible thoracic metastases and has out-dated previous procedures like pneumomediastinography and radio-isotope scanning. In various series, the CT-diagnosis of thymoma was confirmed in 85-90% (131-137), but a false positive diagnosis of thymoma was found in 44% (133), ± 25% (137), 3% (134), or 1.3% (131) of patients with hyperplasia, depending the criterium of abnormality. Particularly in younger patients false positive diagnoses of thymic abnormality were made, because the normal picture was not well known. A systematic study of a large series of normals revealed that the thymus was seen in 100% of patients under the age of 30, in 73% of patients between 30 and 49 years, and in 17% of patients over 49 years of age (138). In younger patients, the density of the thymus was similar to that of muscle. **(Fig. 3.9)** Even with strict criteria the CT-diagnosis of the state of the thymus in MG is not completely reliable. Investigations where MRI, CT of the mediastinum and surgical findings were compared, do not suggest that MRI is superior to CT in terms of sensitivity and specificity (139-141).

If rethymectomy is considered, e.g. after transcervical or thoracoscopic (142) thymectomy, it should be realized that CT and MRI were not reliable: in only one of 5 patients who had thymic tissue removed at operation, MRI was indicative and CT in none (143). Since TH are very rare under the age of 20 (< 2%) a routine CT of the mediastinum is not indicated in this category, except if AMA tests are positive. The prevalence of TH increases with age up to 30% over the age of 40 years. A negative AMA test is found in about 20% of TH patients at *the onset* of the MG. If AChR-Ab are negative, a TH is excluded (3.2).

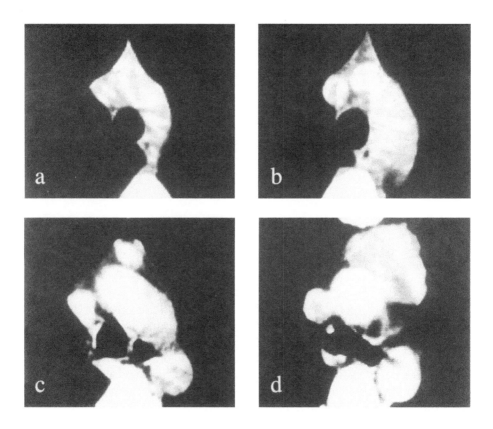

Figure 3.9 Computerized tomography (CT) of the thorax at the level of the aortic arch. **a.** M 16, no MG, thymus in a normal man of 16 years; **b.** W 35, no MG, thymus in a normal woman of 35 years. Compare the density of the thymus with that of the subcutaneous fat; **c.** M 57, MG since 5 years. Small thymoma not detectable on routine X-rays nor on a CT-scan made 2 years previously. Anti-SM were strongly positive from the onset of MG; **d.** W 38, MG since 3 months. Thymoma (5 x 6 x 3 cm) was visible on routine X-rays.

3.6 Summary of diagnostic strategy

The data of the previous chapter may have confounded the general neurologist in choosing the most adequate strategy to confirm his clinical suspicion of MG or to exclude it. Therefore a short summary may be appropriate.

Confirmation of a diagnosis relies on positive tests with high specificity, exclusion on negative tests with a high sensitivity (note 3.3).

The demonstration of rapidly fluctuating weakness is a clinical test with high specificity since rapid fluctuations of weakness rarely occur in other neuromuscular diseases. The additional proof is a positive atropine-neostigmine test, which has a high specificity as well as a high sensitivity. The combination of rapidly fluctivating weakness and a positive atropine-neostigmine test makes the diagnosis certain. Routine EMG is then unnecessary and a waste of effort and money (for the patient and the insurance!). Additional determination of AChR-Ab neither contributes to the diagnosis in this situation. It is possible that the absence of AChR-Ab in the conventional test has implications for the prognosis and management. In these patients the course of MG is in general less severe, a thymoma is absent and the reaction to thymectomy is dubious or absent in our experience, but the latter should be investigated in a clinical trial. So in seronegative MG patients a CT of the mediastinum is not indicated. If the clinical diagnosis is not confirmed by a 'lege artis' **(table 3.4)** performed and repeated atropine-neostigmine or edrophonium test, the determination of AChR-Ab is indicated. If this test is negative in patients with ocular signs only, single fibre EMG of the m.orbicularis oculi may be of diagnostic importance. In a minority of our patients all these 3 tests were negative (5.3.1) so that the diagnosis ocular MG relied upon the clinical features only.

It should be unnecessary to say that a CT-scan of the mediastinium is not indicated if the diagnosis MG is not certain. In patients undergoing thymectomy a CT-scan is indicated to diagnose a thymoma. In early onset patients the presence of AMA largely increases the likelihood of a thymoma, so that this test has some additional diagnostic value. In all older patients a CT of the mediastinum is indicated to detect a possible thymoma which in itself is an indication for operation. In older patients AMA have no additional diagnostic value.

If no thymoma is present on the CT-scan, a periodic cheque-up by repeating CT-scans seems not indicated since I have never seen a thymoma appearing during follow-up.

If a thymoma is diagnosed in a patient not known to have MG, a neurological examination is indicated including tests for AChR-Ab and AMA. MG may be present, which has implications for the use of muscle relaxants and the risk for postoperative ventilatory insufficiency. Patients without clinical signs with antibodies have a higher risk to develop MG later on.

Because MG patients have a high lifetime prevalence of other autoimmune diseases, particularly of the thyroid gland routine thyroid function tests including autoantibodies are a defendable diagnostic strategy. A routine screening of other antibodies, or HLA types is not recommended.

A final comment is the importance of the parenteral atropine-neostigmine test. Some neurologists try oral Mestinon as a diagnostic test and base their final judgement of the effect on the opinion of the patient. In this way a placebo effect in non-MG patients is difficult to exclude so that a false positive diagnosis is made. On the other hand oral Mestinon may fail to have a useful effect e.g. on diplopia,, whereas the intramuscular test would have been positive. The second reason to perform initially an intramuscular test is that the maximum effect of anti-AChE may be estimated. For instance if eye muscle pareses and diplopia fail to react, but the limb muscles do, it is of no use to increase the dosage of oral anti-AChE in order to alleviate the eye muscle pareses.

NOTES

[1] The hand-held dynamometer can be purchased at C.I.T. Technics BV, Bieslookstraat, 9731 HH Groningen. Fax +50.5424286. Price about 2,000.-- Dutch guilders.

[2] Since 1978 dr P.C. Limburg, biochemist in the department of Rheumatology Academic Hospital Groningen, has carried out and supervised the immunoprecipitation test for the detection of AChR-ab. The antigen (AChR) is extracted from amputated legs of which the chronic ischemic muscles are partly denervated and form extrajunctional AChR. To guarantee a reasonably stable concentration of antigen, the muscle tissue of at least 3 legs is mixed in one batch. The limit for a positive test is ≥ 1 nMol/L, with a sensitivity of 0.93 for generalized MG. To compare antibody concentration in the course of the disease in individual patients the same batch of antigen is preferable. In the last 5 years 1200 tests were performed per year of which only 10% of newly examined patients was positive. In the Central Laboratory of the Blood Transfusion Service Amsterdam also denervated muscle tissue is used as an antigen. Of the 1200 tests per year about 10% was positive. The costs of the test is Dfl. 93.--. (Courtesy of Dr R. Geertzen.)

Since denervated muscle tissue is not easily obtainable another source of antigen would be attractive. Human rhabdomyosarcoma cells (TE 671) express the fetal AChR and extracts may be used as antigen. The sensitivity of these extrajunctional AChR is lower than those from ischemic muscle which express both extrajunctional and junctional receptors. Low AChR-Ab levels (< 2 nMol) cannot be detected with this test (151). By transfecting TE 671 cells with cDNA encoding the human muscle AChR epsilon subunit (junctional receptor) it was possible to express the adult AChR subtype on the TE 671 cell membrane which enhances the sensitvity of the test considerably (152). From the reports of the External Quality Assessment Schemes (Sheffield GB) it appears that about $2/3$ of the 34 European laboratories which perform the AChR-Ab test are using denervated human muscle as antigen and $1/3$ the TE 671 cell line.

[3] The predictive value of a diagnostic test is determined by its sensitivity (the proportion of positive tests in the disease population) and its specificity (1 minus the proportion of positive tests in a comparable normal population), combined in the likelihood ratio (LR). The LR of a positive test (LR+) is defined as

$\dfrac{\text{sens}}{1\text{-spec.}}$; the LR of a negative test (LR-) as: $\dfrac{1\text{-sens.}}{\text{spec.}}$.

The relationship between pretest or clinical probability and post-test probability is given in Bayes' theorem, which can be remodeled in the odds ratio form

$$\dfrac{p}{1\text{-}p} \; x \, LR \; = \dfrac{P}{1\text{-}P} \qquad \begin{array}{l} p = \text{pretest probability} \\ P = \text{post-test probability} \end{array}$$

The LR's of the 3 most used tests for MG can be accounted from table 3.1. The use of multiple tests requires that they measure independent features. This is probably not entirely true for the effect of anticholinesterases and the repetitive nerve stimulation test that are both measuring the function of neuromuscular transmission.

[4] There are many arguments that also "seronegative" patients (SNMG) have circulating antibodies that interfere with neuromuscular transmission. Plasma-exchange may be effective in SNMG (144). Passive transfer studies of serum from SNMG to mice resulted in deficits of neuromuscular transmission, though to a lesser degree than was the case with serum of AChR-ab positive patients (145). Degradation of AChR in tissue cultures were comparable between seropositive and seronegative MG, and related to the severity of MG (146). If peripheral lymphocytes of SNMG patients were transferred to immunodeficient mice, these developed circulating AChR-ab and changes of their postsynaptic membranes (147).

[5] If a patient with MG is subjected to a routine needle EMG because the diagnosis myopathy is surmised, a frequent finding is a myopathic pattern, consisting of short and polyphasic muscle unit potentials (MUP). It was shown that the duration of the MUPs became normal after administration of anticholinesterases (148).
A shortening and loss of amplitude was also found in the eye muscles after sustained effort, becoming normal after edrophonium (149). In longstanding myasthenic ophthalmoplegia without visible reaction to anticholinesterases this method may reveal the activation of fibres which are nevertheless unable to move the eye. This method is also useful for the differentiation with ocular myopathies in which electric activity is increased in discrepancy with the paralysis. Also single fibre EMG of the superior rectus and levator palpebrae complex revealed abnormal jitter in 17 MG patients with purely ocular signs and not in 9 control patients with other (not further specified) ocular disease (150). The specificity of this method should be investigated in a larger patient group.

4

TREATMENTS

4.1 General remarks

MG is a chronic and even for half of the adequately treated patients, a lifelong disease. The course is inpredictable in the individual patients. As in all chronic diseases the patient has to live with her[1] disability and most patients succeed in doing so. Many however have to go through a period of uncertainty in which the diagnosis is not made (1, 2) and emotional problems are thought to be the cause of their symptoms. After the diagnosis is made, the patient needs a thorough explanation of the nature of the disease and frequent contact with a doctor who is able to treat her. Many patients complain that their doctors know less of MG than they do themselves, especially if they have become a member of a MG-patient association[2.] Problems may arise if they are treated for other diseases (3). Many patients know that certain drugs may enhance their symptoms **(table 4.3)**, and are critical if a new drug is prescribed or are inclined not to take it. Patients should know that emotions and stress though not the cause of their disease are likely to have great influence upon it, that short periods of rest are effective and vigourous exercise is to be avoided, and that MG has spontaneous fluctuations, particularly in the first 3 to 5 years. The same knowledge will make doctors somewhat reluctant to change a therapy too soon, or to ascribe any improvement to a new way of treatment. Symptoms may be exacerbated during infections with fever, extreme environmental temperatures (avoid hot baths, sauna, sunbathing), hot foods and in the premenstrual period in about one third of the women. Operations and other medical interventions may also be followed by an exacerbation.[3] Patients should be advised to do what they feel they are able to, without a priori restrictions. Keeping a diary is very helpful for doctor and patient to get a better insight into the factors that influence the symptoms and the effect of therapy. A general outline of treatment is given in **table 4.1**.

Table 4.1 GENERAL PLAN OF TREATMENT IN MG

---

1 a. Give adequate explanation, consider psychological factors
  b. Pyridostigmine (Mestinon®) 5-6 dd 20-90 mg; increase gradually; add atropine sulfate $^1/_8$-$^1/_4$ mg to each dose if parasympathetic side effects. Try additionally 3-5 dd prostigmine 7.5-15 mg or ephedrine 2-3 dd 25 mg.[4]
  c. In premenstrual exacerbation try an ovulatory pill
  d. Be cautious with certain medicaments (see table 4.3)

2 Thymectomy, if no spontaneous remission has occurred within 6-12 months after onset in patients with generalized MG:
  a. in all patients aged 10-40, irrespective the effect of anti-AChE and severity
  b. in patients aged 40-50 if MG is of short duration (< 3 years) and not responding well to anticholinesterases.
  c. Undelayed operation of thymoma, as soon as this can be done safely.

3 Prednisone, starting with 1-1.5 mg/kg/day, gradually tapered to 0.5 mg/kg on alternate days in severe MG (stages 3, 4 and 5).
In purely ocular MG if other measures (eyelid-support, occlusion, prisms) fail, start with 0.5-1 mg/kg/day.

4 Azathioprine 2.5 mg/kg/day
  a. in moderate MG, if prednisone is contraindicated or not wel tolerated
  b. in severe MG, combined with prednisone

5 Cyclosporine 2-5 mg/kg/day if prednisone combined with azathioprine fail or are not well tolerated.

6 Plasmapheresis 3-6 times 1.5 - 2.5 L
  a. in emergency: e.g. respiratory crisis (without infection), before thymectomy, preceding prednisone treatment to avoid the initial deterioration.
  b. if 1-5 fail, 1-2 sessions every 2-4 weeks, combined with IS therapy.

4.2 Anticholinesterases (anti AChE)

The drug of choice is pyridostigmine-Br (Mestinon®) available in tablets (10 mg, 60 mg and 180 mg time span = retard), a syrup (12 mg/ml), or a 5‰ solution.[5] If given by mouth, its effect begins after 15-30 minutes, reaches a peak at 1-2 hours and lasts to 3-4 hours. Most patients need 5-6 doses per day, which usually range from 30-120 mg and rarely higher. In my experience only a few patients had benefit from higher dosages of Mestinon® than 120 mg 5-6 times a day. As cholinergic side effects are sometimes embarrassing at onset, it is wise to start with 20 mg 5 times, to increase the dosage every second day with 10 mg until the optimum is reached. The maximum achievable strength can be determined as the effect of 1.5-2.0 mg neostigmine administered intramuscularly. Most patients prefer to take their morning dose in bed, but not on an empty stomach. The appropriate dosage in children would be about $n/(n+12)$ (n = age in years) of the adult dosage, with the same interindividual differences. Neonates may receive 2-3 mg pyridostigmine orally per dose.

Although it is possible to measure the concentration of pyridostigmine in the serum, there is no simple relationship between plasma levels and dosage, nor between the plasma level and the therapeutic effect.[6]

The patient should be instructed to keep a diary concerning the fluctuation of the symptoms and eventually perform some simple tests at fixed times in order to know when the effect of the previous dose is wearing off. The timing and the height of the dose should be adjusted to individual needs, with special attention to meals and other peak activities. The 5-6 times a day regime interferes with the common times of drug administration in the hospital, where MG patients should be given these drugs under their own control. The parasympathetic (muscarinic) side effects, diarrhoea, gastric discomfort, salivation, frequent micturition and bronchorrhoea, if present, commonly disappear in a few weeks. If they persist or increase they may be antagonized with $1/8$ - $1/4$ mg of atropinesulfate or $7^1/2$ - 15 mg probantine (Propantheline) per dose of Mestinon. Atropine should not be given as a routine from the start. Bronchoconstriction may be problematic in COPD patients (2). In a recent survey 39% of 100 patients reported one or more side effects even while using atropine or an equivalent anticholinergic drug (probantine). However in only 1% anti-AChE were withdrawn (2a).

The optimum dosage is not always the maximum dosage that is supported by the patient. Moreover the optimum dosage may be different in various muscle groups. (**Fig. 4.1**) In that case one has to choose which muscle group is to be treated most effectively even if this results in an underdosage for other muscles. If it is not obvious whether an increase of the dosage has a beneficial effect, an injection of edrophonium-Cl (Tensilon®) administered about 2 hours after the last oral medication, may reveal this. Tensilon is a short acting (2-5 minutes) antiAChE. When given intravenously it works within 30 seconds: if the patient's symptoms are alleviated, the dose of Mestinon may be increased. If there is no effect, the dose of Mestinon is probably appropriate, if the symptoms increase the patient has an overdose. Tensilon can best be titrated in portions of 2 mg (= 0.2 cc) with 30 seconds interval with a maximum of 10 mg. The clinical signs of overdosage are fasciculations, particularly in the face, and feelings of stiffness and weakness.

In some patients, Mestinon may be combined with neostigmine, which acts within a shorter interval and has a shorter duration (**table 4.2**) and a more pronounced peak activity. Thus it may be used prior to meals or other activities. Neostigmine usually has more parasympathetic side effects than Mestinon.

(Table 4.2) If pyridostigmine is combined with alcohol a red flushing of the face may occur. Interaction with other drugs is not reported. There are no clinical suspicions in man that anti-AChE have a deleterious effect on muscle or nerve in the long term. Also can they be used safely in pregnancy. The concentration of pyridostigmine in breast milk varied from 36-113% of the maternal plasma concentration. There is <u>no</u> contraindication to breast feeding if the daily maternal dosage is not exceeding 300 mg (4).

Ambenonium-Cl (Mytelase®) is not widely used. Its action is longer than that of Mestinon and its side effects are perhaps less than those of neostigmine but adequate comparisons are scarce (5, 6). Others reported the narrow margin between the therapeutic and intoxicating dosage (7), which may be due to the absence of warning muscarinic side effects. It may be prescribed for patients who are hypersensitive to bromide (acne). Long-acting compounds available are Mestinon retard® (timespan) 0.180 per tablet and distigmine (Ubretid®) 5 mg per tablet. The action of Mestinon-retard lasts 6-8 hours because about 60 mg is released immediately and the remainder gradually. It may be given before the night sleep if patients are severely disabled and cannot swallow in the morning. Since these patients are treated with prednisone, this indication is rare nowadays. There is little advantage in giving Mestinon-retard during the

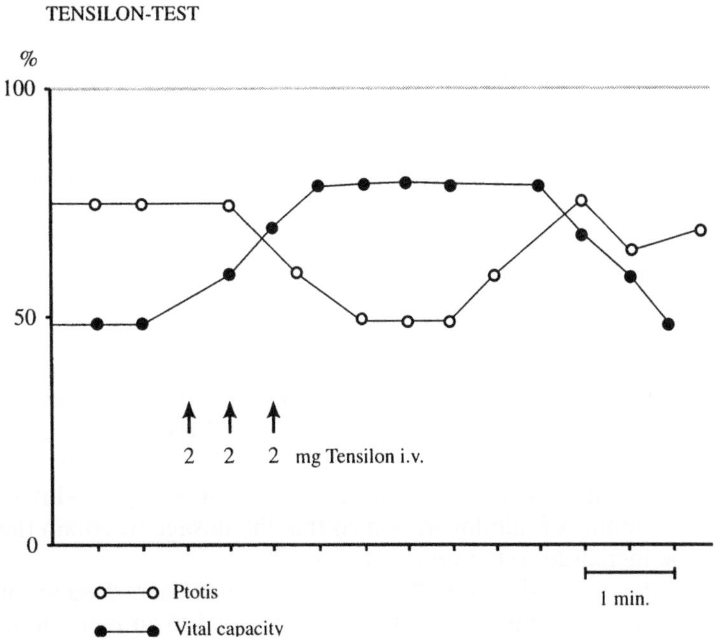

TENSILON-TEST

Figure 4.1

Tensilon test to assess the optimal therapy with anti-cholinesterases. The patients had received Mestinon 2 hours previously. Vital capacity increases but ptosis tends to become worse following 4-6 mg of Tensilon. The effect wears off after 2-3 minutes.

Table 4.2 DRUGS COMMONLY USED IN MG

GENERIC AND TRADE NAMES	ORAL DOSE IN MG	DURATION OF ACTION	EQUIVALENT DOSAGES IN MG		
			PER OS	I.V.	I.M.
1. Pyridostigmine-BR.			60	2	2
Mestinon®	10, 60	2.5-4 h			
Mestinon retard	180	6-8 h			
2. Prostigmine-BR					
Neostigmine®[2]	15	2-3 h	15	0.5[1]	1.5[1]
3. Ambenomium-Cl[2]					
Mytelase®	10	4-8 h	10	--	--
4. Edrophonium-Cl	--	2-5 min.	--	2-10	2-10
Tensilon					
5. Distigmine					
Ubretid®	5	24-48 h	--	--	--
6. Atropine sulfate[2]	0.25-0.5	3-4 h	0.25	0.25	0.25-0.5
7. Propantheline	7.5-15	3-4 h	--	--	--
Probantine					
8. Ephedrine (HCl or					
sulphate)	25	3-4 h	--	--	--

[1] neostigmine methyl sulphate

[2] tablets are no more registered in most European countries since 1995 but pharmacists can make capsules of the rough substance

The intestinal absorbtion of anti-AChE is only 5-10%, so the oral dosage is much higher than the parenteral. In case of accidental parenteral overdosage, atropine should be administered to counteract muscarinic side effects and the patient should be observed in an intensive care unit because of the increase in muscle weakness that may develop due to a cholinergic block.

day. If not available 2 tablets of Mestinon 60 mg probably have the same effect. Distigmine acts 24-48 hours and is more commonly used as a bladder-stimulant (8). In my experience few patients prefer it over Mestinon, because of the side effects.

It is a common experience that the effect of anticholinesterases slowly decreases in the first months of administration so that the dosage to obtain the same effect has to be increased to the optimum described.

The patient should be warned explicitly not to increase her dosage of anticholinesterases on her own initiative, since this may lead to an increase in weakness. It is of no use to increase the dosage still more in a patient who is left with diplopia, if other muscles have reacted reasonably well. In fact I have seen many patients who were overtreated and suffered more from the side

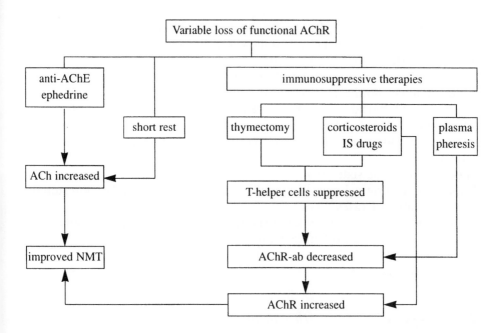

Figure 4.2 PRINCIPLES OF TREATMENT IN MG. Anti-cholinesterases (anti-AChE) prolong the effect of acetylcholine (ACh) on the acetylcholine receptors (AChR) by inhibiting the breakdown by the enzym acetylcholinesterase present in the synaptic cleft. If enough AChR are left at the postsynaptic membrane, the underlying muscle fibre will be able to contract, but the effect will diminish if the concentration of AChR further decreases by the immunological attack. A larger amount of ACh is physiologically present following rest at the first contraction, which explains the beneficial effect of short (seconds to minutes) rest. Ephedrine probably enhances the release of ACh at the nerve terminals.

The other branch indicates the measures able to suppress the immunological attack on the AChR. Thymectomy causes an effect by a decrease of specific T-helper cells, corticosteroids by the anti-inflammatory action and lymphocytolysis, azathioprine and other immunosuppressive (IS) drugs by leukocytolysis and plasma pheresis by decreasing circulating AChR-Ab and leukokines. The effect is an increase of active AChR by a more positive balance between the physiological production and pathological destruction of AChR.

effects than from their ocular symptoms. In patients with only ocular MG 5-6 dd 60-90 mg Mestinon is usually the maximum.

If oral medication is prohibited e.g. on the day(s) following an operation, Mestinon may be given intravenously or subcutaneously. The parenteral dosage is much lower than the oral one (**table 4.1**), but in my experience it is difficult to predict the parenteral need from the equivalence 60 mg per os = 2 mg parenterally. It seems wise to start with a relatively low dose e.g. ¹/₄ mg Mestinon i.v. or i.m per hour to ensure the vital functions (respiration, swallowing, coughing) and to adjust the dosage according to the need of the patient. A Tensilon-test may be of some value. In patients who cannot swallow their tablets subcutaneous administration of neostigmine or Mestinon may be tried with use of a syringe driver (9). Administration of nebulized pyridostigmine (80 mg in 2 cc sterile water) by an aerosol mask had a good effect on oculobulbar signs in one patient, suggesting local absorption and diffusion (10). This favourable effect was confirmed in 18 out of 20 patients by intranasal neostigmine sulfate (6 g/100 ml, 4-6 mg/puff) administered by an aerosol (11).

In general it can be stated that:

1. the patient's original muscle strength and endurance is mostly not restored by anticholinesterases
2. most patients have more or less benefit from anticholinesterases; only the extra-ocular muscles often do not respond sufficiently
3. very rarely patients show no reaction to anticholinesterases (12, 13) (personal experience).

4.3 Drugs to be used with caution

Certain medicaments are reported to increase or provoke myasthenic weakness[7]. (**Table 4.3**) Most cases concern patients who were not yet diagnosed as having MG or who were not yet treated adequately. In most drugs the contraindiation is only relative: they may aggravate MG signs in a minority of patients but are the most suited in a certain situation e.g. aminoglycosides in specific infection. The published incidents in individual patients might unnecessarily lead to withholding appropriate therapies e.g. anti-arrhythmics or beta-blockers in cardiac emergencies. In a group moderately affected MG patients intravenous administration of a beta-blocker or a calcium-influx antagonist had no adverse influence on MG symptoms or on the decrement in nerve stimulation tests (57). Also diazepam i.v. did not increase weakness in 11 patients (58).

In my own patients the most reported (mild) side effects were due to the use of tetracyclines, beta-blockers, and quinidine derivates but many patients must have received these drugs without influence of their myasthenic symptoms. Even d-penicillamin, although provoking MG in about 1.5% of rheumatoid arthritis (RA) patients could be given in severe RA patients whose MG was in remission. Also low dose benzodiazepines had no adverse effect on MG signs. It is remarkable in the official Dutch "Farmacotherapeutisch Kompas" only benzodiazepines are mentioned as a contraindication in MG. The message must be that many old and probably new drugs, including radiocontrast agents, may aggravate MG weakness in some patients, particularly in those who are not yet adequately treated for their MG.

Table 4.3 DRUGS TO BE USED WITH CAUTION (14, 15, 16)

---

1 Quinine and related agents used as
   a. antimalaria drugs e.g. chloroquine* (17, 18)
   b. antiarrhythmics: procainamide (19, 20), quinidine
   c. antihelmintics: piperazine (21), pyrantelpamoate (22)
   d. local anaesthetics e.g. lidocaine

2 Antibiotics
   a. aminoglycosides: streptomycin (23, 24), kanamycine (25), gentamicin (26)
   b. lyncomycines: erythromycin (27)
   c. polypeptides: colistin (14), polymyxine (28)
   d. tetracyclines: doxacycline (29)
   e. chinolones: ciprofloxacine (30), norfloxacine (31)
   f. penicillines: Ampiciline (32, 33)

3 Cardiovascular agents
   a. beta-adrenergic blockers: labetalol (34), propranolol (35), timolol, timol eye drops
      (36-38), acebutolol (39)
   b. calcium influx inhibitors: verapamil (40), propafenon (41)
   c. diuretics: acetazolamide

4 Psychotropic drugs
   Chlorpromazine (42), lithiumcarbonate (43, 44)
   diphylhydantoin (45-48), trimethadione (49, 50), diazepam (14), trihexyphenidyl (51)

5 Corticosteroids: deterioration 3rd-10th day after onset

6 Iodinated contrast agents: gadolinium (52-56)

7 Interferon-alpha (57)

---

* also anti-rheumatic

4.4 Thymectomy

4.4.1 Patients without thymoma

The indication for thymectomy in early onset patients was found by clinical intuition (Ch. 1.5). Although no controlled clinical trials have been performed, it is generally excepted that thymectomy improves the prognosis of early onset generalized MG.
In 1984 I summarized the reported experience (59). The best results were seen

in early onset patients with a duration of illness shorter than 3 years. Complete remissions at the end of the follow-up were varying from 18 to 38% and 7.5 to 24% in comparable (but not matched) nonthymectomized controls. An additional 30-50% were found to be improved. It was not evident that thymectomy in the first year of onset gave a better result than if performed in the second or third year. The results were the same in men and women. The rate of improvement was not related to the severity of the MG shortly before the operation. Improvement was thought to go on for 3-5 years or even longer, but it was difficult to separate the effect of thymectomy from the natural history. Contradictory data were reported in patients between the ages of 40 to 60 years. In many series patients over the age of 40 were included but not analysed as a separate group. Nevertheless the indication for thymectomy in nonthymoma patients was gradually extended in some centres to 60 years or even older. Patients with purely ocular signs were usually not operated but if they were the effect remained uncertain.

In the newer series (60-65a) the results are sometimes contaminated by the pre- and postoperative use of immunosuppressive drugs. In some series (60, 61, 63, 64) results were better with a shorter preoperative duration of MG, but not in others (62, 65). Complete remissions are reported ranging from 23 to 46% and additional improvement in 30-50%. The best results are claimed if maximal thymectomy with transsternal cervical exploration was performed (66) although the results are probably comparable with extended thymectomy by only transsternal approach (68). The latter procedure would be safer in regard to the possible damage to the phrenic and recurrent nerves (67).

The specific effect of thymectomy over the age of 40 remains unsettled. In a preliminary report from Scandinavia a somewhat better outcome was found in the thymectomized group but the definite publication of this retrospective study is not available (69). No difference in outcome was found in the remission rate or need for IS drugs in a retrospective study in Rome (70).

A prospective European study was attempted but failed to raise enough patients. One study indicating some benefit in patients with purely ocular MG was without comparable controls (71). Also a systematic study in seronegative patients is lacking but the impression is that thymectomy is less effective than in MG with AChR-Ab (142, own experience).

It is still not possible to predict the effect of thymectomy in the individual patient. A main factor however appears the total removal of the thymus. This is proved by the beneficial effect of rethymectomy in patients who had failed to improve by the first operation and in whom residual thymus was removed during the second operation (72-74). Incomplete removal may occur in transcervical thymectomy (73) but also in transsternal thymectomy by experienced surgeons. Thymic tissue can be localized in the neck region (74a), in the region of the diaphragm (75), even behind the carina (76) and in the mediastinal fat where it is not well recognizable at operation. If a patient improves after thymectomy AChR-Ab gradually tend to decrease (77); this was not the case in 4 of my patients after a partial (3 transcervical, one transsternal) thymectomy, but occurred after rethymectomy with concomitant improvement (fig. 5.11).

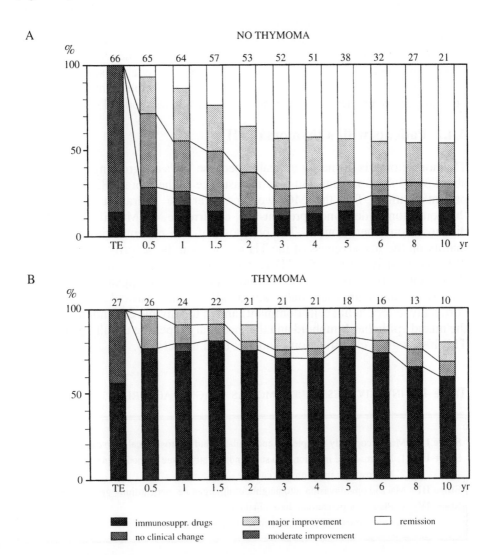

Figure 4.3 Follow-up after thymectomy in non-thymoma (A) and thymoma patients (B). The numbers of patients available at each point of time are depicted on the top. A remission is defined as no signs or symptoms without immunomodulating medication. A major and moderate imptovement are defined as a shift of 2 and 1 points respectively on the disability scale. Patients on immunomodulating drugs are not considered to be improved (65a). Courtesy of Dr J.B.M. Kuks.

If AChR-Ab were not decreased by 25% after thymectomy, clinical improvement was less pronounced (78). A difference in thymic lymphoid subsets was found between patients who reacted favourably to thymectomy and who did not: in the nonreacting group also the ratio of CD8 cells in the peripheral blood was increased (79). In another study CD4 T subsets did not reflect the severity of MG nor the influence of thymectomy and azathioprine (80). Further work is needed to find indications for the completeness of thymectomy because CT and MRI are not completely reliable (see 3.5). Unless proven otherwise, it remains to be doubted whether complete thymectomy can be achieved by the newly developed thoracoscopic method (81).

4.4.2 Patients with a thymoma (TH)

Thymomectomy is primarily indicated because TH's are growing invasively in about 30-45% of patients and may metastasize in the thorax (82, 83). In most patients with a TH, the MG worsens after the operation (82, 84) and thymomectomy does not prevent the occurrence of MG if the TH was diagnosed on other grounds. The prognosis of MG patients with TH depends mainly on the invasiveness of the TH and less on the severity of the MG (85, 86). The invasiveness of the TH is commonly scored according to Masaoka (87) (**Table 4.4**) mainly on macroscopic criteria; it also appears related to the microscopical picture (88): malignant growth is found particularly in TH of the cortical type (epithelial cells dominant) and in the thymic carcinomas, whereas the mixed epithelial-lymphoid and the medullary types are usually benign (89). This histological classification is not yet used universally.

Table 4.4 INVASIVENESS OF THYMOMAS, STAGING ACCORDING TO MASAOKA

Stage I	Macroscopically completely encapsulated and microscopically no capsular invasion
Stage II	1. Macroscopic invasion into surrounding fatty tissue or mediastinal pleura
	2. Microscopic invasion into capsule
Stage III	Macroscopic invasion into neighbouring organ i.e. pericardium, great vessels, lung
Stage IV	1. Pleural or pericardial dissemination
	2. Lymphogenous or hematogenous metastasis

Controlled clinical studies are lacking, but most authors advocate high dose radiation therapy in all patients with TH stage III and IV. Patients with TH stage I usually do not receive radiotherapy but the results of one study following 83 TH patients (25 with MG) lead to the conclusion that all TH patients should have radiotherapy except those with the mixed type stage I and the medullary types stage I and II (88). If all patients (also stage I) received postoperative radiotherapy, the 5-year survival was respectively 100%, 91%, 88% and 47% in the stages I-IV (90), but it is difficult to know if this result is better for stage II than the operation alone and this regime is not recommended as a general policy.

If the TH recurs without previous radiotherapy the decision is difficult: reoperation possibly followed by radiation therapy and, or chemotherapy (91, 92). A combination of cisplatin, doxorubicin and cyclophosphamide in 2-4 cycles followed by 54 Gy radiation to the tumor and regional lymph nodes yielded a 5 years survival of 52% in 26 patients, compared with 25% in previous series (93). Prednisone therapy may also reduce tumor size even when chemotherapy has failed (94). In one reported case, combined chemotherapy was effective in a patient who had a recurrence of a previously operated and irradiated TH (95). In another study 16 patients were treated with cisplatin and etoposide: 5 complete and 4 partial responses were obtained with a median response duration of 3.4 years (96). The poor prognosis of these patients is further determined by the possible occurrence of TH associated auto-immune diseases (see 2.6.5 and table 5.18).

4.5 Immunosuppressive drugs

4.5.1 Corticosteroids and azathioprine

The beneficial effect on MG of relatively high dosage of prednisone (PR) is known from the early 1970s (97). Earlier attempts in the 1950s were first abandoned because of the risk of an initial exacerbation; in severely affected patients this could lead to respiratory insufficiency which could not be managed adequately at that time (Ch. 1.7). This initial exacerbation[8] is still an important and not always foreseeable risk but it can often be prevented by preceding and concomitant plasmapheresis (PP) (4.6).

The effect of PR is gradual and may start after a few days but is usually obvious after two weeks, exceptionnally only after 4-6 weeks (98, 99). In one study the initial exacerbation started between day 1-17 (mean day 5) and lasted 1-20 days (mean 4 days); it occurred in 48% of patients, in 9% with respiratory failure (100). The maximum improvement is usually reached after 6-12 months but variations are considerable. Improvement starts earlier when high daily dosages are given and this regime is usually chosen, combined with PP in patients in (impending) crisis in an intensive care unit. A slowly increasing alternate day (AD) schedule (start with 30 mg, increase with 10 mg AD) may be used in less severe patients to avoid the initial exacerbation (101) but this may still occur (99). The effect is reached in this regime with a longer delay. Patients on an AD schedule usually start to improve on the PR day. If the MG signs are severe on the off-day, a small dose (5-20 mg) may prevent too large fluctuations. The dose should be kept high until this on-off effect has disappeared. Some patients are weakest in the afternoon of the 'off'-day but start to improve in the same evening and are already optimal before they take their next PR dose! (102) If the patient improves during PR therapy, anti-AChE may be reduced or omitted. It is recommended that the full (AD) dose of PR be taken between 6-8 a.m. in order to diminish the influence on cortisol production which is nevertheless suppressed at the day of administration. In case of sudden stress (e.g. operation, high fever) hydrocortisone should be supplied additionally. Signs of infection (sinusitis, appendicitis even peritonitis) may be masked by high PR and only appear on the off-day. Patients on an AD regime because of their MG are sometimes dysregulated if they receive short courses of PR for intercurrent diseases e.g. chronic obstructive pulmonary disease.

On the other hand short courses of high dosages (2 g) methylprednisolon intravenously were employed with good results to manage exacerbations (103). In 1984 I reviewed the result of PR treatment (104). In 6 series comprising 330 patients the remission rate was 20% (range 9-42%), the rate of marked improvement 32% (range 15-51%) and failures occurred in 18% (range 8-24%). The difference might be attributed to the different definitions of the categories of clinical outcome, the age of the patients, the severity of MG and the dosage schedules used. These restrictions still apply to the newer series. There seems a tendency to use IS more frequently in the mildly or moderately affected patients,

Azathioprine (AZA) as a single treatment is effective in amounts of 2.5-3 mg/kg (tablets 50 and 25 mg, Imuran®, Imurek®) (105-107). The effect starts 3-6 months after onset and reaches its maximum after 12-24 months; therefore it is as a single drug not the first choice in severely affected patients. It is useful however in moderately affected and particularly in older patients (107). In retrospectively analysed series (107, 108) and in two controlled studies (109, 110)[9] AZA enhanced the effect of PR and reduced the dosage of PR needed to reach a steady improvement or remission. In some of the severe patients PR could not be withdrawn completely, as is my own experience. When the response to AZA is good, the dosage may be reduced to 1.5-2 mg/kg; a lower dosage is usually followed by an exacerbation if the therapy is really needed. It seems reasonable to try a dosage reduction every 2-3 years in chronically treated patients (100, 107, 111-114).

In more recent series pharmacological remissions are reported in 12-37% by using PR as a single drug, in 25-33% by using AZA as a single drug, and 6-32% in a combined therapy. (**Table 4.5**) These series comprise a relatively large number of patients having or having been operated upon a thymoma and late onset patients. Pharmacological remissions were less frequent in early onset patients who had not reacted to thymectomy (112). PR as a single therapy is also effective in patients with ocular MG in whom the effect of combined therapy or AZA as a single drug is usually not attempted.

Table 4.5 THERAPEUTIC EFFECTS OF PREDNISONE (PR) AND AZATHIOPRINE (A) IN SEVERE MG

	A	PR+A	PR	PR/A/PR+A	PR	PR+A	A	A	A*+PR
Remission	25**	32	37	38	28	12	6	33	0
Much improved	28	26	18	35	53	41	57	24	10
Improved	22	12	12	22	15	15	20	33	25
No effect	16	18	13	5	5	32	17	10	65
Number of patients studied	32	57	60	106	116	34	35	21	20
Reference	111	111	111	112	100	113	113	114	114

* Patients were initially treated with PR alone but is treatment failure occurred AZA was added.
** percentages

The beneficial effect of IS drugs is counterbalanced by the side effects which are most prominent in PR therapy and much lower in AZA. **(Table 4.6 and 4.7)** The incidence and the severity of side effects as reported are rather variable, ranging from 22-67% (113, 100, 2) in PR and 12-39% in AZA (2, 116, 117). In the latter leucopenia is commonly included although this is a direct dosage related effect and not a side effect sensu stricto. It is not clear whether the IS effect is dependent on the peripheral blood changes. In one study a better effect was found in patients who had a leucopenia ($< 4 \times 10^9$/L), but the therapeutic effect was not related to the occurrence of a macrocytosis (MCV > 96) present in 63% or a relative lymphopenia (< 15%) present in 67% (114). However the mean duration of therapy which is obviously an important factor is frequently not stated, nor the percentage of patients that have to be withdrawn because of side effects. In 100 consecutive patients referred to our centre side effects of PR were present in 65% but necessitated withdrawal in only 10%; for AZA the percentages were respectively 39% (leukopenia not included) and 18% (2). In another study (116) AZA had to be withdrawn in 11%.

In my review of 6 older series severe side effects of PR varied from 0.44 to 1.36 per 100 treatment months so that one in four treated patients could expect a severe side effect in 4 treatment years (102).

There is no indication that AZA increased the incidence of carcinomas (114) or other malignancies in patients with AI-diseases (118); two patients developing non Hodgkin lymphomas are reported in 2 series (114, 116) including 145 patients, but not in other series so that coincidence is not excluded. An increase in basal cell carcinomas of the skin is reported in patients treated with AZA for other diseases. For further details see next chapter.

Table 4.6 SIDE EFFECTS OF PREDNISONE

COMMON (mentioned in large series)
- Cushing face, girdle fat (Buffalo hump), thinning extremities
- Obesity (hunger $\rightarrow$ increase calory intake)[1]
- Cataract (only of the posterior subcapsular type!)[2]
- Diabetes mellitus (2-12%)
- Hypertension (3-12%)
- Osteoporotic fractures: vertebral, femoral head[3]
- Skin changes: impaired wound healing, easy bleeding, atrophy, hirsutism
- Opportunistic infections: herpes zoster, candidiasis, acne,
                           fungal infections of the skin
- Mood changes: depression, irritability, overactivity, sleeplessness
- Gastrointestinal disturbances, peptic ulcer

UNCOMMON
- Proximal myopathy (fluocorticoids!) (120, 120a)
- Fatal bacterial (opportunistic) infections
- Gastric hemorrhage, bowel perforation
- Pancreatitis
- Benign intra cranial hypertension
- Intraspinal liposis with myelum compression (121)
- Psychosis
- Venous or arterial thrombosis, lung embolism

[1] many patients gain 5-10 kg after the start of PR, therewith regaining their previous loss of weight due to swallowing impairment!

[2] not all cataracts in older patients are due to PR; in the literature the difference between specific PR cataract and common old-day cataract is not made, so that cataract as a side effect of PR is probably overestimated

[3] these occurred in respectively 9% (113), 7% (119) and 6% (2); radiological osteoporosis and decreased bone density measured with the dexa-method are probably more common but the relation with impending fractures is uncertain. Treatment with oestrogens or recalcification promoting drugs may be indicated.

4.5.2 Details of treatment

Prednisone (PR) (or prednisolone in which PR is metabolized) is started in a daily dose of 1.0 - 1.5 mg/kg which is maintained for 2-4 weeks, in which period a definite improvement is to be expected. PR is then tapered off by 10 mg/2d until an AD dose is reached in 3 weeks. A further decrease of the AD dose should be slower (5 mg/2 weeks) until about 14 weeks after the start a dosage of 60 mg/2 d is reached. For some patients may this be a critical dose

Table 4.7 SIDE EFFECTS OF AZATHIOPRINE

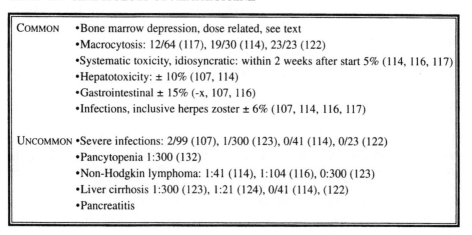

COMMON	•Bone marrow depression, dose related, see text
	•Macrocytosis: 12/64 (117), 19/30 (114), 23/23 (122)
	•Systematic toxicity, idiosyncratic: within 2 weeks after start 5% (114, 116, 117)
	•Hepatotoxicity: ± 10% (107, 114)
	•Gastrointestinal ± 15% (-x, 107, 116)
	•Infections, inclusive herpes zoster ± 6% (107, 114, 116, 117)
UNCOMMON	•Severe infections: 2/99 (107), 1/300 (123), 0/41 (114), 0/23 (122)
	•Pancytopenia 1:300 (132)
	•Non-Hodgkin lymphoma: 1:41 (114), 1:104 (116), 0:300 (123)
	•Liver cirrhosis 1:300 (123), 1:21 (124), 0/41 (114), (122)
	•Pancreatitis

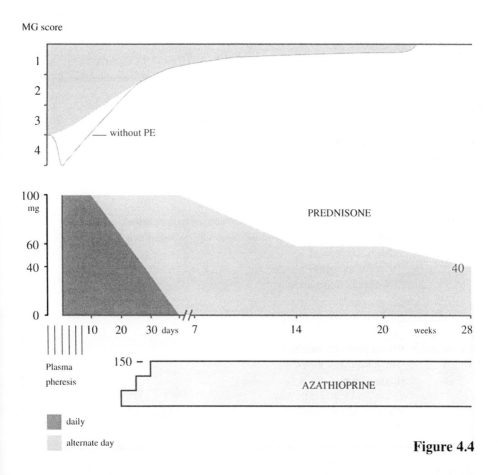

Figure 4.4

so that a 4-6 week pause is made in dosis reduction. Depending on the clinical signs PR is further reduced with 5 mg/2 weeks until a dosage of 1/2 mg/kg/2d is reached. In my experience this is the minimal effective dosage if AZA is not yet active. In patients with bulbar signs not reacting to AChE, or with a vital capacity ≤ 75%, plasmapheresis (PP) is started so that 3 phereses are done before the start of PR and 3 in the first week of PR. The PR exacerbation occurs in about 50% of the patients without PP, although not always life-threatening. AZA 2.5 mg/kg is started after 2 weeks, to distinguish the possible gastro-intestinal side effects common to PR and AZA, and increased with 50 mg/3d. This scheme may be altered if MG signs reappear or exacerbate during dose reduction or in case of severe side effects. It is mandatory to start this regime in hospital and to see the patient frequently thereafter to make up the clinical state by history and standardized tests (3.2) and to monitor side effects.

Before starting this therapy the patient gets a general check-up with special attention to risk factors (see **table 4.8**) and possible additional preventive therapies. As a prevention of osteoporosis additional Ca^{++} (1 g) is prescribed and the advice of regular walking is given. Specific osteoporosis therapy is a

Table 4.8 ROUTINE EXAMINATION BEFORE STARTING IS THERAPY

HISTORY: •Tuberculosis (possibly INH profylaxis)
    •Hypertension (treatment)
    •Peptic ulcers (preventively ranitidine)
    •(Latent) infections: bladder, skin (mucosis, acne)
    •Diabetes
    •Osteoporosis (bone densimetry)
    •Psychosis

LABORATORY: •Blood: Hb, leukocytes, differential counts, liver enzymes, glycose,
        renal function, renal creatinine clearance (cyclosporine), BSE, CRP,
        Na-K, cholesterol
    •Bone densimetry
    •X-Thorax (tuberculosis)

CONSULTATION: •Cataract, intraocular-pressure

FOLLOW-UP: •Blood pressure, weight
    •Hb, leukocytes, differential count
    •Liver enzymes, Na-K (cholesterol)
    •Bone densimetry after 3 and 12 months
    •Control cataract, intraocular pressure at 3 and 12 months
    •MG-function tests

matter of controverse, in our routine only given on indication. The patient should be warned for unwanted weight gain, even if feelings of hunger are not prominent. Except for calories no diet restrictions (salt) are recommended except in case of hypertension. Additional potassium is rarely indicated. The patient should be warned for mood changes (overactivity, lack of control, but also depressive feelings) which particularly occur when the prednisone dosage is high. There is an increase in common fungal and staphylococcal (acne!) infections of the skin which should be treated prophylactically if present before the start. Rarely severe bacterial, particularly opportunistic, infections develop. The incidence of herpes zoster seems increased and should be treated with acyclovir. Diabetes is relatively rare, but more frequent in patients who also have had diabetes in pregnancy or who have a familial history; it may appear acutely. Patients with peptic ulcers should be treated with H_2-receptor antagonists.

Withdrawal of PR is frequently associated with arthralgias and occasionally with a temporary carpal tunnel syndrome (own experience). The most reported side effects of AZA are gastrointestinal (nausea, loss of appetite, sometimes regarding special foods, diarrhoea); in most patients they disappear in a few weeks, eventually after increasing the intake to 6 times a day and by taking it after the meal. In about 5% of patients fever, general malaise and lymphadenopathy occurs as an idiosyncratic reaction which forces withdrawal. Also pancreatitis or acute hepatotoxicity may rarely occur. Leukopenia and thrombocytopenia are dosage dependent side effects which are in fact the primary goal of the therapy. They are especially common at onset and may necessitate dosage adjustment in some patients. Control of leukocytes and thrombocytes is advocated at week 1, 2, 4, 8, 12, 16 and every 3 months. If leukocytes fall $> 2.5 - < 3.5 \times 10^9/L$ a dose reduction of 50% is necessary, if $< 2.5 \times 10^9/L$ a temporary withdrawal of 2-3 weeks, with reinstitution of a 50 mg lower dosage. Thrombocytes would only fall if there is also a leukopenia (105) and do not have to be controlled routinely. Macrocytosis is not uncommon (Mean corpuscular volume > 96) but does not need treatment. PR commonly causes leukocytosis so that leukopenia may become a problem during or after withdrawal of PR. Liver toxicity is reflected in a mild increase in liver enzymes which is usually transient. If persistent and not due to other causes (alcohol!) a dose reduction may be needed. An increase in bacterial infections is difficult to assess but may play a role in otherwise debilitated and older patients; viral infections seem to be reduced (107) except herpes zoster. Since AZA is degraded by xanthine oxidase to 6-mercaptopurine, it should not be given in combination with xanthine oxidase inhibitors such as allopurinol (anti-gout) in which case toxic levels of the drug may develop (107). Also INH (tuberculose prophylaxis) has this effect. It is adviced to postpone pregnancy until 3 months after discontinuation of azathioprine and to assure adequate anticonception in fertile women who have to use the drug. However experience with renal transplant receivers treated with PR + AZA does not point to a higher risk of congenital malformations (125-127). Because the incidence of basal cell carcinomas in sun-exposed areas of the skin was increased in patients treated with AZA for other diseases, sunbathing should be disencouraged.

Vaccinations are not contraindicated during immunosuppressive therapy except if living virus is used.

4.5.3 Management of crisis

Respiratory insufficiency (crisis) is a life threatening event occurring in about 20% (115, 139, 229, 230) of MG patients and in about half of the patients with thymomas (115, 230). If not adequately treated the mortality rate is 50% or still higher (139, 231, 232). A rare cause of MG death is a cardiac rhythm disturbance, either due to anoxia or to myocarditis. The latter condition occurs predominantly in patients with a thymoma (233).

The management of MG crisis relies upon: 1. early recognition of impending crisis, 2. immediate transfer to an intensive care unit with respiratory support, 3. treatment of possible infection, 4. plasmapheresis (PP) (4.6) or intravenous gammaglobulin.

A problem actual in the period before IS therapies and PP was the distinction between a myasthenic and a cholinergic crisis by a relative overdosage of anti-AChE. Apart from an accidental overdosage of anti-AChE, it was soon recognized that in many patients increasing MG weakness lead to an overdosage of anti-AChE, so that a mixed crisis resulted. Aspiration of food and saliva, increased bronchial secretion or a mild upper respiratory infection caused a further exhaustion of the respiratory muscles in vain attempts to cough. Bronchial obstruction with atelectasis and bronchopneumonia would then follow. Other crisis precipitating mechanisms could be emotional stress, infections with sudden elevation of body temperature, notably in childhood, hyperthyroidism, surgery (139, 229, 231, 232, 234) or ionidated contrast administration (55). An impending crisis should be recognized by the occurrence of short attacks of dyspnoea frequently with inspiratory stridor and sometimes leading to a short lasting loss of consciousness, increasing bulbar weakness (dysphagia, salivation), restlessness and insomnia, tachycardia and hypertension (due to CO_2-retention). In hospital, a careful observation of the patient and measurement of clinical parameters (vital capacity, peak flow measurement, pulse frequency and bloodpressure) are more important than repeated measuring of 'blood-gas values' by arterial puncture. The latter may give a false impression of security as they may remain normal until a sudden decompensation takes place. Chronic hypoventilation is very uncommon in MG (235) probably because acidosis increases MG weakness. In general the intercostal and auxiliary respiratory muscles become paralysed first and the diaphragm later. This course of events is similar to that of partial curarization. Patients in a myasthenic crisis commonly have signs of autonomic disturbance: sweating, salivation, urge to urinate and to defaecate, tachycardia, which make its distincion from a cholinergic crisis difficult. Only dilated pupils would be a specific sign, as cholinergic overdosage invariably causes miosis.

Patients in a myasthenic crisis are anxious and restless in so far as the weakness enables them to move. The weakness may be generalized, preventing the patient from showing facial expression of distress (234) or to use his auxiliary respiratory muscles. On the other hand, I have seen patients who had full strength in their limb muscles, but who could not breath, and in whom neostigmine intravenously restored breathing but caused widespread fasciculations in the limb muscles. This apparent dissociation of muscle weakness is another difficulty if the Tensilon test is used to distinguish between myasthenic and cholinergic weakness. No definite diagnosis of either a myasthenic or cholinergic crisis should be made before the patient's respiration is supported and the patient is transferred to an intensive care unit. In fact this means that the patient has to be intubated, preferably through the nose after a short narcosis, and ventilated artifically. Anticholinesterases should be omitted and the underlying cause of the crisis explored. The most effective way to terminate a crisis i.e. to restore the patient's respiratory capacity is to combine PP with a high dosage (1.5 -2.0 mg/kg) prednisone daily. Improvement usually starts after the second or third PE but depends on the amounts of plasma that can be substituted without side effects. High daily dosages of prednisone may produce an initial deterioration, but this will be prevented by the simultaneous PP. The effect of this prednisone schedule usually starts on the 7th to 10th day from onset, so that PP may be omitted at that time. This approach shortens the period of artifical respiration to a minimum, thereby reducing the risk of pulmonary complications and avoiding tracheostomy, which may be needed if spontaneous recovery would be awaited.

Prednisone may be withheld to patients whose crisis was due to intercurrent infection, thyrotoxicosis, severe emotions or an obvious under- or overdosage of anticholinesterases, whereas their MG had been moderate and stable. In these patients crisis intervention with a short period of artificial respiration, possibly combined with PP and cure of the underlying cause of exacerbation is sufficient. In crises due to infections, cephalosporins can be given without adverse effect on MG symptoms. Many antibiotics (see table 4.3) may have adverse effects on neuromuscular transmission, but in an intensive care setting these effects are less important (236).

It was stated (139) that crises will cease spontaneously after a shorter or longer time even without an adequate dose of anticholinesterases, providing the underlying cause (e.g. pulmonary infection) has subsided. This is in general not my own experience. In the years 1960-1970, before the use of ACTH or prednisone, I followed several patients with severe MG who could not be disconnected from their respirators and finally died from complications.

With the use of high dosages of prednisone, artificial ventilation could always be terminated after 2-3 weeks.

4.6 *Plasmapheresis and immunoadsorbtion*

Plasmapheresis (PP) was introduced in 1976 to treat MG patients in (impending) crises (128) and later also used as an intermittent supportative treatment in patients who responded insufficiently to IS therapy (129). It also has a place in improving the condition of patients to be prepared for an operation i.c. thymectomy (130). Initially PP was performed by replacing the patient's serum by fresh frozen plasma or by a solution of albumen and globulins. Administration of fresh frozen plasma caused more side effects than that of human albumine and had no clear advantage so that the latter is now commonly used.[9]

In general a series of 6 PP within 2 weeks is carried out but the result of one study indicate that if combined with IS therapy 1-2 PP on subsequent days would have the same effect (131). Side effects may occur by the use of citrate; some transient hypotension is not uncommon, rarely are circulatory shock and infections reported (132).

Good results are reported in 60-70% of patients, particularly in those with acute exacerbations and less in chronic stable patients (129, 133-136). Improvement rarely occurs following the first PP but more commonly after the second or third procedure or even later (137). Improvement lasts from 3-4 weeks to months (138) but in most series the specific effect is difficult to guess because most patients receive IS regimes started or changed concomitant with PP. It is probable that the long-term effect in some patients is due to the spontaneous recovery in a crisis (139) which may be self limiting. Even a placebo effect should not be excluded, as was exemplified by the "beneficial effect" of imaginary PP in 6 patients with severe generalized MG over three weeks of treatment (140).

The effect is only partly related to the decrease of AChR-Ab, which is usually maximal after 3 PP. The time elapsed between the end of the PP series and the moment at which AChR-Ab have reached half of the pretreatment value (T $^1/_2$) is 8-9 days (133). **(Fig. 4.5)** It has been suggested that removal of cytokines and interleukines or an activation and consumption of complement factors and IgM (141) may be important, though a long lasting decrease of complement factors was not found in an other study (147). That the removal of AChR-Ab is not the decisive factor is adstructed by the beneficial effect in patients without detectable antibodies (141-143).

The immunoadsorption technique uses the adsorption of IgG autoantibodies in columns coated with an affinity gel based on tryptophane linked polyvinyl alcohol resin (144). These columns may be reused in the same patient after regeneration by 40% glycerol. The procedure is semiselective.

AChR-Ab concentrations were reduced by 45-60% in each run compared to pretreatment values (145-147) while total IgG and total protein were only reduced by 20% and 10% respectively, but serum fibrinogen by 40%. The main advantage of this procedure is that no foreign albumin has to be reinfused.

Serious side effects were not reported. The overall effects are comparable (148) with that of PP or better (147). In one study (149) the use of a protein A-Sepharose gel was highly effective while the tryptophan polyvinyl alcohol gel was not. This technique however was not yet applicable to patients at the time of report because of the leakage of protein A.

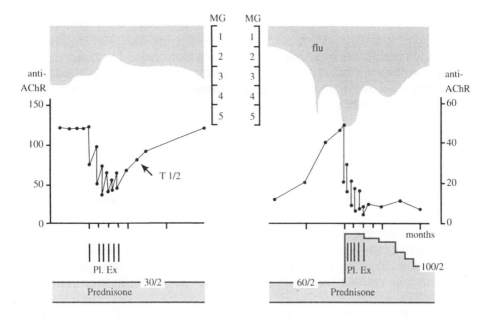

Figure 4.5 Examples of AChR-Ab during PP in 2 patients.
a. M 23: Prednisone treatment since 18 months. Stabilized at 30 mg/2 days. Clinical effect not impressive. AChR-Ab decreased to 32% and increased with T¹/₂ of 14 days.
b. W 48: Deterioration during prednisone 60 mg/2 days. Crisis treated with PP and increase of prednisone to 100 mg daily. AChR-Ab decreased to 10% and remained at this level. After PP a redistribution of IgG and of AChR-Ab occurs within the extracellular space, with a delay of 24 hours. So the AChR-Ab values measured at the end of a PE procedure are much lower than the values before the onset of the subsequent one.

4.7 Other immunosuppressive drugs and measures

4.7.1 Cyclosporine A (CSA)

CSA probably acts by a selective inhibition of the production of interleukine 2 and other factors essential for the proliferation of T-helper cells. It is mainly used as a prophylactic drug in organ transplant patients.
In MG it is used in some open studies with a small number of patients who

were relatively resistent to other IS therapies (150-152) and in two controlled clinical trials (153, 154). In this category of therapy resistent patients improvement was variable but significant although a complete remission was never induced. Concomitant PR could be reduced in most patients (154) but rarely completely withdrawn. In one study comparing CSA with AZA the improvement was comparable (153): some patients not reacting to CSA did so to AZA and vice versa. The effect became apparent after 2-6 months and maximal after 12 months (154). Initial exacerbations are not reported. The dosage used initially was 5-6 mg/kg in 2 dosages but had to be adjusted in relation to renal function, which usually tended to decrease. Other side effects like paraesthesias, hirsutism, gum hypertrophy, mild tremor, headache, gastrointerstinal disturbances, arterial hypertension were variably reported and were not infrequently a reason to stop the drug. The risk on malignancies in auto-immune diseases treated with CsA is unknown. An increase of lymphoproliferative and virus mediated tumors in transplant patients has been reported (155). Since side effects are dose dependent future trials using smaller dosages of CSA combined with AZA compared with PR + AZA might be tried.

4.7.2 Cyclophosphamide, methotrexate, 6-mercaptopurine

Cytostatic drugs like mercaptopurine, actinomycine, methotrexate were found to be effective but were abandoned in favour of AZA because the latter had less side effects (105). One of my patients has obtained a complete remission by treatment with chlorambucil after pancreatis developed during treatment with combined PR and AZA (102).

Cyclophosphamide induced clinical remissions in 60% of 42 patients (156) most of whom were treated with PR at the same time. The effects were particularly good in patients with a thymoma (TH) which was also reported in two other studies (157, 158) and confirmed by my own experience. In a retrospective study of 27 thymectomized and PR resistant patients who received 1-2 mg/kg, 4 patients reached a remission and 18 improved. Improvement started within 1 month in most patients. In this series side effects were mild and transient (158). In the first study of 42 patients side effects included alopecia (75%), leucopenia (35%), gastrointestinal symptoms (25%), discoloration of the skin (17%) or of the nails (12%), arthralgia (10%), haemorrhagic cystitis (8%). This discrepancy in the incidence of side effects is probably due to the higher dosages in the first series (156). An increase of malignancies is known from other studies (159, 107), particularly concerning lymphoma and leukemia. Permanent infertility may occur both in men and in women. Rare side effects are myocardial damage and pulmonary fibrosis. Notwithstanding possible side effects it may be considered to treat PR + AZA-resistent TH-patients with cyclophosphamide or methotrexate; the latter is not studied in larger series. My own experiences are described in Chapter 5.

4.7.3 Antilymphocyte globulines

Antilymphocyte globulins (160, 161) have been employed to treat patients with progressive and therapy resistent MG with favourable responses of varying degree in two thirds. The production of the antisera is difficult and anaphylactic reaction may be problematic and no reports since 1979 could be found.
A more promising approach was the reduction of T-helper cell activity with use of a monoclonal anti-CD4 antibody produced in mice. A woman of 57 who was previously operated for a thymoma received anti-CD4 mAb for seven days. Improvement started on day 4, was maximal between days 16 and 58 and lasted 3 months. CD4 + lymphocytes decreased in peripheral blood and recovered slowly during the first year of follow-up and did not correlate with disease severity. AChR-Ab were not decreased by the treatment (162).

4.7.4 Partial or total body irradiation

Irridiation of the spleen (1000 rads per 2 weeks repeated up to 3 courses) induced a definite improvement in 3 out of 5 patients and total body irradiation (150 rads in 5 weeks) had a favourable effect in one patient. The improvement was transient and accompanied by a temporary lymphocytopenia in patients with spleen irradiation and by a permanent lymphocytopenia in the patient with total body irradiation (163).
A total body irradiation (0.1 Gy 2-3/week up to 1.8-2.3 Gy) resulted in a moderate improvement in 6 out of 12 patients, who were previously thymectomized and who were refractory to IS therapy. The procedure caused a decrease in CD4+ cells but not of CD8+ cells and in a lymphocytopenia. The CD4+ decrease was more prominent in the patients who improved. This procedure was well tolerated (164).

4.7.5 Intravenous immunoglobulins

Intravenous administration of immunoglobulines (IVIG) was found to improve patients with various immunohematological and autoimmune diseases. The mechanism of action is not completely understood (165, 166). Like all new therapies it was initially used in severely affected patients. In MG the first results were reported in 1982 (167) and several small series soon followed (168-170). The usual dosage is 0.4 mg/kg/day on 5-6 consecutive days or in 2-3 weeks. A global impression (171) is that considerable improvement followed in 40%, moderate improvement in 30% and no effect was obtained in 30%. Improvement started after 1-2 weeks, rarely in a few days. The maximum effect was reached in 10-20 days and lasted up to 6 months (168, 172, 173). In two series (174, 175) an initial exacerbation occurred comparable with that after the start of PR. Patients in a crisis reacted favourably (176) or insufficiently (177, 178). Mild side effects i.c. fever, myalgias and headache are sporadically mentioned but acute renal failure was a severe complication (179).

In about half of the series a decrease of AChR-Ab was measured, but no decrease occurred in the others. In 2 series (169, 177) AChR-Ab decrease had a delay of 10-15 days following clinical improvement suggesting an influence on the balance between idiotype and anti-idiotype antibodies (180). An increase of T-suppressor cells was measured on day 6 and 21 with a decrease of the T-helper - T-suppressor cell ratio (172, 175).

IVIG therapy is comparable with PP but easier to apply. The costs however are considerable and higher than PP.[9] Controlled studies comparing IVIG and PP in acute exacerbations and in periodic intermittent use are needed.

4.8 Physical therapy and speech-training

Before the diagnosis is made, MG patients are not infrequently referred to physiotherapists or speech therapists, who sometimes suggest the right diagnosis. Obviously the nature of MG makes active exercises useless because they induce further weakness. Most patients learn themselves how to live with their restricted muscle strength and know what they are able to do and what not. Short (minutes) periods of rest are beneficial. Physiotherapists should know this principle in treating MG patients for other ailments. They should also know that extreme, particularly high temperatures may increase the MG weakness. If weak neck muscles become painful a soft neck collar may give relief. **(Fig. 4.6)**

Speech training is occasionally useful in patients with severe dysarthria and dysphagia. Verbal communication may be improved by learning the patient to speak intermittently and slowly, and by giving feedback by making her listen to her own speech with a tape recorder. Patients with dysphagia should learn not to speak unnecessarily during their meals; foods should be ground and smooth, and preferably cold. A device for sucking saliva may be indicated.

In general there is no reason to disencourage physical activities such as walking, bicycling, swimming, if a patient feels she is able to. Physical training is usually not indicated except in patients who are reluctant to perform the muscle activities they should be able to do. In a study of 11 patients with mild or moderate signs a program of 3 training sessions per week during 10 weeks resulted in a 23% increase in quadriceps function (compared with 5% in the not trained side used as control) but no increase occurred in the upper arm muscles. Fatiguability was not influenced in any muscle group (181).

Figure 4.6

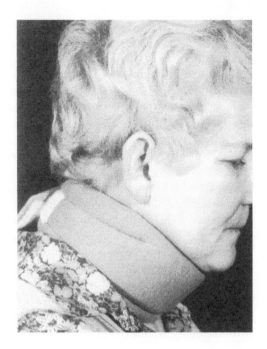

Soft collar sustaining the head in a
patient (W 47) with severe weakness
of the neck muscles.

4.9 Psychological aspects

4.9.1 Reaction to a chronic illness

Treatment of MG patients is impossible without considering the mutual
influence of psychological mechanisms and chronic disability. Sudden
emotions, particularly anxiety and feelings of aggression and envy, increase
myasthenic weakness (1, 182-186) and chronic weakness may influence the
development of the personality (185, 187) and aggravate a pre-existent
neurosis (186, 188).
No specific premorbid personality traits seem to exist (189, 190), but this is a
clinical impression rather than a conclusion based on the outcome of
personality tests. If patients are given such tests after many (5-10) years of
illness they often show increased indexes of neuroticism (185), anxiety (189,
191, 192), depression and hypochondriasis (190), but these findings may be
interpreted as the result of their chronic illness and not as the cause. In one
study no difference from the average German population was found (193).

Patients react to their illness in various ways obviously depending on their
personality. Traits of dependence and passivity may be enhanced in some
individuals, while others display a certain denial of illness leading to a poor
compliance and a tendency to take their own initiatives to change the

medication or to omit it suddenly. It is of utmost importance that these factors are taken into consideration. Emotions or stressful periods are reported to precede the onset of the first signs in about one third (185) to one half (1) of the patients. Patients who had improved in the last year reported a significant lower number of stressful life events than patients who did not improve or worsened (206). This fact and the fluctuation of symptoms, which may have disappeared during rest in the doctor's waiting room, lead to the initial diagnosis of psychosomatic illness or hysteria in 20-30% of patients (1, 185, 207). If the diagnosis is finally made, this greatly relieves the feelings of uncertainty (208) in those patients who have been considered neurotics or even malingerers. It is important to explain the nature of the disease not only to the patient but also to the spouse and to members of the immediate family. Many patients have difficulties in doing this themselves.

In other patients the diagnosis leads to reactions of depression or confusion. The initial explanation will not include the final prognosis which is essentially unknown to the doctor himself. So the patient has to live with her uncertainty, which not only includes the natural history of her disease, but also the unpredictable reaction to thymectomy or other therapies. If the doctor tells her that 60-70% of patients react favourably to thymectomy, but 30% do not she will obviously wonder which group she will belong to.

4.9.2 Uncertain doctors

The uncertainty of the doctor himself may preclude a sufficient explanation of the disease (183) or the outline of a plan of treatment. Most patients nowadays want to know the name of their disease and they are able to seek information elsewhere, but this does not always lead to reassurance. They return to their doctor with many questions that are not easily answered. It seems to depend largely on the personality of the doctor as to which future perspectives will be suggested: lifelong drug dependence and invalidism, therapeutic optimism, with early use of thymectomy, prednisone, immunosuppressives and plasmapheresis or a more expectant and supporting attitude. The modern patient, in touch with an MG association, will soon get the whole range of information brochures and will learn more of her disease than the average doctor has retained from his studies. So the patient has a more specific knowledge of the disease in general and particularly of her own symptoms, a fact that is not always appreciated by the doctor and may give rise to considerable misunderstanding and irritation, resulting in a nonoptimal treatment. Good communication between doctor and patient is of paramount importance. The patient should learn to cope with her own myasthenic symptoms, the doctor with the way in which the patient succeeds in doing so. At the start of treatment the patient should see her doctor when anything acute interferes with the therapeutic plans.

As is the case with many chronic diseases, many patients don't continue to consult their doctors after a certain period, but find their own adaptations and restrictions (182). This may give the false impression that the disease has been 'cured'. The real condition can be evaluated only by careful history taking and by testing the patient's muscle force and endurance. Therefore the problems of daily living are not easily understood by those in the patient's surroundings, in many cases even not by her doctor or nurse, and the patient often senses a slight mistrust in others.

4.9.3 Communication problems

Patients with more apparent ocular and bulbar symptoms have problems of communication, not only in the plain inability to speak intelligibly but also by their inadequate facial expression. They don't like to meet strangers who are unable to see whether they are laughing or crying or who believe that they are always angry because of their inability to smile (190). Weakness of the legs causing sudden falls may induce street phobia. Another aspect of dysarthria is the inability to express aggression verbally, the more so as aggressive or anxious feelings often lead to an increase of the dysarthria. This may be a factor in the development of unpleasant somatic feelings including nonspecific psychogenic 'fatigue'.

Neurotic states in reaction to MG in otherwise normal individuals were reported in 20% of 80 patients, and hysterical or hypochondriacal reactions occurred in another 17.5% of the patients with a premorbid neurosis (186). One may expect more severe psychological and psychiatric problems in patients who are totally dependent or treated by artificial respiration. In this situation communication is restricted to writing short sentences or spelling words by pointing to each letter. Psychotic periods may occur, usually with paranoid features. When patients were interviewed afterwards about these periods they usually had partial or even complete amnesia. In general, patients who have been treated for longer periods by artificial respiration have a very patchy recall of that period, and the events that led eventually to their admission to the intensive care unit may not have been retained at all. Sudden dyspnoea leading to coma is not remembered, and only if the dyspnoea is more or less chronic will it contribute to later feelings of anxiety. In some patients, psychotic periods may be accompanied by a considerable amelioration of MG symptoms (102).

4.9.4 Central nervous system involvement?

Clinical experience with MG patients does not raise the suspicion of central nervous system involvement, nonetheless indications for organic brain affection have been found concerning visual attention and reaction times (194). Also memory function was found to be impaired in a series of 12 MG patients when tested with visual as well as auditory tests and lower than in disease controls. An unexplained observation was the improvement of memory function during plasmapheresis, in line with the increase of muscle strength (195). In another study the presence of memory defects could not be confirmed (192). An auditory vigilance test in 5 patients did not reveal any abnormality (196). These contradictions are not well explained. Other arguments for a central nervous deficit were the putative increase of epilepsy in some older series (197, 198) but not confirmed in others (199, 200), and mild EEG abnormalities, found in 37% of 94 MG patients (controls 11%) in one older study (201) which was recently confirmed in an uncontrolled study (192).

Another line of investigations to detect a possible dysfunction of central cholinergic systems were all night sleep registrations showing a deficit in REM-sleep periods (202, 203), apparently without complaints. Also central sleep-apnoea periods were reported in 6 out of 10 well controlled MG patients (204). A decrement in the amplitude of the late (central) response in the brainstem auditory evoked potentials at repetitive stimulation was also interpreted as due to a dysfunction of central cholinergic neurons (203). An important finding was that AChR-Ab from MG patients did <u>not</u> bind to nicotine AChR-receptors extracted from human brain (205), which makes it unlikely that central AChR are the target of an autoimmune process.

4.9.5 Possible effect of medications

It has been suggested that restlessness, anxiety and agitation may be due to a toxic effect of the anticholinesterase medication and are the first signs of a cholinergic crisis. However quarternary ammonium-bases to which neostigmine, pyridostigmine and ambenomium belong, have no access to the central nervous system. The central effects are probably due to hypoxia and to the unpleasant side effects on the autonomic nervous system. If only the latter exist, the patient may feel agitated and irritable. Severe mood changes are occasionally seen in patients treated with prednisone. In others, mood changes are mild, to be characterized as depersonalisation, euphoria or depression and they may only be reported retrospectively when the drug is omitted. Some of my patients preferred moderate localized myasthenic symptoms (e.g. dysarthria, ptosis) to these undefinable feelings of not being themselves.

If depressions are the result of the relative severity of the MG condition there may be a good reason to change the therapeutic plan (e.g. to a treatment with prednisone or azathioprine) but a psychiatric consultation and an exploration of the social and relational conditions will not infrequently reveal problems that are amenable to specific interventions (190, 193). If the depression is accompanied by vital signs (e.g. loss of appetite, sleeplessness), a treatment with antidepressive drugs may be indicated (184). Mild sedation may be helpful in a difficult period. Although benzodiazepines are "officially" contraindicated, it is certainly not my experience that this is justified and small doses of chlordiazepoxide or meprobamate may be tried with caution.

4.9.6 MG is not a lifelong disease.

There is still a lot of misunderstanding among family doctors and even neurologists about the prognosis which is often estimated too pessimistically. Thymectomized young patients achieve a complete remission in at least 40% and another 40% improve considerably. Also in nonthymectomized patients complete remissions are possible after a longer delay. This obviously implies that they do not need to take their anticholinesterase medications. Some patients have the conviction that their well-being is still drug dependent, which is implicitly confirmed by their family doctor, who automatically prolongs the prescription. At least 70% of patients will be able to live a normal life 3 to 5 years after onset of their disease, with minimal restrictions. Unfortunately some of them will have lost their jobs and are not aided to make a new start, because of the 'dubious prognosis'. Problems may also arise in the higher prices for life-insurances, which are not reasonable in thymectomized patients who have considerably improved and are not treated with immunosuppressive therapies.

NOTES

[1] The female form will be used on statistical grounds; her implies also his, she also he etc.

[2] MG patient associations are active in holding meetings where information is given by experts and patients find support in mutual contact. Also manuals are provided with practical advice (do's and don'ts). A list of European MG associations is given on page.....

[3] Several factors are important: emotional disturbance, omission or inappropriate scheduling of anti AChE, infections and the use of certain medicaments (table 4.3). Many patients still have the fear of postoperative paralysis or prolonged apnoea due to muscle relaxants, which is of course unnecessary in modern anaesthesiological practice. Anaesthesiologists will know that suxamethonium has to be given in relatively high amounts (1 mg/kg) to produce sufficient relaxation thereby producing a nondepolarizing block (209) at intubation. Short lasting nondepolarizing agents such as atracurium (210) or vencuronium (211) may be used safely in MG patients. The dosage of vencuronium needed to maintain muscle relaxation was about 25% of that required in normals and was inversely related to the concentration of AChR-Ab (212). Halotane and still more isoflurane have a depressing effect on NMT (213).

4 The therapeutic effect of ephedrine is not generally accepted in MG in spite of early reports (Ch 1.4). It was shown however that ephedrine and aminophylline increased the twitch height of MG intercostal muscle preparations (220). In alpha-bungarotoxin induced experimental MG in the rat no specific effect of ephedrine could be demonstrated (221).

5 In 1995 tablets of Neostigmine and Mytelase®, the 5‰ Mestinon solution and the Mestinon syrup were suddenly no more commercially available in most European countries. In the Netherlands no official announcement or informal information of the patients or their organisations took place. Also tablets of atropine 1/4 mg were withdrawn. In hospital the parenteral Mestinon solution can be provided by the pharmacist.

6 Plasma concentrations of pyridostigmine and prostigmine can be determined by gas (liquid) chromatography (214, 215).
Plasma concentrations after single oral doses of 120 mg pyridostigmine reached a peak after 1-2 hours in fasting subjects (215, 216) ranging from 40-70 microg/L, the half time being 1.74 hours. A half life of 1.5 hours was found after intramuscular (216) or intravenous (215) administration. When taken together with food the time to reach the peak concentration was prolonged to 3.2 hours. Bioavailability was calculated to be 7.6 ±2.4%, which was not influenced by concomitant food intake (215). In another study bioavailability of oral pyridostigmine was 10-20% (217). Patients taking their usual dosis and in a steady state had only mild fluctuations in their pyridostigmine concentrations but these were not related to the height of the dose and only poorly to the clinical effect (217, 218).
Methylcellulose was found to prevent the absorption of the drug (218). In my own experience plasma levels are very variable even if measured repeatedly in the same patient under the same conditions. Before 1970 the dosage of pyridostigmine (60 mg) or prostigmine (15 mg) mounted to 20-25 tablets per day with considerable side effects. Today the maximum dosage used rarely exceeds 600 mg (10 tablets). Pyridostigmine and prostigmine are bromides. Exceptionally brome hypersensitivity may occur. Also bromide intoxication (psychosis) is possible if large dosages of pyridostigmine are used over a long period and chloride intake is low (219).

7 The normal neuromuscular transmission (NMT) has a large (400%) safety factor by an abundance of transmitter (ACh) release and of AChR. Clinical weakness will develop only if 25% of the AChR or of the ACh production at a coherent group of muscle fibres is lost. Many drugs have the potency to influence NMT either by inhibiting ACh release (chloroquine [223], beta-blockers [224], gadolinium [225] or by binding to the postsynaptic side (polymyxines, tetracyclines, procainamide, pymantelpalmoate [226], lithium [228]) or by both mechanisms (aminoglycosides, phenytoin, chlorpromazine, verapamil [227]). The induction of a myasthenic syndrome (c.q. MG) has been reported in patients without subsequent MG by chloroquine (223), a high dosage of beta-blockers (224), and gentamycin (26) and also occurred in one of

my patients by kinine. One may speculate that some nonmyasthenics have a reduced safety factor of NMT (223). The sudden exacerbation during stressful situations may also be caused by an increase of adrenocorticoids and catecholamines.

[8] The initial deterioration in prednisone therapy is not well explained. The latent interval with a mean of 5 days suggests an immunological influence, because suppressor cells would be influenced earlier than T-helper cells (223). In various laboratory experiments a direct action of prednisone on NTM was reported but the results were contradictory possibly depending on the acuteness of the experiment and the dosages used (review 102). The action of pancuronium (curare-like) was diminished in a non-MG patient who was treated with 100 mg prednisone per day and underwent splenectomy (222).

[9] Controlled randomized trials are apparently difficult in MG. A North-European study concerning cyclosporine versus azathioprine was cancelled because no more than 6 patients could be included in the first year in 9 participating centres. The French study (109) in 6 centres comparing prednisone and azathioprine recruited only 41 patients in 7 years. An English multicentre study comparing prednisone and azathioprine with prednisone raised 34 patients in 3 years (110).

[10] The common procedure is to remove 2-3 L of plasma in repeated 200 cc runs by an indwelling catheter in an arm vein but the volume exchangeable is dependent upon the accessibility of the veins and the general condition of the patient. In some chronic patients transfemoral catheterization or the construction of an arteriovenous shunt is necessary with a higher chance of thromboembolic complications and infections.

In the last 3 years PP was performed in 19 MG patients in the neurological department of the Academic Hospital Groningen. In most patients 6 procedures were done in 2 weeks; one patient was treated once per month for more than one year. The mean exchange per procedure was 1900 (range 1400-2700) ml. The replacement fluid was 4% albumin. The costs per procedure are about Dfl. 1,000.--. (Courtesy of dr. A. Westerterp-Maas, Stichting Rode Kruis Bloedbank Noord-Nederland) The costs for treatment with intravenous immunoglobulins is about Dfl. 700.-- per 10 gr. Mean dosage per patient 70 x 0.4 gr. per procedure. A series of 5 treatments costs about Dfl. 10,500.-- compared with Dfl. 6,000.-- per series of PP.

5

Eight Hundred Patients With MG

1960-1994

5.1 Patients and methods

Since 1960 when I became resident in the Neurological Department of the University Hospital (head Prof. Dr A. Biemond) in Amsterdam, I examined about 900 patients with MG of whom 813 are included in this survey.

The inclusion criteria were:

a. Diagnosis according to generally accepted criteria (3.1);

b. Follow-up of at least 3 years, or to the patient's death;

c. Medical data confirmed by specialists or family doctor.

In the first years an active search was made in the archives of several other large neurological centres[1] and all traceable patients were personally examined and sera were collected for immunological studies (1-7). Gradually the acquisition of patients came from referrals from other neurologists to the Neurological Department in Amsterdam until 1976 and to the University Hospital Groningen from 1976 to 1994.

About one half of these patients have been under my treatment during one or more periods of their MG; the other half were seen in consultation, often more than once.

Details of the history of the disease were always more reliable and exact when obtained from the patient than from the referring doctor. As onset of the disease was taken as the moment of the first specific signs (e.g. diplopia) and not of unspecific symptoms like fatigue.

The clinical examination was standardized by means of tests that could measure muscle force and endurance, and to make a disability score (DS) at fixed moments during the follow-up (0.5, 1, 2, 3, 4, 5, 7, 10, 12, 15, 20, 25, 30, 40 years after onset). If patients were not under my regular treatment, they were followed by telephone calls and if appropriate by obtaining information from their own doctors. I always tried to study the original documents (e.g. PA-reports, EMG-descriptions) and to see the original photographs and

100

histological preparations (muscle biopsies, thymus histology). These attempts usually succeeded though not always without tenacity.

Thymectomies were performed in the centres for thoracic surgery, mainly in the University Hospitals, by transsternal approach. Apart from the surgical skills the postoperative management was of utmost importance; for this reason a relatively large number of thymectomies was performed in Leiden between 1965 and 1975. Of the patients included after 1976 most thymectomies were performed in the Academic Hospital Groningen. From 1984 dr J. B. M. Kuks was my associate and companion in patient care and research.

Reports concerning the outcome of treatments in several patient groups have been published elsewhere (8-11).

5.2 General features of the 4 subgroups (see 2.1)

5.2.1 Epidemiology

The distributions of age at onset, gender and type are given in fig. 2.24. The relative prevalence for each age group and gender compared with the total population in the same age groups is given in **table 5.1**. Also after this correction the highest incidence occurred in young women, but in men the relative incidence was highest in the late onset group. The incidence in children was relatively low. The relative incidence of thymoma was not significantly different between the sexes.

The first signs are given in table 2.1. Part of the patients who started with ocular signs became generalized after a certain delay. **(Fig. 5.1)** Although most patients reached their definite type within 3 years after onset, a late conversion

Table 5.1 RELATIVE PREVALENCE OF MG (per 100.000)*

Men	Age at onset	Women
1.26	0-9	1.30
4.00	10-19	11.65
3.22	20-29	10.09
2.71	30-39	7.13
3.84	40-49	7.24
5.42	50-59	6.35
6.48	60-69	4.88
9.7	70-79	4.88
--	80-	1.57

* adjusted to the Dutch population 1992

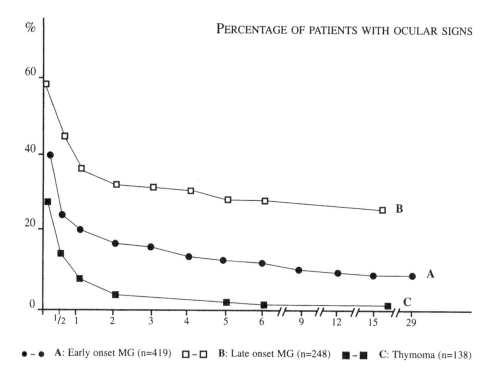

● - ● A: Early onset MG (n=419) □ - □ B: Late onset MG (n=248) ■ - ■ C: Thymoma (n=138)

Figure 5.1 Only ocular signs at onset were present in 39%, 58% and 27% of patients with early onset, late onset and thymoma respectively. After 3 years also other muscle groups were involved in 84%, 68% and 96%. at the end of the follow-up 9.6%, 26.6% and 1% remained purely ocular.

from ocular to generalized could occur after 10-20 years. The diagnosis ocular MG was based in clinical findings: no weakness in other muscle groups could be demonstrated by quantified tests (3.2), while the presence of EMG abnormalities in skeletal muscles although rare, was not decisive.

Apart from 805 patients with acquired MG, 8 patients were diagnosed as suffering from a congenital myasthenic syndrome (5.7).

Familial MG was found in 14 patients or 1.7%. (**Table 5.2**)

5.2.2 Diagnosis

The delay of the diagnosis could be considerable, particularly in early onset women. For instance after 1 year the diagnosis was made in 52% of early onset (EO) women, in 65% of EO men, in 65% of late onset (LO) women and in 72% of LO men. After 2 years these percentages were 72, 80, 78 and 88 and after 5 years 80, 95, 92 and 99. One factor for this delay was the more protracted course in women which was found in the analysis of 100 consecutive patients

Table 5.2 ACQUIRED FAMILIAL MG 1960-1994

PROBAND				FAMILY MEMBER			
sex	age at onset	MG	AChR-Ab		Age at onset	MG	AChR-Ab
M	10	gen.	neg.	Son	15	oc.	pos.
W	14	gen.	pos.	Sister	35	gen.	pos.
M	1	gen.	neg.	Brother[1]	1	gen.	--
W	24	gen.	pos.	Sister	41	gen.	pos.
W	37	gen.	neg.	Father	67	oc.	pos.
W	55	TH	pos.	Daughter	38	TH	pos.
W	35	gen.	pos.	Brother of Father	74	oc.	neg.

[1] Twin brother died in crisis during chickenpox (see note 5.10).

seen in our department between 1985 and 1989 (11). Another factor could have been a different diagnostic approach of men and women in EO patients. This was also reflected in the referrals to a psychiatry department before the diagnosis was made: 8% in women and none in men. Patients with only or mainly limb muscle weakness had a higher risk for the diagnosis to be missed. At least 4 young females made the diagnosis themselves after they had read about MG in a popular magazine. In several girls the diagnosis anorexia nervosa was made although their mentrual cycle was normal. In some patients the speech therapist suggested the diagnosis, being aware of the fluctuation of the dysarthria.

Before the AChR-Ab test became available (in 1978), the confirmation of the surmised diagnosis relied upon the effect of anticholinesterases (anti AChE), or on repetitive nerve stimulation. Both tests could be negative in 10-15% of patients in the first year of illness, part of them only later becoming positive. The sensitivity and specificity of the main diagnostic tests, calculated from part of this material are given in table 3.1.

Other confounding factors were the presentation with muscle atrophy (5.2.5) in an early stage, and concomitant other diseases or emotional stress. Reflections about diagnostic reasoning were not always prominent in medical correspondence, which makes retrospective inferences difficult. If the diagnosis was made by the neurologist it was not unusual that additional investigations were first used to exclude other diseases (11).

5.2.3 Severity and death

For the 3 groups of generalized MG the maximum disability score at any moment of the disease is given in **table 5.3**. The categories 5 and myasthenic

Table 5.3 MAXIMUM DISABILITY SCORE AND MORTALITY
IN 3 CATEGORIES OF MG (%)

maximum disability score*	EARLY ONSET 10-39 years n=353	LATE ONSET 40-85 years 180	THYMOMA All ages 138
1	2	1	4
2	25	26	13
3	45	40	32
4	9	14	9
5	17	14	25
died in MG crisis	1.4	5	17

* maximum DS (see table 2.3) at any moment of course of MG

death comprise patients with the same basic severity, the outcome depending upon a successful intervention or not. An analysis of the subgroups revealed that in the group of 1-14 years the percentage with a MG crisis was 30%, but there were no deaths. The median DS seems to be somewhat higher in the late onset (LO) than in the early onset (EO) group, but only the patients with TH had a definitely higher DS. Nearly all deaths occurred in the time before steroids were used or were caused by a deliberate withdrawal of corticosteroids (n=2). In the TH-group 9% of patients died from the invasive TH and 3% from complications of IS therapies (see 5.6.3).

5.2.4 AChR-Ab and AMA

From a survey of our 250 patients (fig. 3.3) it was concluded that AChR-Ab levels did not correspond significantly to individual differences in disease activity at the moment of serum sampling. AChR-Ab values varied from 0-1100 nMol/L with a median of 46 nMol/L and a mean of 18 nMol/L. EO patients had higher Ab-levels than LO patients; the lowest values were found in patients with ocular MG. Patients with TH had the same Ab-levels as the EO group but were always seropositive. Steroid therapy lowered Ab-levels (12). There was a strong correlation between the change of AChR-Ab levels and the change in clinical condition of the individual patient during treatment with PR or IS and in the periods after thymectomy; a weaker correlation was present in periods without IS. In only 3 out of 75 patients the changes in AChR-Ab concentration preceded the clinical change. No changes in AChR-Ab concentration were found if improvement was due to the effect of anti-AChE or if deterioration was caused by infections or emotions (13).
In the final material AChR-Ab levels were determined in 280 EO patients, 113

LO patients, 103 TH patients and 84 ocular patients. (Table 5.4) Again the Ab-levels varied considerably, with significant lower values in the OMG and a lower mean in the LO group than in the EO group and in the TH-patients. AChR-Ab were found in 87% of EO, in 96% of LO, in 100% of the TH and in 39% of OMG patients. Low values (1-2 nMol/L) were absent in TH patients. In ±100 patients AChR-Ab were measured before and during follow-up after thymectomy: in 2% AChR-Ab became negative without IS therapy. A change from seronegativity to seropositivity was seen in only 4 patients, usually when ocular signs became generalized. The disappearance of AChR-Ab in the LO group was seen in 5 patients: this occurred spontaneously in 1 man with a fluctuating course and a low AChR-Ab titers; the others used PR.

Table 5.4 ACHR-AB TITERS (%)

x10⁻⁹mol	EO[1)	LO	TH	OMG
negative	13	4[2)	--	64
1-2	9	11	4	13
3-10	11	27	24	14
11-20	12	20	18	4
21-50	24	23	27	2
51-100	15	9	19	
101-500	14	5	7	1
501-1000	1			
> 1000	2	1		1
No of patients	292	113	103	84

1) In each titer group about 1/3 of the patients were thymectomized before serum sampling.

2). Three out of 4 patients used PR at serum sampling.

AChR-Ab levels are partly a result of antibody production by peripheral blood lymphocytes (PBL). Spontaneous and pokeweed stimulated in vitro production of AChR-Ab by PBL were measured in 79 patients with EOMG. Spontaneous AChR-Ab production was found in 10 patients, pokeweed stimulated AChR-Ab production in 47 patients of whom 12 were thymectomized. The presence of spontaneous AChR-Ab production before thymectomy and the persistence of pokeweed stimulated AChR-Ab production after thymectomy corresponded with a poor reaction to thymectomy (14).

AMA were determined with the indirect immunofluorescence test in 618 patients (table 5.5)[2]. As was reported previously (12) a high incidence was

Table 5.5 ANTI MUSCLE ANTIBODIES (%)

	EO	LO	TH	Oc.
negative	96	47	10	82
positive 16-64	3	29	42[1]	7
≥ 128	1	24	49	11[2]
n =	299	150	102	67

[1] In 9 patients AMA became positive following thymomectomy.
[2] 1 patient with TH.

found in patients with TH, irrespective of age and also in late onset patients, with an increasing incidence with advancing age (positive findings in age group 40-49 years: 24%, 50-59 years: 47%, 60-69 years: 64%, 70-85 years: 91%). Also in OMG positive findings were related to the actual age of the patient at serum sampling and not to the age of onset.

These findings imply that a TH is improbable in EO patients if AMA are negative. In a minority of TH patients AMA became positive at a later age, usually after thymomectomy. The increase with age in LO and OMG may reflect a general age-dependent deficit in immunoregulation.

5.2.5 Muscle atrophy[3]

Muscle atrophy was always localized e.g. in the tongue (**fig. 5.2**), the shoulder muscles, and some patients had atrophy in more than one muscle group e.g. hand and foot extensors, tongue and face and throat (**table 5.6**). In only one patient, a man aged 25 with a TH (not tabulated), a generalized muscle atrophy developed during three months of artificial ventilation and periods of sepsis. At autopsy signs of focal demyelination of peripheral nerves were found suggesting a metabolic (deficiency) polyneuropathy.

In autopsies of other MG patients no abnormalities in peripheral nerves were found.

If atrophy was present at onset of the disease considerable diagnostic problems could arise: in several EO patients the diagnosis myopathy or peripheral nerve injury was made, in LO patients amyotrophic lateral sclerosis of the bulbar type. Two patients (woman aged 40, man aged 45) developed dropping hands and dropping fingers with severe atrophy of the forearm extensors, later followed by weakness and atrophy of the foot extensors. Three other men (aged 42, 49, 48) had a combination of fluctuating external ophthalmoplegia and neurogenic atrophy of the feet extensors, in one patient also of the hand extensors and upper arm extensors, without other MG signs. This type was described by Garcin et al (15) in one male patient.

Atrophy of the face muscles could be symmetrical (fig 2.16) or very partial **(fig. 5.3)**. In one female patient with a longstanding atrophy, face lifting was

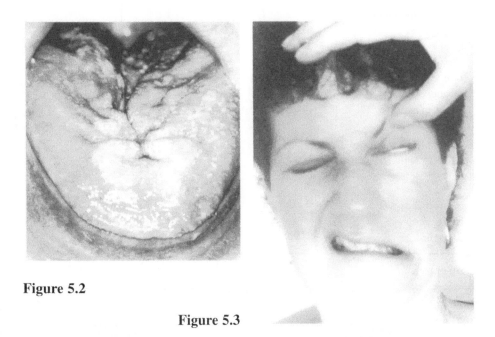

Figure 5.2

Figure 5.3

Figure 5.2 W, onset at age 60. (LO max. DS 5) She gradually developed a severe atrophy of the tongue and a moderate weakness of the facial muscles about 5 years after onset. No change after treatment with PR + AZA since age 66, which improved her ocular and limb weakness. Autopsy at age 75 showed focal neurogenic atrophy in the tongue and skeletal muscles (left).

Figure 5.3 W 34. Onset at age 15; thymectomy followed by IS treatment (PR, PR + AZA). Mild facial weakness since onset but only since five years marked focal weakness of left m.levator labii superioris (right).

performed with subjective improvement. Atrophy of the tongue could be persisting, but also transient, disappearing with other bulbar signs e.g. after thymectomy. In some patients the atrophic tongue became enlarged and protruded outside the mouth **(see case history A)**. In several EO patients a combined atrophy of tongue, throat and face muscles developed, which was resistent to thymectomy and subsequent immunosuppressive therapy. In general, muscle atrophy in MG patients was not influenced by prednisone and could even develop despite prednisone therapy which had a favourable

Table 5.6 LOCALIZED MUSCLE ATROPHY IN MG

	Early Onset	Late Onset	Thymoma
shoulder girdle	12	5	8
in triceps muscles only	1	1	
forearm	4		
hand			1
face	2		2
tongue	6	1	1
face + m.masseter	1	1	
tongue and throat	4	1	2
face + tongue + throat	4	1	
tongue + m.masseter	2		
m.masseter		2	6
m.quadriceps	1		1
foot extensors	3	4	
paraspinal	1	1	
No of patients	32 (9%)	15 (8%)	17 (12%)

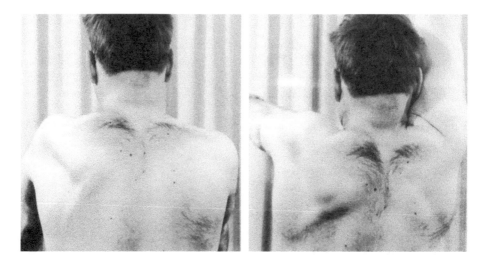

Figure 5.4 M 32. Age at onset 18. Improvement by thymectomy followed by prednisone, until age 26. Residual external ophthalmoplegia, ptosis and gradually developed weakness of left shoulder muscles with marked atrophy.

108

Patient A

Woman, onset with transient diplopia at age 28, followed by limb muscle weakness at age 29 and bulbar signs at age 31. Definite diagnosis at age 38 after MG crisis and Co_2 coma. From that time she needed intermittent ventilatory assistence ('curasse') and never could be weaned off. Therapy with anti-AchE gave many side effects. Thymectomy was thought to be too risky (in 1963). When I saw her at the age of 46, she had a mild atrophy of the face and jaw muscles, a severe atrophy and weakness of the shoulder- and upper arm muscles, but a normal strength in hands and legs. Thoracic excursions were limited with a vital capacity of 1200 cc (normal 4000 cc). She had a mild dysarthria and a normal tongue. She had a partial external ophthalmoplegia but no ptosis. Swallowing was impaired and she needed additonal feeding through a nasal tube. From that time she was treated with PR (100 mg/d tapered off to 30 mg/2d) with some improvement in swallowing and a decrease of the time she needed artificial respiration. In the subsequent years there was a gradual deterioration. I saw here again at the age of 60, when she was treated with PR 25/2d. She was dependent on artifical ventilation for most of the day. The atrophy of her face and jaw muscles had remained the same but she had developed a total immobility of the tongue which was enlarged and protruded through the open mouth. As a matter of fact she could not speak and in the last years also her ability for written communication was impaired by increasing weakness of the hands. I suggested an increase of the PR to 40 mg/2d, which indeed resulted in a gradual improvement in hand function and respiratory capacity. Here severe atrophy remained the same. She died at home at the age of 69 from an arterial bleeding out of the lung, problably due to a tracheal perforation by the ventilation tube.

Comments: 1. Striking was the severe, although still localized muscle atrophy and the beneficial reaction of the not atrophic muscles to a higher dosage of PR.

2. I have seen this extreme protrusion of the tongue in a patient with a chronic polyradiculopathy (M 65) who was completely paralysed and artificially ventilated for 5 years.

influence on other MG signs. (**Fig. 5.4**) On the other hand no proximal leg weakness occurred during prednisone therapy, of the type described in the treatment with high dosage fluorocorticoids.

In the rare cases that a biopsy was taken from an atrophic muscle, this showed neurogenic lesions, occasionally combined with lymphorrhagic infiltrations. Also biopsies from muscles that were not clinically atrophic could show neurogenic changes, with or without lymphorrhagic infiltrations. The latter were highly correlated with TH, the former not (16). In this series of patients one patient (M 40, TH) had the biopsy picture of a polymyositis although the clinical signs were not typical. In the next series one patient (W 54, DS3) developed during AZA therapy a painful proximal leg weakness, elevated CK (10x), general malaise, fever and icterus. She died from cardiac insufficiency. At autopsy extensive inflammatory changes were found in all skeletal muscles

and also in the heart muscle (PA diagnosis polymyositis and myocarditis).
In none of the other 30 autopsies lesions of the heart muscle indicative for
myocarditis were found.[4]

5.2.6 Associated autoimmune diseases

The autoimmune (A.I.) diseases that have been diagnosed in the 4 MG groups
are compared in **table 5.7**. The diagnoses were made by the specialists
concerned, according to official diagnostic criteria.[5] Since the incidence is
apparently influenced by the lengths of the follow-up periods, the latter were
calculated to enable comparison.
As could be expected (5.6) there was a predominance in women; the highest
relative incidence was found in the LO-group.
Some diseases occurred exclusively in the TH group: aplastic anemia,
pancytopenia, hyper- and hypogammaglobulinaemia and polymyositis (5.6).
A.I. thyroid disease was the most frequently associated disorder (± 5%) with a
definite predominance in women. Non A.I.-hyperthyroidism was found in
another 3% of patients. Thyroid disorders could become symptomatic at any
age without a relation with the onset of MG: about 25% before, about 25%
coinciding (within one year) and in 50% following the onset of MG. Malignant
exophthalmus had to be treated in 6 out of 25 patients with A.I. thyroiditis or
dysthyroid ophthalmoplegy.
The next frequent A.I. disease was rheumatoid arthritis (RA) also with a
predominance in women (5% vs 3% in men). Patients with RA induced by d-
penicillamine (5.3) are excluded here. Striking was the absence of RA in TH
patients. The onset of RA coincided with MG in 5 patients, preceded MG in 9
and followed MG in 20 patients.
No difference in prevalence of A.I.-diseases was found between the previously
thymectomized and nonthymectomized patients.
The maximal severity of MG was not related to the prevalence of A.I.-diseases.

5.2.7 Other associated diseases

The prevalence of malignancies in 4 categories of MG patients is given in **table
5.8**. No relation to the onset of MG was apparent. In only one TH-patient (W
70) a carcinoma of the breast and a melanoma were detected when she was
admitted for thymomectomy. This was cancelled; her MG was controlled with
PR but she died from cancer within one year. Nine patients developed a
carcinoma and two patients a lymphoproliferative disorder after having used
azathioprine (n=9), 6-mercaptopurine (n=1) or chlorambucil (n=1). In the EO
group a non-Hodgkin lymphoma (W40 AZA 6y), colon carcinoma (W 67 AZA
10y); in the LO group: prostate carcinoma (M 67, AZA 7y), thyroid carcinoma
(M 66 AZA 6y), abdominal malignancy e.c.i. W 69 AZA 3y); in the TH group:
mammacarcinoma (W 53, AZA 3) basal cell carcinoma (W 58, AZA 10y),

Table 5.7 AUTOIMMUNE DISEASES

	EO		LO		TH		OMG		Total	
	M	W	M	W	M	W	M	W	M	W
Rheumatoid arthritis	4	14	3	11	--	--	1	1	8	26
Primary hyperthyroidism[1]	--	13	--	5	1	3	1	3	2	24
Primary hypothyroidism	1	7	1	4	--	1	--	--	2	12
Systemic lupus erythematosus	--	9	--	1	--	2	--	1	--	13
Nephrotic syndrome	--	3	--	--	--	--	--	--	--	3
Sarcoidosis (Besnier Boeck)	--	4	--	1	--	2	--	--	--	7
Psoriasis	2	5	--	1	--	--	--	--	2	6
Vasculitis (non RA)	--	3	--	--	--	--	--	--	--	3
A.I.-gastritis (pernicious anemia)	--	2	--	3	--	1	1	1	1	7
A.I.-thrombopenia (17)	2	1	--	1	--	--	--	--	2	2
A.I.-hemolytic anemia	--	1	--	--	--	--	--	--	--	1
Secondary amenorrhoe	--	4	--	--	--	--	--	--	--	4
Vitiligo	2	1	--	1	--	--	--	1	2	3
Insuline dependent diabetes	1	--	--	2	--	--	--	--	1	2
m.Sjögren	--	--	--	1	--	--	--	--	--	1
Colitis ulcerosa	--	1	--	2	--	--	--	--	--	3
Ileitis terminalis (M. Crohn)	--	--	1	--	--	1	--	--	1	1
Multiple sclerosis	--	2	--	--	--	1	--	--	--	3
A.I. hepatitis	--	1	--	--	1	--	--	--	1	1
A.I. adrenalitis	--	--	--	--	--	1	--	--	--	1
Hypergammaglobulinemia (18)	--	--	--	--	1	2	--	--	1	2
Hypogammaglobulinemia	--	--	--	--	--	2	--	--	--	2
Aplastic anemia/pancytopenia	--	--	--	--	2	4	--	--	2	4
Polymyositis + myocarditis	--	--	--	--	--	1	--	--	--	1
Polymyalgia rheumatica	--	--	--	--	--	1	--	--	--	1
Hair follicle trichoepithelioma (19)	--	1	--	--	--	--	--	--	--	1
Alopecia totalis	--	1	--	--	1	--	--	--	1	1
No of A.I. diseases	12	73	5	33	6	22	3	7	26	135
No of patients with A.I. diseases	10	61	5	27	5	18	3	5	23	111
≥.2 A.I.-diseases	2	11	--	5	1	4	--	2	3	22
No of MG patients	71	301	88	88	45	90	61	40	265	519
% A.I.-diseases	17	24	6	38	13	24	5	17	10	26
Follow-up, mean	27	26	11	14	11	16	11	15	--	--
range	11-47	2-59	3-28	1-38	1-20	2-37	5-16	6-28	--	--

[1] Non-A.I. hyperthyroidism | -- | 8 | 2 | 9 | -- | 2 | 2 | 2 | 4 | 21

Table 5.8 MALIGNANCIES IN MG

	EO	LO	TH	Oc.
carcinoma/sarcoma	14 (6)*	18***	18 (9)+****	2
lymphoproliferative disease	5 (3)*	2	2 (2)+	2
central nervous system	1 (1)[1]	1[2]	--	--
mean age (y)	50	70	58	59
% of total patients	5	12	12	4

() Number of patients who had been thymectomized   * Patient treated with AZA

[1] Hypophyseal adenoma   + Patient treated with Mercaptopurine

[2] Intramedullary glioma

cervix carcinoma in situ (W 36, AZA 6y) recurrent basal cell carcinoma of the face (M70, chlorambucil 8y), fibrosarcoma and leukaemia (W 53 and 65, 6-mercaptopurine resp. 1 and 13y). Except from the skin and mucosa tumors (n=4) and from the leukemia the relation with the use of AZA is doubtful (20). The influence of a previous thymectomy on tumor growth was improbable.

Neurological disease: Nine patients had epilepsy (5 primary generalized, 3 focal e.c.i., one generalized, cause unknown; the frequency lies within the expected range.

Parkinson's disease was diagnosed in 2 patients; m.Alzheimer in 4 patients.

Focal dystonias were seen in 9 patients : spastic torticollis in 2, blepharospasm in 3, hemifacial spasm in 2, eyelid apraxia in 1, prolonged eye closure (**fig. 5.5**) in 2. The spastic torticollis preceded the MG and was not alleviated by possible MG-weakness; the dystonias of the facial muscles developed in patients whose MG was in (nearly) complete remission, but they were in some patients erroneously interpreted as a recurrence of MG.

Other neurological diseases are not specified here but there is no suspicion of a deviant prevalence than in the total population.

Psychiatric diseases:chronic psychosis or acute psychotic periods occurred in 14 patients: schizophrenia in 2, manic depressive psychosis in 2, severe psychotic depressions in 2, chronic paranoid psychosis in 2, acute psychogenic psychosis in 6, of whom 4 were induced by high PR treatment. In 2 patients severe alcoholism had existed. Apart from the PR induced psychotic periods they had no intrinsic relation to their MG. Striking were improvements of MG during psychotic periods, which were characterized by maniacal features (21). Mild and mainly transient conversion reactions (hemiparesis, abasia) were occasionally observed e.g. following thymectomy; in 4 patients serious problems with the MG treatment emerged (**patient B**).

Patient A

Woman, onset with transient diplopia at age 28, followed by limb muscle weakness at age 29 and bulbar signs at age 31. Definite diagnosis at age 38 after MG crisis and CO_2 coma. From that time she needed intermittent ventilatory assistence ('curasse') and never could be weaned off. Therapy with anti-AchE gave many side effects. Thymectomy was thought to be too risky (in 1963). When I saw her at the age of 46, she had a mild atrophy of the face and jaw muscles, a severe atrophy and weakness of the shoulder- and upper arm muscles, but a normal strength in hands and legs. Thoracic excursions were limited with a vital capacity of 1200 cc (normal 4000 cc). She had a mild dysarthria and a normal tongue. She had a partial external ophthalmoplegia but no ptosis. Swallowing was impaired and she needed additonal feeding through a nasal tube. From that time she was treated with PR (100 mg/d tapered off to 30 mg/2d) with some improvement in swallowing and a decrease of the time she needed artificial respiration. In the subsequent years there was a gradual deterioration. I saw here again at the age of 60, when she was treated with PR 25/2d. She was dependent on artifical ventilation for most of the day. The atrophy of her face and jaw muscles had remained the same but she had developed a total immobility of the tongue which was enlarged and protruded through the open mouth. As a matter of fact she could not speak and in the last years also her ability for written communication was impaired by increasing weakness of the hands. I suggested an increase of the PR to 40 mg/2d, which indeed resulted in a gradual improvement in hand function and respiratory capacity. Here severe atrophy remained the same. She died at home at the age of 69 from an arterial bleeding out of the lung, problably due to a tracheal perforation by the ventilation tube.

Comments: 1. Striking was the severe, although still localized muscle atrophy and the beneficial reaction of the not atrophic muscles to a higher dosage of PR.

2. I have seen this extreme protrusion of the tongue in a patient with a chronic polyradiculopathy (M 65) who was completely paralysed and artificially ventilated for 5 years.

Another problem that was occasionally encountered were nightly anxiety attacks with breathlessness and hyperventilation; particularly patients who had experienced real MG dyspnoea were sometimes acutely admitted to the intensive care unit under suspicion of a MG crisis.

COPD (Chronic obstructive pulmonary disease) is not uncommon and may lead to acute respiratory insufficiency with the need of transient artificial ventilation. COPD probably has the same incidence in MG patients as in the general population which implies that about 5% of MG patients may have propensity to COPD. The bronchoconstrictive action of anti-AChE might even enhance this predisposition. The work load of the respiratory muscles in severe bronchoconstriction is considerably increased so that a mild MG weakness of the ventilatory muscles increases further during a COPD-attack, leading to a

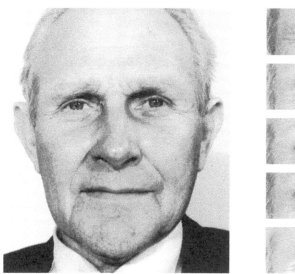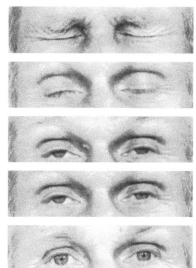

Figure 5.5 M 60, age at onset 53. Thymoma. Max. DS: 5, early severe crises; after complications from PR and AZA treated with chorambucil. Complete remission, but later complaints about 'ptosis', particularly after sneezing. Delayed relaxation after forceful eye closure. This symptom subsided gradually in 5 years.

combined MG and COPD crisis.

Two patients in this cohort have died in a COPD crisis, probably without being influenced by their MG; in at least 8 other patients COPD crises were influenced by concomitant deterioration of MG.

5.3 Ocular Myasthenia (OMG)

5.3.1 Diagnosis

OMG was diagnosed if muscular weakness was restricted to the palpebral levators and/or the eye moving muscles, and fluctuation could be demonstrated or was reported by the patient. A mild weakness of the m.orbicularis oculi was present in about 10%. Since the sensitivity of the conventional diagnostic tests is lower in OMG than in the generalized form (table 3.1), and not all tests were performed, a clinical score was constructed (**table 5.9**).[5] The inclusion was made by a positive anti-AChE test in 81 out of 98 patients (81%), by the presence of AChR-Ab in 16 additional patients, in 3 patients with negative anti-AChE tests and a negative antibody test by specific EMG abnormalities in the m.orbicularis oculi (decrement, increased jitter), in one patient by a positive

Table 5.9 OCULAR MG - CLINICAL SCORE (MAX. 10)

Ptosis: none, one, both eyes	0-2
alternating side	3
Diplopia, eye muscle pareses	0-2
History: fluctuating during the day	0-1
longer periods	0-2
Examination: worse by exertion	0-2
improved by rest	0-2

For the diagnosis OMG the following criteria had to be fulfilled:
• Follow-up ≥ 3 years
• Clinical score ≥ 5/10
• Other diseases reasonably excluded

reaction to 1 mg d-tubocurarine and in 7 patients by a positive clinical score alone (3 patients ≥ 7, 4 patients ≥ 5). **(Fig. 5.6)** Patients with mainly ocular signs but with also a period of bulbar or limb muscle weakness were (re)classified as mild generalized (n=6). All these patients had AChR-Ab. AChR-Ab were found in 39% with concentrations ranging from 1.5-1000 nMol/L (median 5 nMol/L). **(Table 5.10)** In 7 out of 80 patients anti-AChE had an equivocal or negative effect at the first attempt, leading to a sometimes considerable delay of the diagnosis.

5.3.2 Epidemiology

Men, particularly over the age of 40, predominated in OMG (table 2.1, fig. 2.24, table 5.1). OMG started in the first decade in 5 boys and 5 girls and comprised 40% of the total MG patients with onset in that period. Of the patients who started with ocular signs, only a minority remained purely ocular (table 2.1, fig. 5.1) at the end of the follow-up period (3-43 years, mean 12 years). The extension from ocular to generalized signs was most rapid in the TH patients of whom only 1 remained purely ocular (follow-up 20 years).

5.3.3 Clinical signs

Diplopia was the most frequent initial sign (table 2.1). In the course of OMG nearly all patients had a combination of ptosis and eye muscle pareses; only one patient had ptosis without diplopia and 4 patients had diplopia without ptosis. Diplopia was especially embarrassing if vertical and at downward gaze. Complaints of unsteady gait and 'dizziness' were then common in older

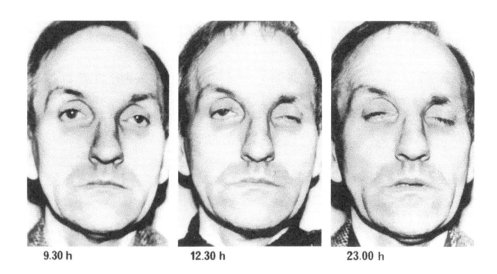

| 9.30 h | 12.30 h | 23.00 h |

Figure 5.6 M 47. Diplopia since age 31. No relief by strabism operation. Ptosis since age 42. Effect of Mestinon equivocal; curaretest (1 mg) negative, AChR-Ab negative, EMG m.orbicularis oculi normal. No diagnosis was made. Photographs at age 47 show a convincing increase of ptosis in the course of the day. An atropine-neostigmine test in the late afternoon was positive.

Table 5.10 OMG-EPIDEMIOLOGICAL DATA

| | A C h R - A b | | | |
	+	−	?	
No of patients	32	53	23	108
M:W	15:17	33:20	15:8	63:45
< 40:≥ 40 y	11:21	25:28	7:16	42:66
AMA positive	10/20	5/32	0/18	15/70
Thymoma	1	--	--	1
A.I. diseases	4[1]	2	2	8
Non-A.I.-hyperthyroidism	--	3	1	4
D-penicillamine induced	2	4	--	6
Malignancies	2	--	2	4

[1] 2 LO patients had malignant exophthalmus

patients. In some patients the extension to a nearly complete external ophthalmoplegia diminished the diplopia.

The course of OMG could be very capricious with periodical exacerbations and remissions without a clear provocative factor e.g. stress or infection. In 14 patients this periodic course was prominent (**fig. 5.7**); in 3 additional older patients a spontaneous remission came within 1 year.

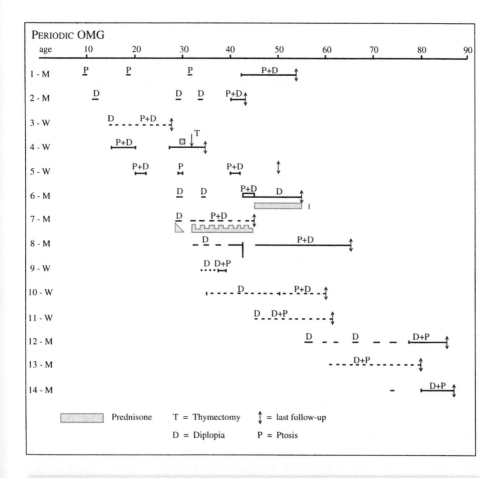

Figure 5.7

Patient 1: M. One year left sided ptosis; recurrence at the age of 18, disappearance after ptosis operation. Recurrence at the age of 35; ptosis disappeared again after ptosis operation. Since the age of 42 fluctuating ptosis and diplopia. The ptosis improved by anti-AChE.

Patient 4: Ptosis R at the age of 17, after 2 months diplopia. Edrophonium test +. Ptosis reacted to Mestinon®. Diplopia returned in periods until the age of 21. No symptoms until the age of 28, then diplopia again and after 1 year also ptosis. Pr 60 mg/2d caused disappearance of ptosis butdiplopia did not disappear entirely. PR was stopped because Cushing face and obesity. Ptosis and diplopia reappeared but fluctuated spontaneously. Thymectomy at the age of 31 (normal thymus) had no efect. OMG had again a fluctuating course: ptosis R > L, multiple eye muscle pareses.

Patient 7: M 29: one week vertical diplopia: after 6 weeks again diplopia, later combined with transient ptosis R. Six months after onset ptosis L, after 3 days also R. Positive edrophonium test but no effect of Mestinon. PR 30 mg/2d: ptosis disappeared after 1 week, diplopia after 3 months. No symptoms with use of PR 10 mg/2d. After 2 years PR was stopped: diplopia returned after 6 weeks. Age 32-45 years: PR varying from 10-30 mg/2d. At a dosage of 10 mg/2d he has 3 times per year a period of diplopia especially during stress. He is able to work as a high school teacher.

Patient 11: W. Since the age of 45 she had periods of 3-6 months with diplopia, sometimes combined with ptosis. At age 53: operation ptosis L; diplopia relieved with prisms. At age 55: diagnosis OMG: diplopia and ptosis R; AChR-Ab +. No effect of Mestinon. At age 61: periods of diplopia 3 weeks to 3 months. No more ptosis.

The particular ocular signs are described in 2.2.1. I found it useful to make a rough sketch of the eye movements in the primary directions and of the ptosis to compare the clinical states more easily. **(Fig. 5.8)** Two patients (M 64, W 71) had a dysthyroid ophthalmoplegia with malignant exophthalmus combined with fluctuating ptosis and AChR-Ab. In both the OMG disappeared spontaneously in 5 years, after treatment for the exophthalmus. Malignant exophthalmus occurred in 4 other patients with generalized MG (2 EO and 2 TH).[7]

5.3.4 Treatments

Anti-AChE were tried in nearly all patients. The effect was often unrewarding, particularly concerning the diplopia. Most neurologists (and patients) tended to increase the dosage of anti-AChE gradually if the results were insufficient. Often patients had more side-effects of the anti-AChE medication than benefits. If parenteral administration of anti-AChE failed to relieve the signs, oral anti-AChE would not do better. But even if parenteral anti-AChE relieved the ocular signs, the effect of oral medication tended to wane gradually.
Overdosage of Mestinon caused sensations of stiffness in the lips and tongue in some patients, which gave the erroneous suspicion of involvement of the bulbar muscles.
Some patients got used to their ocular disability and omitted their anti-AChE medication. They occluded one eye in situations where diplopia was dangerous or embarrassing. Others preferred a permanent occlusion of one eye. A solution for this problem was a 10 diopter positive lens so that the occluded eye remains visible (though somewhat enlarged). This is socially more acceptable than occlusion by an eye-pad. Also occluding contact lenses could serve this purpose. Another way to decrease diplopia was the use of press-on prisms,

which may ensure a normal vision in the central position of the eyes. Ptosis could be relieved by flexible eyelid supports inserted half way the temples of the frame.[8] **(Fig. 5.9)** Patients with diplopia were advised not to use bifocal glasses but to employ separate reading glasses.

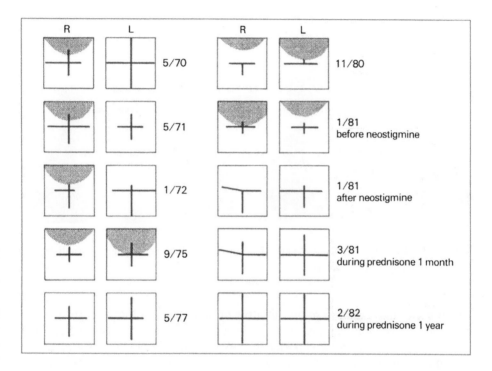

Figure 5.8 W 65. Ten years history of fluctuating diplopia and ptosis. In 1971 negative edrophonium test. Minimal symptoms between 1977 and 1980. In 1980 the atropine-neostigmene test was positive. Complete remission on treatment with PR 40 mg/2d. Range of ocular movements and degree of ptosis are schematized.

Figure 5.9 a

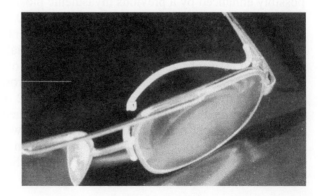

Flexible eyelid support, attached to the temple of the glasses.

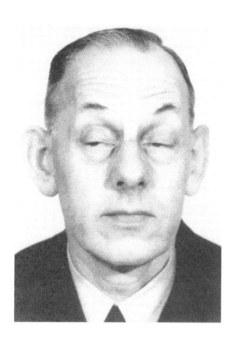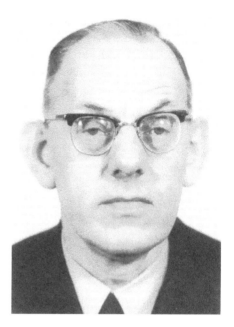

Figure 5.9 b, c M 60. MG onset at age 17. Mainly ocular signs not responding to anti-AChE. Ptosis relieved by eyelid supports.

Eye muscle operations were on initiative of an ophthalmologist, performed in 6 patients before the diagnosis was made and in another 7 patients in a chronic stage. Three of the latter reported a good result within one year after the operation, but in one patient three operations were performed. No lasting positive effect resulted in the early operated group.

Ptosis operations were performed in 5 patients before the diagnosis of MG, without lasting benefit. In a later stage a permanent ptosis could be operated, because it was due to excessive skin folding (dermatochalazis; fig. 6.4) possibly enhanced by a previous myasthenic ptosis.

These measures failed for different reasons in 20 patients, which made them candidates for PR-treatment; another 7 patients received PR on other indications. **(Table 5.11)** The ptosis reacted usually within 1-2 weeks, the diplopia in 3 weeks to 3 months; nearly half of the patients went into a complete remission. The start dosage varied from 0.5-1.0 mg/kg/day; the lowest effective dosage ranged from 10-45 mg/2 days and was found in the individual patients by trial and error. As a spontaneous remission might occur, we adviced to taper off the dosage every one or two years.

Thymectomy was performed in 3 young women with AChR-Ab and EMG abnormalities in their limb muscles, but without clinical weakness. They failed

Table 5.11 THERAPIES IN OMG, FINAL OUTCOME

Treatment	Remission	Improved	No change	Total
Anti-AChE[1]	23	18	32[2]	73
Drug omission[3]	6	2	0	8
Prednisone	15[4]	11	1	27
Total	44	31	33	108

[1] c.q. spontaneous course

[2] Three patients were thymectomized, 1, 15 and 16 years after onset.

[3] In 6 patients, MG was induced by d-penicillamine, in one patient by a calcium influx blocker, in one by a beta-blocker.

[4] Three patients received a short course of steroids with transient improvement (2 malignant exophthalmus, 1 COPD) but later achieved a remission without cortico steroids. Four other patients received prednisone in treatment for their COPD (n=3) or SLE.

to respond, but in 2 the interval between onset and thymectomy was more than 15 years.

A man aged 47 with alternating ptosis and incomplete external ophthalmoplegia with diplopia in all directions, was treated with cyclosporine (300-500 mg/day). It took 9 months before his diplopia had finally disappeared, while the ptosis had reacted in 2 weeks. He was previously treated with PR with the same slow reaction of the diplopia.

5.4 Early onset MG

5.4.1 Epidemiology

Between the ages of 10 and 40 years women were 2-3 times more represented than men (fig. 2.24, table 5.1). The diagnosis had a longer delay in women than in men (5.2.2). Associated autoimmune diseases occurred in 17% of men and 24% of women (table 5.7) and malignancies in 5% (table 5.8).

HLA types were determined in 95 patients (22). HLA-B8 positive were 6 of 11 men and 74 of 84 women ($p < 0.001$). In a series of 40 patients (23) the subtypes HLA-A1, HLA-B8, DRW3 and DQW2 were present in respectively 70%, 78%, 65% and 70% (population controls: 32%, 28%, 25% and 30%). MG in infancy (1-9 years) is described in 5.7.

5.4.2 Thymectomy vs natural course

Thymectomy in patients without thymoma was nearly exclusively done in this age group (262 patients with onset from 10-39 years, 17 with onset from 40-55 years, 3 children aged 8-9 years). In my follow-up series are 107 patients with onset from 10 to 40 years who have not been thymectomized, mainly because thymectomy was an unusual therapy between 1945 and 1965 when their disease had started. The maximum DS of the thymectomized appeared to be somewhat (but not significantly) higher than the non-thymectomized group, possibly due to selection by survival. **(Fig. 5.10)** If the cumulative "remission" rate of both groups were compared, the "remission-rate" of the thymectomized patients was significantly higher at nearly all follow-up points. Three years after disease onset 70% of thymectomies was performed, 90% within 7 years. The same calculation comparing 17 thymectomized and 44 non-thymectomized patients over the age of 40 yielded no difference (Remission rate 10% after 5 years in both groups and 43% vs 35% after 10 years).

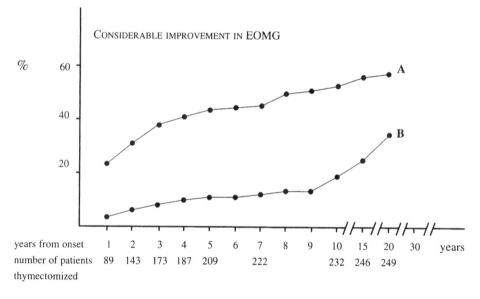

Figure 5.10 Considerable improvement includes complete remission and much improved (decrease of ≥ 2 points on DS [e.g. DS 3 → DS 1], without IS and max. 180 mg Mestinon). Cumulative %.

A: 249 thymectomized patients (M 48; W 201), max. DS (1-5): 0%, 23%, 51%, 9%, 17%.
   Death by MG 5; remissions 39 patients; much improved 18 patients.
B: 107 non-thymectomized patients (M 21; W 86), max. DS (1-5): 7%, 31%, 42%, 9%, 11%.
   Death by MG 2; remissions 108 patients; much improved 36 patients.

By comparing 20 patients in remission after thymectomy with 20 non-responders, no relation between the outcome of thymectomy and HLA-types was found except a higher incidence of DR 4 in the patients with remission (p < 0.05) (23).

A difficult practical problem was to advise patients if their MG existed for more than 5-7 years. Although a previous analysis of the first part of the included patients (8) had shown that the results of thymectomy were better if performed within 3-5 years after onset, in some young patients good results were seen with symptoms since 7-12 years. In general I advised thymectomy, considering that the chance of spontaneous considerable improvement in the period 7-15 years after onset is about 10-15% (8, fig. 5.10).

Late thymectomies (≥ 7 years after onset) were performed in 36 patients. In the group with an interval of 7-10 years (n=18) the results after 5 years were: remission 4, much improved 3, improved 6, no effect 5 patients; in the group with an interval of 11-20 years (n=18) the results were: remission 2 much improved 4, improved 4, no effect 8; in the group with an interval of 15-20 years (n=8) 2 patients improved. These results (42% considerable improvement) were the same as in the early thymectomized patients. **(Fig. 5.10)**

In a previous analysis of the first series of the included patients no relation could be found between the histological picture of the thymus (normal, hypertrophic, atrophic) and the results of thymectomy (24).In 39 recently thymectomized patients a remission occurred sooner in patients with absent or occasional germinal centres (25).[9]

Rethymectomy was performed in 3 patients who had not improved after initial cervical thymectomy **(fig. 5.11)** and in one whose transsternal thymectomy was apparently incomplete (CT-scan). These 4 patients went into remission after the second operation. In 3 other patients who had not improved after transsternal thymectomy and did not respond sufficiently to IS therapy, a rethymectomy was not successful (no thymus found in one patient, normal thymus remnants in 2).

Late exacerbations after initial considerable improvement or remission were rare (8 out of 160); in 3 patients treatment with IS was necessary, in 5 others the symptoms were mild, mainly diplopia or ptosis, and transient. These exacerbations occurred 6-18 (mean 11) years after the postoperative remission.

A not well explained phenomenon was the improvement immediately following thymectomy: this was reported by 45 out of 245 patients who were operated without previous treatment with PR or PP. This improvement ("I could suddenly speak and swallow normally", "my double vision and eyelid drooping had vanished") was permanent in 11% and transient in 7%. The transient improvement lasted 3 days to 3 months (medium 14 days). Five years later 47% of the patients with a transient remission had a permanent remission or considerable impovement which is about the same as the remission rate of the whole group (fig. 5.10). Only one patient was treated with PR for some years before thymectomy was done (fig. 7.3).

123

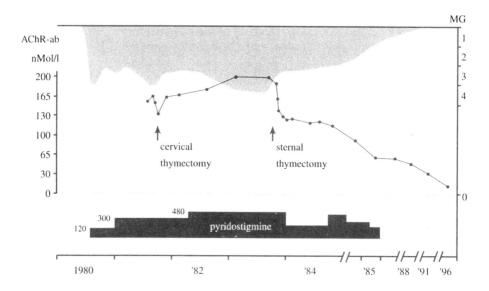

Figure 5.11 W 22. Generalized signs at onset. Insufficient reaction to Mestinon. Cervical thymectomy 15 months after onset (hyperplastic thymus). No clinical improvement and increase of AChR-Ab levels. Transsternal thymectomy 3 years after onset (normal thymus, 50% fat) followed by gradual improvement and decrease of AChR-Ab levels. Complete remission since 5 years after the second operation.

5.4.3 Pre- and postoperative management

In the 1960s thymectomy had to be considered as a riskful operation in patients who had already gone through a period of ventilatory insufficiency or crisis (see 4.5.3) mainly by severe bulbar signs (dysphagia) and the inability to cough vigourously. Since a thoracotomy reduces the ventilatory capacity in the postoperative days, these patients received a tracheostomy before operation and were as routine artificially ventilated during some days or weeks. In severely affected patients with a risk of recurrent crisis, the tracheostoma was kept open by a fenestrated silver canule. They were able to speak by occluding the external orifice by a rubber stop, or by their finger! In the 1980s when soft intubation tubes had become available tracheostomy could be avoided in most patients. One of the frequent problems was the development of an atelectasis, which could be provoked by a transient paralysis of the diaphragm due to a phrenicus lesion by the operation. Anti-AChE were usually omitted or drastically reduced in the postoperative period to avoid bronchosecretion, and later reinstituted as the patient could be weaned from the respirator. The edrophonium test was then useful to adjust the dosage of anti-AChE and was also be used to improve the strength of the expiratory muscles as an aid in the bronchial cleaning.

Since the 1980s patients with moderate or severe bulbar signs and/or previous crises are prepared for thymectomy by PP, usually combined with PR starting 2-3 weeks before operation (see 4.5.1). In this way postoperative crises or the need for postoperative artificial ventilation can be prevented.

Crises occurred in 17% of the thymectomized patients, in 13% only before thymectomy, in 2% as an unforeseen postoperative complication and in another 2% (7 patients) also after the operation. Of these 7 patients, 3 died later in a crisis, without being treated with IS.

5.4.4 Anti-AChE and IS therapies

Nearly all patients were treated with <u>anti-AChE</u>, before 1960 only with prostigmine, later with Mestinon, frequently combined with Neostigmine. These drugs were extremely important in the period before IS were used. In general higher dosages were given than nowadays, with more cholinergic side effects, which could only partly be antagonized by atropine.

Also ephedrine was a valuable auxillary drug in some patients. The effect of anti-AChE was variable, rarely entirely absent but also rarely leading to a complete remission. If this occurred it was my policy to omit the anti-AChE gradually, surmising that the remission was spontaneous, though this advice often raised a psychological resistance in the patient.

In **table 5.12 a** the global results are given of the therapies used in both the EO and LO groups. It should be emphasized that these treatments were initiated and followed by many neurologists whose individual strategies varied, so that comparison is only possible on the main points. The effect of IS therapies (PR, AZA, rarely cyclosporine) is given in **table 5.12 b**. Nearly 80% of the EO group improved considerably (remission or decrease of ≥ 2 points on DS) but only 24% achieved a complete remission; this is significantly lower than the 66% remissions in the LO group. The numbers are too small to compare the effect in the operated and nonoperated groups. Patients who received PR only pre- or postoperatively are omitted, since they were finally not dependent on this therapy. If the effects of IS treatment are added to the outcome after thymectomy or the spontaneous course, considerable improvement was reached in 70% of the operated EO group, in 59% of the non-operated EO group, in 76% of the operated LO patients and in 70% of the (non-operated) LO patients. Though these results are rewarding, they implicate a "life-long" treatment for a certain category of patients. This is particularly a psychological burden for young patients, as is exemplified in the history of **patient D and E.**

Patient D

Man aged 14 (1977). Onset with diplopia and ptosis, after 3 months followed by weakness of the limbs and the face. Thymectomy 5 months after onset (normal

20 mg o.a.d. Gradual but definite improvement (DS2: O_2, B_0, U_2, L_1, V_0) in 1979 and 1980, with decrease of AChR-Ab. Deterioration 3 months after omission of AZA and increase of AChR-Ab. It took 2 years to regain a stable state by transient increase of PR and AZA. In this period (1983-85) he could perform his university studies with mild impairment (DS2), due to intermittent ptosis and proximal arm muscle weakness and not hindered by his symmetrical external ophthalmoplegia. Exacerbations followed in 1985 by tapering and omission of PR and later in 1987 by withdrawal of AZA. The same occurred in 1991 and also in 1994 when withdrawal of PR on his own initiative was followed by a severe exacerbation (not shown in the figure). At this time he had given his confidence to an "alternative" medical doctor who had incriminated his amalgame tooth fillings combined with a (not radiologically verified) chronic frontal sinusitis as the cause of his MG. Acupuncture had no effect, though he felt an improvement of his general condition. After reinstitution of PR 60 mg/d combined with PP he improved gradually but it took one year to reach his former condition. At the end of 1996 he informed me that he was married and wished again to taper off the AZA, because he desired to get healthy children. This was the advice of another acupuncturist who was willing to treat his possibly evolving MG signs.

Comments: 1. Experimental evidence from the previous treatment and the high intellect of the patient did not lead to the acceptance of the necessary IS treatment of which he had no side effects.
2. The alternative doctors did not answer my letters.
3. There is no evidence that AZA influences male fertility or the health of the child.

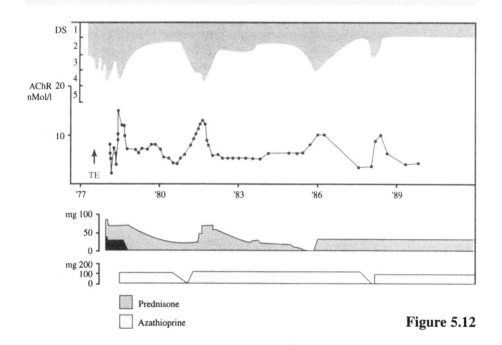

Figure 5.12

126

Table 5.12 a FINAL GLOBAL OUTCOME IN EO MG AND LO MG

Outcome %	EO thymectomy +	EO thymectomy −	LO thymectomy +	LO thymectomy −
Remission	48	37	29	25
Much improved*	15	18	12	7
Improved**	14	20	18	9
Not improved	9	16	--	12
Not improved - IS	13	5	41	42
MG-death	1.4	2	--	6
Number of patients	249	107	17	164

* Much improved: decrease of ≥ 2 points on DS.

** Improved decrease ≥ 1 point on DS.

The category not improved IS comprises patients with DS ≥ 3 who were not improved after thymectomy or had this condition in the natural history of their disease.

Table 5.12 b EFFECT OF IMMUNOSUPPRESSIVE THERAPY

	EO Thx*	EO non-Thx	LO Thx	LO non-Thx	Total
Remission	7	--	4	46	57
Much improved	21	4	2	16	43
Improved	2	4	1	5	12
No effect	3	--	--	2	5
No of patients	33	8	7	69	117

* Thx = thymectomized

5.4.5 Pregnancy and neonatal MG (NMG)

One hundred forty four patients had had 215 pregnancies resulting in 209 living children. The causes of death were neonatal MG (diagnosed retrospectively) 1, immaturity 2, congenital heart failure 1, unknown 2. The reported period ranges from 1940-1992; so some of the data had a long history and may not be remembered exactly.

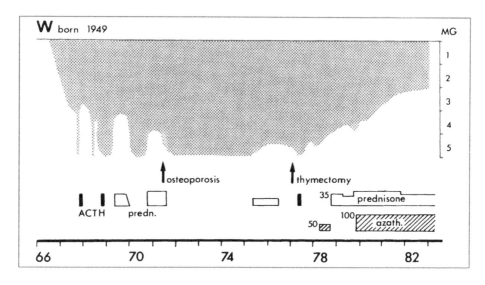

Figure 5.13 a

Patient E

Woman born in 1949. Onset of MG at age 17 with diplopia, soon becoming generalized. Crisis 15 months after onset, responding to ACTH (100 E/d during 10d) and PR (30-50 mg/d). PR was omitted in 1970 because of vertebral collapse. Continuous assisted ventilation (in wheel chair) from 1970 until 1978. I advised thymectomy in 1978 (hyperplastic thymus), which was followed by a gradual improvement though PR and AZA were still needed. She had developed a permanent facial weakness and atrophy of the tongue that did not respond to IS **(fig. 5.13 b and c)**. From 1980 she had been living independently and working part time (MG score O_1, B_2, U_1, L_1, V_1). In 1986 a non-Hodgkin lymphoma (NHL) of the coecum was diagnosed, treated with operation and chemotherapy. She had then used AZA for 6 years. Six months later an intracerebral localization of the NHL was treated with radiotherapy and metothrexate but she died one year later. The MG did not change.

Comments: 1. The previous vertebral collapse when she was immobilized in a wheel chair was no contraindication to treat her later with PR. In fact AZA alone had insufficient effect.

2. The question arises whether thymectomy 12 years after onset finally reversed the course of her disease.

3. The NHL may have been caused by AZA.

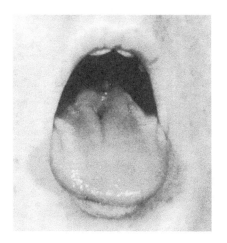
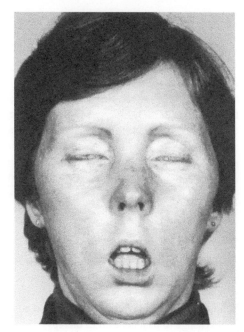

Figure 5.13 b, c

NMG was reported in 22 children born to 19 mothers, but it was not always possible to get a confirmation from a pediatrician. Three women had 2 children with NMG. The retrospective diagnosis relied upon a postnatal period of poor crying and sucking which subsided spontaneously and for which no other cause was probable. The duration was some days to maximal 3 weeks; some children were treated with neostigmine or pyridostigmine through a feeding tube. All women with a child with NMG had a mild or moderate MG (DS 2-3) at the time that their child was born.

NMG occurred in 8 out of 84 patients who had been thymectomized and in 14 out of 131 patients who had not (no difference). As far as AChR-Ab had been determined the values ranged from 20-50 nMol/L (n=15); in the umbilical cord blood of the child these antibodies were present in the same concentrations, but AChR-Ab were also found in children without NMG.

The relationship between the course of MG and pregnancy was complex. **(Table 5.13)**

In general, improvement of MG was more frequent than deterioration although crises during pregnancy were reported in 2 patients. In 3 women the diagnosis of MG was made after the birth of a child with NMG (**patient F**).

In general the parturition itself had not given problems, as far as the patients reported. Obstetrical details were not available in most patients.

Patient F

Woman aged 40. Since the age of 12 ptosis, diplopia, mild proximal arm weakness. These signs were fluctuating with periods of near remission. Exacerbation after the delivery of her first child at age 26. This child had shown signs compatible with NMG as was analyzed later. At the age of 28 a second child was born by Cesarean section, that also had NMG. She had to be ventilated artificially for 2 days, probably because of the prolonged action of muscle relaxants. The diagnosis was then made in mother and child. She improved spontaneously until the preoperative condition and also reacted favourably on pyridostigmine. She refused thymectomy. At the age of 41 she wears prisms to suppress her diplopia; she has no medication. Her muscle strength is normal in rest but she is unable to carry heavy loads (DS 1).

Table 5.13 PREGNANCY AND MG

MG in remission, no change	28
Improvement (mild to remission)	44
Improvement in pregnancy, exacerbation post partem	26
No change (6 patients with IS therapy)	28
Deterioration (2 patients crisis)	25
Deterioration post partem (2 patients sectio)	5
Deterioration in first term, improvement in second and third term	4
Onset MG post partem	19
Onset in pregnancy	12
Unknown	24

Five women had used IS drugs in 7 pregnancies: PR: 2, AZA: 1, PR + AZA: 2. The 7 children were delivered à terme, with a normal weight, without abnormalities except one child, with NMG who also appeared to have the syndrome of Rubinstein-Taybi (**patient G**).

Patient G

Woman aged 41. MG since the age of 17, thymectomy six months after onset, followed by PR at age 18, combined with AZA at age 23 and PP at age 24. DS score varied from 2-4. AZA was withdrawn but PR 30 mg/2 d was continued at age 25 because she wanted a child. No pregnancy followed but an exacerbation of her MG (DS 4)which was treated with PP and reinstitution of AZA. At age 30 she became pregnant and had a complete remission of her MG from the first month of pregnancy. After childbirth MG relapsed to DS 2; medication: AZA 125 mg/d + PR 15 mg/2 d. At the age of 34 she had a second pregnancy without change in her DS (2). Her second child had congenital anomalies of the face and fingers, no NMG. As the child was also mentally retarded, the diagnosis syndrome of Rubinstein-Taybi was made. At the age of 41 her MG is much improved (DS 1) with PR 15/2 d and AZA 125 mg/d.

Comment: The relation of the syndrome of Rubinstein-Taybi and the use of AZA is unknown.

5.4.6 Infantile MG

Acquired MG was rare in childhood (first decade) (table 5.1, fig. 2.24), and relatively frequent confined to the ocular muscles (10/25 = 40%). The 10 infantile patients with only ocular signs are included in the OMG group (5.3). Five patients came into a remission after 1, 3, 3, 15 and 15 years respectively; three patients improved, 3 did not change. In 15 patients the signs were generalized; the onset was precipitous during a childhood infection in 5 patients with need of ventilatory support in 4. One of these patients had a identical twin brother who died in the same period.[10] In the others the onset was more gradual. A particular course was seen in 2 Antillian patients who had only ocular signs from the age of 6 with generalization at the ages of 19 and 21. Subsequent thymectomy had no effect. Three other patients with onset at age 9 were thymectomized; an immediate remission occurred in one patient, but the other 2 had to be treated with IS therapy. Six patients went into remission after respectively 1, 3, 5, 12, 15, 25 years but improved much sooner, and 3 others improved considerably. The general policy was not to advice thymectomy in patients younger than 8-9 years and to await the spontaneous course.

AChR-Ab were present in none of the 7 generalized patients with onset from 1-3 years and in 5 out of 8 patients with onset from 4-9 years.

Patient H

W 71. From the age of 6 years drooping of the upper eye lids visible at photographs. No medical consultations. Between the age of 14 and 20 years frequent falls, particularly in attempts to run or in bicycling. As a teacher in primary school she could not read aloud for more than 3 minutes because she would become unintelligible. From the age of 38 years she had increased ptosis and loss of arm strength; she could no longer function as a teacher. Also dysarthria increased. At the age of 51 the diagnosis was made following a prolonged apnoea by muscle relaxants in an abdominal operation. After a positive Tensilon test she was treated with pyridostigmine 5 dd 60 mg combined with 3 dd neostigmine 15 mg. I saw her at the age of 52 years. Her main signs were ptosis on both eyes, and slight diplopia, no limb muscle weakness or bulbar signs. She improved gradually, withdrawing her medication to 120 mg pyridostigmine.

At the age of 71 she travels alone, has no further symptoms than diplopia at night. AChR-Ab: 60 nMol/L.

5.5 Late onset MG

5.5.1 Epidemiology

The prevalence was the same in men and women (table 5.1), and the maximal DS was the same as in the EO group (table 5.3). Associated A.I.-diseases were diagnosed in 6% of men and 38% of women (table 5.7) and malignancies in 12% of patients of whom 2% had used AZA (5.2.7).
MG weakness was most often maximal 2-5 years after onset but late exacerbations (> 5 years) occurred in 9% of patients of whom 6% after 10 years.

5.5.2 Therapies

Thymectomy was performed in 17 patients. In 9 patients aged 41-45 years at onset the results were about as good as in the EO group: remissions in 3 patients, considerable improvement in 2 patients, improvement in 2 patients, no improvement in 2 patients. In 8 patients aged 49-58 years at onset the results were: remissions in 2 patients, no impovement and PR dependency in 6 patients. Two patients were operated on suspicion of a TH (false positive CT scan). The outcome of the entire group was not different from the one of the patients in the age group 40-59 who were not thymectomized. The thymus was normal in 2, hyperplastic in 3, and atrophic in 10 and unknown in 2 patients.
A spontaneous remission or considerable improvement was reached in 20-25% of patients. IS-treatment was given to 25% of the 83 non-thymectomized patients aged 40-59 years, and in 60% of the patients over the age of 60. The beneficial effect of I.S. treatment was not related to the duration of the disease. Patients with a long period of severe signs or late exacerbations reacted equally well as the patients with a short history. In general eye muscle paresis reacted well to PR but not to AZA.
During withdrawal of PR arthralgic pains were common which often made a slower withdrawal or even reinstitution necessary. Also a carpal tunnel syndrome could occur in this situation; this was always transient and was treated by immobilisation during sleep.
D-penicillamine induced MG was present in 5 RA patients; one patient was in remission one year after withdrawal of the drug but in 4 patients mild symptoms persisted.
Ten patients died from MG, of whom 7 in the period before 1965 and 3 later

after a sudden withdrawal of PR which had induced a remission. No deaths were attributable to the side effects of IS in this group.

Plasmapheresis (PP) was carried in 17 EO, 12 LO and 11 TH patients, usually as an acute intervention combined with high-dose prednisone (4.6). In 4 LO and 1 TH patients PP was used as a support of IS therapy (PR + AZA) which at that time had an insufficient effect. In one man (age at onset 19 years, thymectomized) who reacted insufficiently to PR 50 mg/d, and in whom AZA 150 mg/d had no additional effect a monthly PP was needed to improve his condition (extended arms 10" → 3', kneebends 2 → 20 times). An attempt to replace PP by intravenous gammaglobulin failed. AChR-Ab decreased by PP from 1.6 to 0.6 nMol/L (!). He has been receiving monthly PP now for 18 years. An analysis of 24 patients (DS 3-5) showed a considerable improvement in 71% in the first week (3PP) and 88% at the end of the second week (6 PP). These patients were also treated with high-dose PR without initial deterioration. A comparison was made with the effect of high-dose PR as monotherapy in 13 patients with the same clinical condition. Four patients had an initial deterioration, 2 patients had improved after one week (15%) and 8 (69%) patients after 2 weeks (26).

5.5.3 Side effects of IS treatment

Side effects were more prominent in older patients and more frequent in patients treated with PR than with AZA. (**Tables 5.14 a, b, c**)
They necessitated adaptations or change of IS drugs. In only 7 patients of the LO group, complete withdrawal was needed (Cushing 2, vertebral fracture 2, urosepsis 1, diabetes 1, psychosis 1). Exacerbations at the start of PR were seen in about half of the patients without concomitant PP who were closely followed. Most side effects emerged in the first weeks (AZA) or months (PR) after onset, except cataract, and severe infections. A critical note might be made about the specificity of certain side effects: the prevalences of cataract, herpes zoster and osteoporotic fractures all increase with advancing age and

Table 5.14 a SIDE EFFECTS OF PREDNISONE AND AZATHIOPRINE

MG	Total patients	Patients treated with IS	SIDE EFFECTS		
			PR or AZA	PR	AZA
EO	374	91	39%	39%	14%
LO	180	84	68%	54%	28%
OC	108	24	42%	42%	--
TH	138	91	47%	41%	21%

Table 5.14 b SIDE EFFECTS OF PREDNISONE*

	EO	LO	TH	OC	Total
Cushing syndrome	11	8	7	3	29
Gastrointestinal bleeding/ulcers	4	2	1	1	8
Diabetes	--	12	4	--	16
Cataract[1]	3	7(5)	7(3)	3(1)	20
Arterial thrombosis in the leg	1	--	1	--	2
Vertebral collapse	4	6	1	-	11
Limb fracture	--	5	3	-	8
Herpes Zoster	2	4	9	--	15
Skin infections[2]	3	8	3	--	14
Mood changes[3]	2	3	3	3	11
Severe infections [4]	3(1)	1	3(2)	--	7
Benign intracranial hypertension	1	--	--	--	1
Arterial hypertension	--	--	1	--	1
Excessive weight gain	--	3	--	2	5
Psychosis	--	2	--	--	2
Skin bleedings	--	2	--	--	2
Number side effects	34	63	43	12	152
Patients with side effects	32	44	34	10	120

* Mild transient side effects at high dosage are not noticed.

[1] In brackets the number of patients over 70 years of age in whom the cataract was possibly of the senile type.

[2] Acne, candida, herpes simplex, fungal infections.

[3] Depersonalisation, depression, irritation, sleeplessness.

[4] In brackets the number of patients who died; one TH patient also had chronic alcoholism.

also occur in older patients who are not treated with PR or AZA. For instance herpes zoster had the same prevalence in the LO patients treated with IS as in the patients not treated with IS (7/84 vs 9/96 mean follow-up 10.3 and 12.5 year). In the TH patients a higher prevalence of herpes zoster was found if treated with IS (9/91 vs 1/47, possibly due to a longer period of exposure. In some patients osteopenia was found by bone density measurements, without clinical signs.[11]

In patients who did not tolerate PR or AZA other IS therapies were tried. Cyclosporine (2-5 mg/kg) was given to 26 patients as a single drug or combined with PR. Major improvement followed in 8 patients and moderate improvement in 3, but in 4 out of the 11 patients the drug had to be stopped

Table 5.14 c SIDE EFFECTS OF AZATHIOPRINE

	EO	LO	TH	Total
gastrointestinal discomfort	2	2	1	5
general malaise, fever	1	3	3	7
increased liver enzymes	2	1	2	5
leukopenia[1]	--	3	--	3
herpes zoster[2]	--	2	1	3
non-Hodgkin lymphoma (patients)	1	--	--	1
skin reaction	--	1	--	1
basal cell carcinoma[3]	--	1	--	1
icterus	--	--	2	2
pancreatis[4]	--	--	1	1
no of patients treated	44	47	57	148
Patients with side effects	6	13	12	31

[1] only if severe and not corrected by dosage adjustment

[2] in patients with AZA as a single drug; if combined with PR herpes zoster is listed under side effects of PR

[3] except localization in the face

[4] pancreatis and colon perforation in a patient also treated with PR

because of side effects (decreased renal function, tremor, hirsutism, gingivitis, hypertension, headache, gastrointestinal disturbance). These caused omission of the drug in 3 other patients before the clinical effect could be evaluated. Mild side effects occurred in another 8 patients. This experience is somewhat disappointing, but some of these patients had not responded to PR.
Metothrexate, cyclophosphamide and chlorambucil were indicated in a few patients for other diseases (RA, vasculitis, nephrotic syndrome) and could also improve the MG. They could also have a surprisingly good effect when given primarily for the MG (see 5.6.3 and **patient I**).

5.6 Patients with a thymoma

5.6.1 Epidemiology

Thymomas were diagnosed in 17% of 248 men and in 17% of 530 women (fig. 2.24) with the highest relative prevalence in women between 50 and 70 years and in men between the ages of 40 and 60 years. The maximum DS was higher than in any of the other groups (table 5.3) which was reflected in the higher incidence of bulbar signs in the first three months (table 2.1). If the first signs

Patient I

A 35 year old woman developed within one month a severe generalized weakness and in 5 months a respiratory insufficiency. A thymectomy was performed six months after onset whereby a normal thymus and small encapsulated thymoma were removed. The latter had not been visible on planigrams (1969). Before the operation a tracheostoma was made, which was kept open thereafter. Two months later she went into a crisis and had to be ventilated artificially during three months. Improvement was reached by 200 mg spironolactone but deterioration occurred again after this drug was stopped. Again respiratory insufficiency, coma and cardiac arrest occurred which she survived followed by one month of artificial respiration and improvement during spironolactone treatment. She improved gradually, oculobulbar signs disappeared but she had severe limb weakness (DS: O_0, B_0, U_3, L_2, V_1). Treatment with Mestinon 0.120-5 dd, Mestinon Retard at night 0,180, neostigmine 3 dd 15 mg and spironolactone 200 mg. In the next year oculobulbar weakness reappeared (DS: O_2, B_1, U_3, L_2, V_1). At the age of 37 (1971), PR was started 45 mg on alternate days with gradual increase to 90 mg/2d. She deteriorated at day 5 but gradually improved considerably (DS: O_0, B_0, L_2, U_1, V_1). In the next years exacerbations occurred when PR was tapered under 100 mg/2d, coinciding with emotional stress (husband psychotic, death of her mother). AZA 200 mg during one year gave no appreciable benefit and no side effects. Respiratory problems did not occur so that the tracheostoma was closed in 1979 (age 45). She remained severely myasthenic with spontaneous fluctuations. An attempt to taper the PR in 1983 because she had developed hypertension and Cushing signs again resulted in anoxic attacks with coma. She improved by PE and received AZA 150 in addition to PP. In 1985 after 18 months AZA therapy she became icteric, had severe diarrhoea and fever, attributed to AZA which was omitted. A myasthenic crisis developed again which resided after one month with appropriate treatment. She was then treated with PR combined with cyclophosphamide (75 mg/d) and improved in one year considerably so that she could live a normal life for the first time since disease onset despite some proximal arm and leg muscle weakness. Prednisone was tapered off in the next year. In 1989 she lost progressively blood with the stools. The diagnosis m.Crohn was made by biopsies of the sigmoid and she was treated with salazopyrine. In 1991 also her limb muscle weakness had disappeared and until now (1997) she has been in complete remission using cyclophoshamide 75 mg dd without side effects. Also her m.Crohn is in remission since 1989. AChR-Ab decreased from 46 nMol/L in 1983 to 6 nMol/L in 1987 and 1.5 nMol/L in 1997.

Comments: 1. This dramatic history suggests that the final remission is due to cyclophophamide and not spontaneous.

2. She was one of several patients who possibly reacted favourably to spironolactone (28).

3. Severe side effects of AZA only emerged during the second period of treatment and not in the first.

were ocular an extension to other muscle groups took place earlier than in the other groups and in only one patient MG remained confined to the ocular muscles (fig. 5.1).

AChR-Ab were present in all TH patients and also AMA had the highest prevalence (table 5.5).

Two patients were mother (age 55) and daughter (age 28); in the daughter the detection and operation of the TH preceded the signs of MG by two years.

Associated auto-immune diseases were diagnosed in 13% of men and 24% of women, with a striking absence of rheumatoid arthritis. If a correction was made for the TH-associated A.I. diseases (aplastic anaemia, hyper- and hypogammaglobulinaemia, polymyositis) associated A.I. diseases occurred in 6% of men and 14% of women, which is half of the prevalence in the generalized non-TH patients (11% in men, 27% in women).

In 24 TH patients HLA-determinations were made of the A and B locus; 75% had HLA-A2 compared with 55% of the general Dutch population (significance $0.10 \geq p \geq 0.05$).

Malignancies evolved in 8% of the men and 14% of the women compared with 6% and 6% in the nonthymoma groups.

5.6.2 Diagnosis of thymoma

Thymomas were most often detected by radiological examination indicated by the MG or by routine radiological screening. In the latter category 17 thymomas were diagnosed and operated in 16 patients before the onset of their MG and in 2 patients another TH was diagnosed thereafter (table 5.15) with an interval of 6 months to 28(!) years (median 3 years). It was exceptional that the TH itself was symptomatic: only in one young woman a tumor became visible above the clavicula 3 years before onset of the MG; operation followed 7 years later when the tumor had given compression of the trachea. In the majority of patients the diagnosis of TH was made within a year of the diagnosis MG, but in 29 patients there was a delay of more than one year. In the period before 1976 when CT scanning was not available, pneumomediastinography was the method of choice to demonstrate a thymoma that was not visible on plain X-rays (AP and 10° oblique sidewards). Since inflation of air could give rise to an exacerbation of the MG, it was often preferred to perform the mediastinal exploration 'blindly' in young patients. Also the CT-scan was sometimes insufficient to predict the finding of a small thymoma at operation.

In 3 patients in whom a TH was removed respectively 11, 6 and 5 years before the onset of MG, a second TH was diagnosed six months before and six months and 2 years after the onset of MG. In the first patient, a man of 30 years, the first TH had already invaded the lung, but could be removed completely and was not irradiated. The second TH, detected 8 years later could also be removed completely and had not recurred when he died 14 years later from the complications of prednisone therapy. In the other 2 patients the first TH was

Table 5.15 DIAGNOSIS OF THYMOMA

	1960-70	1971-84	1985-94	total
preceding MG	3	5(1)	8(2)	16(3)
within 1 year of MG	21	40	33	93
2-5 years after MG	7	7	5	19
> 6 years after MG	5	4	1	10
X-rays	20	26	20	66
planigraphy (incl. CT)	6	18	22	46
operation	8	11	3	22
autopsy	1	1		2
tumor in jugulo	1			1
unknown			1	1
total	36	56	46	138

() patients with 2 TH

encapsulated and completely removed so that the growth of a second thymoma must be surmised.

Recurrence of completely removed thymomas occurred in 3 other patients with thymoma stage I, in one patient with thymoma stage II and in 4 patients with stage III. (**Fig. 5.14 a** and **b**) Because removal was considered as complete by the surgeon no postoperative irradiation was given. Treatments in these patients were different but 7 out of 11 patients died from their thymoma, while the MG was well controlled by prednisone or in spontaneous remission . (**Table 5.16**) Of the 119 patients in whom the histology of the tumor was known, about half were in stage I and one third in stages III or IV (**table 5.17**). There was no good relation between the time elapsed from the diagnosis of thymoma and the stage, even if the group of the pre-MG thymomas was excluded (27).

Postoperative radiation therapy was performed in 3 of 5 patients in stage II, in 7 of 25 patients in stage III and in 4 of 11 patients in stage IVa thymomas, and primary irradiation in 6 patients. In none of these irradiated patients a recurrence of the thymoma was seen. Seven patients had side effect of the radiation: oesophagitis in 2 patients (one with severe exacerbation of MG despite PR), pneumonitis in 2 older patients who died by pulmonary insufficiency (in one patient probably also caused by PR withdrawal), lung fibrosis with decreased vital capacity in 2 patients and cardiomyopathy in one patient.

Figure 5.14 a

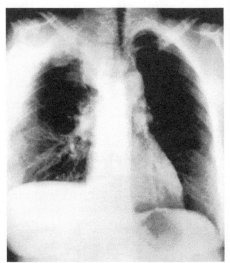 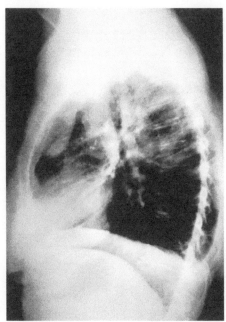

W 62. Age at onset 41 with bulbar weakness, later generalized. Crisis at age 43. Thymomectomy (thymoma stage II, thymus: involution with germinal centres). No postoperative irradiation. DS 2-3. Exacerbation at age 44, treatment with PR improved her to DS 1-2. Age 52: recurrent TH with pleural metastases and cava superior syndrome. (Fig. 5.14 a) Favourable reaction to high dose PR. Age 54: progression TH; radiation therapy 25x2.0 Gy, oesophagitis. Still progression, chemotherapy. MG: DS 1; pulmonary condition stabile but decreased VC. Age 58: pleural exsudate, again chemotherapy. Age 62: invasive growth into the trachea (fig. 5.14 b), laser therapy and irradiation (38 Gy), no complications. MG: DS 0-1. PR 15/2d + AZA 100 mg/d. Age 64: recurrent tracheal invasion, no further therapy. She died at age 64.

5.6.3 Outcome of treatment

The effect of various therapies on the MG at the end of the follow-up period is summarized in **table 5.18**. The effect of anticholinesterases was not considered separately and was relatively unimportant as compared with the IS-therapies. Complete remissions occurred in 44% of patients and considerable improvement in another 22%; two thirds were IS dependent.

Twenty patients died from MG, of whom only two under treatment with IS (both 100 mg azathioprine); 9 died from the invasion of the TH and 3 from TH related diseases (pancytopenia in 2, myocarditis with ventricular fibrillation in one (12), 4 patients died from the complications of IS therapy (2 infections by prednisone, one myeloid leukaemia by 6 mercaptopurine) and one patient died

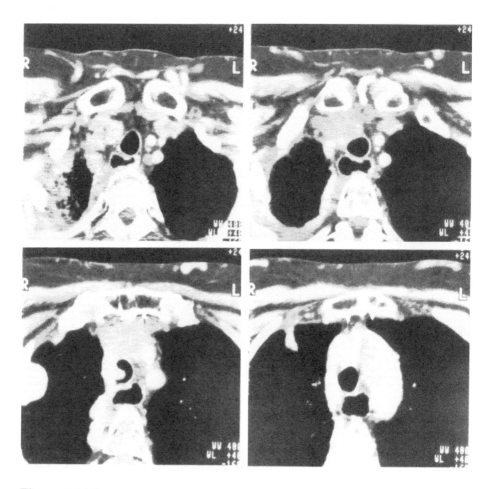

Figure 5.14 b

shortly after the irradiation for the TH from respiratory insufficiency. There was no difference between men and women but death by MG, by TH or by the complications of treatment was more frequent under the age of 50 years (25/80 vs 10/58 p < 0.05). The more efficient treatment of MG in the subsequent periods has resulted in a decrease of death rate due to MG, but the complications of treatment, an invasive growth of the TH and TH-related blood dyscrasies have become now the most prevalent causes of death. (**Table 5.18**) It was difficult to assess the specific effects of thymectomy or irradiation of the TH on the MG. From table 5.18 it is not obvious that patients who were not operated did less well than the operated ones. Patients who went into remission without IS therapy never had a crisis before operation, indicating that their MG was relatively mild. Most patients had to be treated with IS before and after the

Table 5.16 RECURRENT THYMOMAS

STAGE	SEX	AGE AT ONSET MG	FIRST THYMOMA age	FIRST THYMOMA stage	SECOND THYMOMA age	SECOND THYMOMA stage	SECOND THYMOMA therapy	FOLLOW UP UNTIL	DEAD/ ALIVE	MG
1	W	35	24	I	35	IV	O+Rad	42	alive	R
2	M	36	30	III	38	III	O	52	†PR	FR
3	W	37	31	I	36	I	O	42	alive	R
4	W	41	43	I	53	III	Rad+Ch	64	†TH	FR
5	W	32	32	I	37	III	O	38	alive	M
6	M	58	64	II	70	IVa	--	74	†TH	R
7	M	40	41	III	46	IVb	Rad	46	†TH	R
8	W	46	45	I	49	IVa	Rad	49	†TH	M
9	W	40	40	III	58	IVa	O+Ch	60	alive	M
10	W	29	30	III	35	IVb	predn.	35	†TH	M
11	W	38	40	III	46	IVa	predn.	46	†TH	FR

Stages according to Masaoka (   ), O = operation; Rad = Radiation therapy; Ch = Chemotherapy; (F)R = farmacological remission: M = mild, †TH: died by thymoma, †PR: died by complications of prednisone.

Table 5.17 STAGING OF THYMOMA ACCORDING TO MASAOKA (Table 4.4)

	DIAGNOSIS THYMOMA before MG	within 1 y	after 2-5 y	after > 6 y	Total
Operation Stage I	9(2)	41(2)	6	4(1)	60(6)
Stage IIa	1	9	1	--	11
Stage IIb	--	4	1	--	5
Stage III	3	19(4)	1	2	25(4)
Stage IV	2(1)	4	4	1	11(1)
Unknown	1	--	--	--	1
Autopsy	--	5*	1**	1***	7
No operation	--	11	2	5	18
Total	16(3)	93(6)	16	13(1)	138(11)

() recurrent thymoma

* 3 patients stage I; 1 patient stage IIa; 1 patient stage III

** 1 patient stage IVb

*** 1 patient stage I

Table 5.18 FINAL OUTCOME OF THERAPIES IN PATIENTS WITH THYMOMA

	PERIODS OF OBSERVATION			
	-1970	**1971-84**	**1985-94**	**Total**
No immuno suppression*				
Remission	5(4)	9(9)	4(4)	18
Mild (DS 1)	1	7(5)	3(3)	11
Moderate (DS 2)	3(1)	2(2)	1(1)	6
Died from MG	13(10)	5(4)	--	18
Immuno suppression				
Remission	3(3)	9(9)	25(18)	37
Mild (DS 1)	5(2)	7(7)	8(7)	20
Moderate (DS 2)	2(1)	5(4)	3(3)	10
Died from MG	--	2(1)	--	2
Died from thymoma	3(2)	7(7)	2(2)	12**
Died from complications	1(1)	3(2)	--	4
Total	36(25)	56(50)	46(38)	138(113)

() Number of patients who underwent thymomectomy

* No IS therapy was given in 50 patients of whom 44 are listed under 'spontaneous course' and 6 under 'died from thymoma'. Prednisone given in a short period around the operation, is not included.

** 6 patients in remission with IS.

operation and only in a minority the IS medication could be stopped within 2 years. In 80 patients of whom pathological reports were available beside the thymoma, a hyperplastic thymus was found in 13 patients, a normal thymus in 17, an involuted (atrophic) thymus in 19 and no thymus in 31. There was no relation between the presence and the histology of the thymic remnants and the clinical outcome.

In at least 17 of the patients who did not receive immunosuppression or plasma exchange prior to the operation because of mild signs, the MG deteriorated in the 3-6 months following the operation, and necessitated the use of IS. This deterioration was accompanied by an increase of antibodies to acetylcholine receptors and also of anti-striated muscle antibodies as is exemplified in **fig. 5.15**.

Irradiation was given as a single therapy in 6 patients before 1970 without appreciable benefit for the MG. It does not seem that thymectomy, even if the

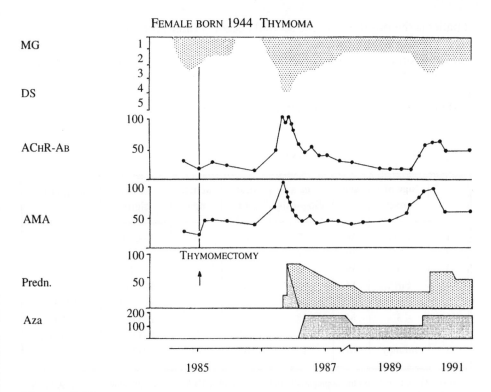

Figure 5.15 Woman age 44. Initially remission after thymomectomy followed by an exacerbation concomitant with increase of levels of AChR-Ab and AMA.

hyperplastic or normal thymus is removed improves the the signs of MG in patients with a TH.

In case history I the dramatic history of a patient is described who finally went into remission using cyclophosphamide (Endoxan®). In one other TH patient chlorambucil (Leukeran®) had the same beneficial effect.

5.7 Congenital myasthenic syndromes

In 8 patients with MG signs the diagnosis congenital myasthenic syndrome (CMS) was made. In 7 patients intercostal biopsies were taken.

Neurophysiological examinations were performed by Dr P. Molenaar, dpt of Physiology, State University Leiden (patient 3-8) and Dr D Wray, Royal Free Hospital School, London (patient 2). Histological and EM examinations were performed by Prof. Dr F. Jennekens and Prof. Dr J. Wokke, dpt Neurology, State University Utrecht.

In most patients the symptoms were present from birth or early infancy but in

143

2 patients the onset was in the second decade. (**Table 5.19**). In most patients the signs fluctuated except the external ophthalmoplegia; if present the latter did not cause diplopia. In some patients bulbar signs were present in early infancy but rarely thereafter. In all patients AChR-Ab were absent (not determined in patient 1).

A short description of these patients will follow.

Table 5.19 CONGENITAL MYASTHENIC SYNDROMES

	age at onset	sex	age at diagnosis	first sign	actual age	actual signs	diagnosis
1	birth	W	7	P	40	P+O+L	F.I.MG
2	12	W	24	L	41	L	SCS
3	16	W	21	P	36	P+L	SCS
4	birth	M	4	B	16	P+O+L	CPSC
5	1	W	54	P	66	general	CPSC
6	3	M	38	P	72	P+O+L	CPSC
7	birth	M	8	B+P	30	P+O+L	AChR-def.
8	infancy	M	18	B	24	P+O+L	?

P: ptosis; O: external ophthalmoplegia; B: bulbar; L: limbs; F.I.MG: familial infantile MG; SCS: slow channel syndrome; CPCS: congenital paucity of synaptic clefts syndrome; AChR-def.: acetylcholine-receptor deficiency.

CMS 1 Congenital infantile myasthenia. W born 1956.

From early infancy this woman had drooping of the eyelids (visible on photographs at age 3 months and 1 year). She could never run as a child. The diagnosis MG was made at age 6; improvement by Mestinon. Thymectomy at age 7 without problems; the thymus was histologically normal with a weight of 29 gr. She had always used Mestinon 10 mg. 5 dd, but after the thymectomy she was never seen by a neurologist. Her muscle strength remained reduced, she could not do sports or gymnastics and has always had some fluctuating ptosis. Her voice became nasal if she had to read aloud.

I saw her at age 23: she had a fluctuating ptosis of both eyes, a nearly complete external ophthalmoplegia with some downward movement left, a mild facial weakness and a mild weakness of the limbs. She refused detailed examination and has not followed my suggestion to increase the dosage of Mestinon. Information at the age of 40 learned that she had got a normal child at age 37. Her symptoms were unchanged.

Her unrelated parents had 2 other children who probably have had the same disease. The eldest child, a girl born in 1951 à terme without complications, birth weight 3,000 gr., had feeble crying and feeding difficulties from birth. Later she could not lift her head, could not open her eyes normally and had to be fed artificially. The diagnosis

esophageal hernia was considered but not confirmed. She was kept 7 months in the hospital. Swallowing remained difficult. At the age of 11 months she had an upper airway infection, which was treated with penicilline in the hospital, but she suddenly died. At autopsy no esophageal hernia was found and only a mild tracheo bronchitis.
The second child, a boy born 1952, also had drooping eyelids, noticed in his first year (present on photographs). He never walked normally, could not run and was weak in his arms. As a schoolboy his friends brought him home from school at the rear of their bicycles.
He suddenly died at the age of nine.
Comment: Although the data concerning the 2 deceased children are mainly based on history and the diagnosis was only made in the third child, the diagnosis familial infantile myasthenia of the autosomal recessive type seems rather certain. The thymectomy was adviced in 1963 by the neurologist referred to in note 5.9.

CMS 2 Slow Channel syndrome (SCS). W born 1955 (29).
At age 23 in the last month of her first pregnancy her upper-arms became weak and three months later she could not lift her child. In the next year also weakness of proximal leg muscles developed and she might fall through the knees after a short distance walking. In the same period she had had 2 periods of 2 weeks in which her right eyelid was completely drooping at awakening but gradually opened in the next hour. In the evening she had sometimes diplopia and difficult chewing. She remembered a period of upper arm weekness at the age of 12 and she would always have had less strength and endurance than others. She was nevertheless employed as a nurse in an eldery home. In 1981 I found weakness at rest in the upper arms and shoulders with mild atrophy of the hand muscles; to a lesser degree also the muscles of the legs and the trunk were weak with evident exhaustibility (arm test 45", knee bends 5 x) but ocular and bulbar signs were not present and could not be provoked. The EMG showed a decrement of 25% of the CMAP in the hand muscles. Although AChR-ab were absent, and she did not react to neostigmine (except side effects), she was thymectomized and later treated with PR (60mg/2d), both without effect. The possible diagnosis CMS was surmised and confirmed by prof. J. Newsom-Davis, London, by the double response to a single nerve stimulation (fig 5.16) and by the prolonged channel open time found in the intercostal muscle biopsy. The subsequent course of her illness is characterised by a progressive weakness of all limb muscles with diurnal and periodical fluctuations. Further muscle atrophy was not obvious at clinical examination. Recently she complained about some diplopia in the evening but no other ocular or bulbar signes or neck weakness were present. She is moderately incapacitated, particularly by the weakness of her proximal leg muscles. In 1986 she was treated for paroxismal ventricular tachycardia with a calcium influx inhibitor, which had no adverse effect on her muscle weakness. Her parents and daughter have no clinical nor EMG signs.
Since age 28 she complained about a progressive forgetfulness. Neuropsychiological examination confirmed a mild disturbance of visual and verbal memory capacity with

intact general intelligence, the memory disturbance was not progressive. CT scan of the brain and the EEG did not show abnormalities.

A mutation in the alpha-subunit of the AChR was demonstrated (30) resulting in a single aminoacid substitution (S2691) in the extracellular loop between M2 and M3 (see fig. 1.10).

Comment: In this patient the initial diagnosis was seronegative MG because of the rather typical fluctuating course, the onset in pregnancy, the transient ocular signs and the EMG decrement. Failure to respond to anti-AChE, thymectomy and prednisone lead to suspicion of CMS, which could be easily confirmed by the double response to nerve stimulation. It is imaginable that the memory disorder is part of the disease.

CMS 3 Slow channel syndrome. W born 1960.

Her first complaints were intermittent weakness of the finger extensors that interfered with her employment as a maternity nurse at age 21. Gradually she also noticed a weakness of her proximal leg muscles so that she had to stop her work. Since the age of 17 years she also had drooping of both upper eyelids, visible on photographs, which had not bothered her very much.

Examination at age 23 revealed a mild weakness of the shoulder- and knee extensors, but she could extend her arms no longer than 20 seconds and perform only 3 deep knee bends. She had a symmetrical ptosis of 25%, which somewhat increased by looking to one side. Also foot- and finger extensors were paretic. Neostigmine per injection and pyridostigmine per os did not improve her weakness and even made it worse. AChR-ab were absent. The EMG showed the typical double response of the CMAP by single stimulation (**fig. 5.16**) and also a decrement of the CMAP by 3/sec stimulation; the diagnosis was confirmed by morphological and electrophysiological examinations of an intercostal biopsy (**fig. 5.17**). In the next 7 years she gradually developed a more permanent weakness of other muscle groups, without clinical atrophy. She was weaker in the second half of her 2 pregnancies but recovered afterwards. Until the age of 36 no further progression occurred. To alleviate her neck muscle weakness she wears a soft neck collar at the end of the day. The ptosis increases at the end of the day: she then wears spectacles with flexible eyelid supports (fig. 5.9a).

Her father, brother and son (age 7) also had the double response by single nerve stimulation but no clinical signs. The intercostal biopsy of the father showed typical neurophysiological abnormalities (29).

Because quinine and quinidine in animal experiments reduce quantal release, interfere with channel opening by ACh and decrease the single channel open time (which is increased in SCS!) (31) we tried the effect of quinidine in the patient, initially in an open trial. She reported and showed considerable improvement in endurance (knee bends 3 to 15 times, arm raising 30 to 90s) and also the amplitude of the second response on single nerve stimulation decreased. However when a n=1 trial was done (4 periods placebo, 4 periods quinidine 2 dd 500 mg) no differences in muscle strength or endurance could be observed in the quinidine and placebo periods.

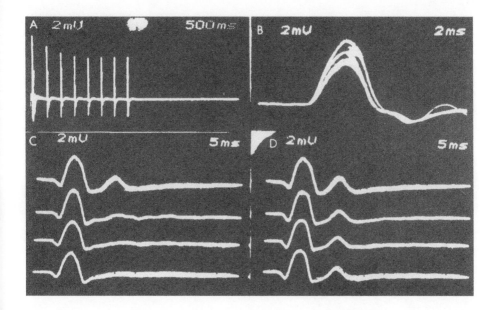

Figure 5.16 a. Routine 3/sec EMG of patient 1 shows a decrement but the second response, (**b.**) can easily be overlooked. **c.** The second response at 3/sec is only visible after the first stimulus. **d.** With a lower stimulation rate (0.2 Hz) the second response remains visible. (Courtesy Dr T. van Weerden.)

Comments: 1. Though rare, the slow-channel syndrome should be considered in seronegative "MG" patients.
2. In this family there is clearly a dominant hereditary pattern, which remained subclinical in three male members in three generations.
3. The need for an objective assessment of a possible effect of a new medication by means of a controled (n=1) trial should be emphasized.

CMS 4 Congenital paucity of synaptic clefts syndrome (CPSC). M born 1980.
His mother told me that he had difficulty in swallowing and weak crying from birth onwards. In the first year ptosis became apparent. His motor development was delayed, probably due to muscle weakness. The diagnosis MG was made at age 2. His symptoms were not appreciably influenced by Mytelase 3 dd 10 mg. At age 4 he had a ptosis of 50% which shortly disappeared after 3 minutes eye-closure, a nearly complete external ophthalmoplegia without diplopia, some weakness of the face, no dysarthria. Chewing was difficult and he often choked in solid foods causing chronic bronchial irritation. His motor pattern was clumsy, he could not run, had sudden falls and his arms were weak.
After omission of Mytelase the ptosis and the limb weakness improved by Mestinon but not the ophthalmoplegia. The diagnosis: mild form of CPCS, was made by an

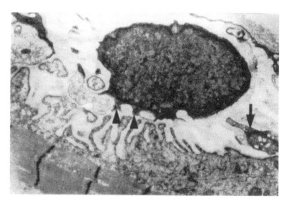

Figure 5.17a

Electronmicrograph. Biopsy from CMS 3. Postsynaptic folds are degenerated at some places causing focal widening of the primary and secondary clefts. The nerve terminal is invaded by Schwann cell processes (arrowheads). At the right a satellite cell (arrow) is seen which extends towards the Schwann cell, covering the axon terminal. Bar is 1 µm.

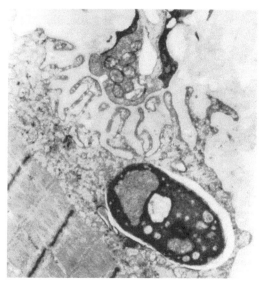

Figure 5.17 b

Electronmicrograph. Same biopsy from CMS 3. The nucleus in the junctional sarcoplasm is degenerated. Widened endoplasmatic reticulum in the nerve terminal Bar is 1 µm.

intercostal biopsy. He was further treated with Mestinon and ephedrine with reasonable effect. At age 12 and 16 he had a ptosis of 25%, a nearly complete external ophthalmoplegia, some facial weakness, a normal articulation, no difficulties in swallowing and chewing and a mild weakness of his extremities (about 2/3 of the 5% percentile value measured with the dynamometer). He did not feel impaired by his weakness if he took his Mestinon regularly and started every morning at 5 a.m. with his work as a newsboy!

Comment: The bulbar signs that were prominent in his first year of life declined gradually. The limb weakness was not progressive.

CMS 5 and 6. CPSM syndrome in M born 1924 and W born 1930.

These patients, brother and sister, were extensively described by Wokke et al. (32).

148

I examined them in 1972 and 1979. In short their history is as follows. Both patients had ptosis from early childhood (documented by photographs) and had to turn their head to be able to look sidewards. They also had limb weakness, could not run or lift heavy objects. The woman also had a mild dysarthria and nasality from age 15 at which time the diagnosis MG was made. She improved partially by taking anti-AChE. In the man the diagnosis was made at age 38 after a prolonged apnoea following a stomach operation and a strongly positive curare test. Curiously he had never used anti-AChE. He felt only slightly disabled and was employed in a shop with bamboo furniture. In the woman the symptoms were gradually progressive. She developed visible atrophy and permanent weakness of the shoulder and arm muscles. A biopsy out of the quadriceps muscle showed neurogenic changes with a type II fibre atrophy. (Courtesy of Prof. Dr H. Busch.) Both patients had a ptosis of 50%, an incomplete external ophthalmoplegia with intact downward movements and generalized muscle weakness, which was more striking in the woman than in the man. Now, at age 66 the woman is still living on her own. She can walk some steps at home with help of her arms but out of doors she is wheelchair dependent. She has no more bulbar symptoms. Her ptosis and arm weakness improve by Neostigmine, but insufficiently.

Her brother, now age 72, lives independently, his symptoms are unchanged but he is now using Mestinon 4 dd 60 mg.

CMS 7 ACh-R deficiency. M born 1966.
His mother has noticed from his birth his weak voice, drooping of the eyelids, a strange facial expression so that she did not know whether he was laughing or crying, difficulties in swallowing especially of warm foods and later frequent falling after some walking and inability to climb stairs. In spite of the mother's uneasiness and many medical (non-neurological) consultations the diagnosis was not made until the age of 8 years. He reacted favourably to Mytelase, which helped him to adapt to his persisting limb weakness.

I saw him at age 15 and age 30 when I found essentially the same abnormalities. He had a ptosis of 50% with very rapid fluctuations, giving the impression of eyelid flutter. This disappeared following 3 minutes of eye closure. He had an external ophthalmoplegia, with symmetrical impairment in horizontal direction but more to the left than to the right; he could not look upwards but downward movements were intact. He had some weakness of the lips and complaints of occasional difficulties in chewing and swallowing, which could not be provoked at examination. He had a mild weakness of the proximal limb muscles (about 60% of normal measured with the dynamometer) but a normal distal strength.Extended arm test: 30-40 seconds. No deep knee bends were possible. He increased the dosage of Mestinon on my advice with some improvement of his endurance.

His intercostal biopsy showed a patchy deficiency of AChR, a shortening of the postsynaptic membrane and an increase of the number of end-plates per muscle fibre (2.7 vs 1.0) (Courtesy of Prof. Dr F.G.I. Jennekens). The miniature end-plate potentials were decreased (0.4 mV, normal 0.7-1.0) at neurophysiological examination. (Courtesy of Dr P. Molenaar.)

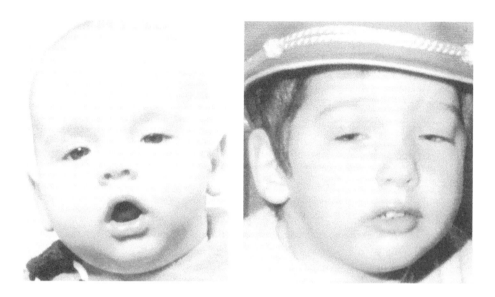

Figure 5.18 Congenital Myasthenic Syndrome. Man 5 months / 4 years. Moderate symmetrical ptosis.

CMS 8 Man born 1972.

Shortly after birth he had feeding difficulties due to insufficient sucking for which he was observed clinically for 3 months. At the end of his first year drooping of his eyelids became apparent; also his face lacked a normal expression. Swallowing was normal. Normal motor development until age 4 when limb muscle weakness was noticed. He could never come up from squatting without aid of his hands, could not run or carry heavy weights but he was socially well adapted. At age 17 he for the first time complained of double vision, especially in the evening. At age 18 he had a mild ptosis increasing by looking upwards and sidewards. Diplopia and nystagmoid movements emerged by looking upwards and sidewards after 15". He had a generalized proximal weakness of the arms and legs and of the wrist extensors and a mild weakness of his face. Extended arm test 2 minutes, no deep knee bends possible. EMG: decrement at 3/sec.; no second response at single stimulation. Atropine-neostigmine test: positive. Anti-AChR negative. Considerable improvement by Mestinon 60 mg 5 dd. Additional examinations (EMG, thyroid function, lactate) were normal. To solve the diagnostic problem: CMS or seronegative MG he was treated with prednisone (1 mg/kg) during 3 months without any effect on his residual weakness. At age 23 an intercostal biopsy was taken. The amplitude of the miniature endplate potentials was reduced to 20% and the ACh-quantal content increased to 280%. Reduction of alpha-BTX binding. The histological picture showed enlarged endplates and sprouting.

Comment: Both neurophysiological and histological data indicate a postsynaptic defect but the distinction between CMS and acquired MG (or both) is still uncertain.

5.8 *Short summary*

5.8.1 General features

1. MG had the highest relative prevalence in EO women over the age of 10 and in LO men.
2. Familial acquired MG occurred in 1.7%.
3. Generalization after initial ocular signs occurred in nearly all TH patients and more often in EO than in the LO patients.
4. A delay in diagnosis was longer in women than in men, and longer in EO than in LO patients.
5. The maximum disability scores were higher in TH patients than in the EO and LO patients.
6. Death rate due to MG has declined since the introduction of IS therapies, plasmapheresis and modern intensive care facilities.
7. a) Mean AChR-Ab levels were higher in EO patients than in LO and TH patients and lowest in OMG.
   b) AChR-Ab were absent in 13% of EO patients, in 4% of LO patients and in none of TH patients.
   c) AChR-Ab rarely became undetectable as a result of thymectomy or IS therapy (< 5%).
   d) AChR-Ab levels had a relation to disease severity in individual patients.
8. AMA were present in only 4% of EO patients and increased with age in LO patients. AMA were present in 90% before thymomectomy in TH patients and in 99% following thymomectomy.
9. Localized muscle atrophy, often symmetrical, developed in about 10% of all 3 categories of generalized MG.
10. Associated A.I.-diseases had an increased frequency in all categories of patients, particularly rheumatoid arthritis and thyroid diseases. Rheumatoid arthritis did not occur in TH patients.
11. Malignancies had a similar frequency as could be expected in the general population (except malignant TH). A causative role of azathioprine was unlikely.
12. No other neurological diseases had an increased frequency.

5.8.2 Ocular MG (OMG)

1. MG remained confined to the ocular muscles in 13% of patients with a relative predominance in children (40%) and LO males (26%).
2. Generalization after onset with ocular signs took place in 20% later than 2 years after onset and in 16% later than 3 years.
3. OMG had often a capricious course with spontaneous fluctuations over short and long periods; this hampered the evaluation of therapies.

4. The diagnosis was difficult in some seronegative patients if the response to anti-AChE was negative or equivocal (7%).
5. The reaction to anti-AChE was poor, particularly of the extra-ocular muscles. Patients had the risk to be overtreated with anti-AChE.
6. Treatment with prednisone lead to remission in 50% of patients and improved another 30% considerably. The ptosis reacted in days to weeks, the extra-ocular muscles in weeks to months.
7. OMG patients may benefit from the use of mechanical devices (flexible eyelid support, prisms, occluding contact lenses) but rarely from a surgical correction of eye muscle pareses or ptosis.
8. Patients with MG may acquire ptosis or pseudo-ptosis due to other diseases (blepharospasm, dermatochalazis, senile ptosis, delayed eyelid relaxation).

5.8.3 Early onset MG (EOMG)

1. The initial diagnosis was psychiatric in 8% of women and in none of men.
2. Thymectomy accelerated the naturally occurring improvement in patients up to age 45 and up to 15 years after onset.
3. Immediate improvement after thymectomy occurred in 10%, transient improvement in another 7%.
4. Improvement after thymectomy was not related to HLA-types.
5. Late exacerbations after initially successful thymectomy occurred in 5%; in most patients these were transient.
6. Twenty three % of patients did not respond sufficiently to thymectomy; 13% were subsequently treated with IS therapy, but this treatment failed in 1.3% of the total group. In general EO patients had a less favourable reaction to IS therapy than LO patients.
7. Side effects of IS therapy occurred in 40%, more often by prednisone than by azathioprine.
8. Neonatal MG was reported in 10% of children. Their mothers had mild or moderate (DS 2-3) signs. The incidence was not dependent on previous thymectomy.
9. During pregnancy MG tended to improve. Onset or exacerbation of MG in the puerperium was common.

5.8.4 Late onset MG (LOMG)

1. Thymectomy had the same effect as in EOMG in patients up to 45 years, but probably no effect in older patients.
2. Spontaneous improvement after a variable delay was seen in 25% of patients.
3. IS treatment had a more favourable effect than in EO patients but the frequency of side effects was considerably higher (nearly 70%).
4. Azathioprine had no effect on ocular signs,

5. Plasmapheresis was effective in 80% of patients with (impending) crises: in some patients who reacted insufficiently to IS therapy periodic plasmapheresis was of additional benefit.

5.8.5 Patients with thymoma (TH)

1. Patients with TH had the highest mean disability score; bulbar signs were more frequent at onset than in patients with EOMG or LOMG.
2. In most patients thymomectomy had no beneficial effect; in patients not treated with IS therapy exacerbations following thymectomy were common.
3. Thymomas preceded MG in 10% of patients.
4. IS therapy induced a remission in 50% of patients and considerable improvement in another 25%.
5. The patho-histological stage of the TH at operation or autopsy was not related to the duration of the MG.
6. Irradiation of incompletely removed TH's prevented recurrence.
7. Since MG could be effectively treated, the main therapeutic problems were invasive growth of TH and TH related blood dyscrasies (pancytopenia).
8. Some patients got a second TH.

5.8.6 Congenital myasthenic syndromes (CMS)

1. About 10% of generalized MG without AChR-Ab had a CMS (= 1% of the MG population).
2. The most frequent CMS were: familial infantile MG, the Congenital Paucity of synaptic Clefts Syndrome and the Slow Channel Syndrome.
3. Most patients with a CMS had a nonprogressive weakness partly reacting to anti-AChE except the patients with the Slow Channel Syndrome.

NOTES

[1] Academic Hospital Leiden (A. Kramer), Valerius Kliniek Amsterdam (J.F. Folkerts), Municipal Hospital Den Haag (A. Verjaal), St Ursulakliniek Wassenaar (J.M.J. Tans), St. Elisabeth Ziekenhuis Tilburg (J.H. van Luyk), Academic Hospital Nijmegen (J.J.G. Prick), Regional Hospital Heerlen (J.G.Y. de Jong).
In a later stage patients could be included from the Academic Hospital Rotterdam (H. Busch, Ch. Loonen, A. van Vliet), the Academic Hospital Utrecht (A. Kemp, F.J.G. Jennekens, J.H.J Wokke), the Academic Hospital Leiden (A.R. Wintzen) and het St. Elisabeth Ziekenhuis Tilburg (A. Op de Coul).

[2] AMA and other autoantibodies were in the 1960s studied by Hugo van der Geld (†1967) and Bert Feltkamp, with help of Arie van Rossum, working in the Central

Laboratory of the Red Cross in Amsterdam. After 1976 the determination of autoantibodies was part of the routine service of the "Streeklaboratorium voor de Volksgezondheid Groningen-Drenthe". AChR-Ab were from 1978 determined with the immunoprecipitation assay (12) under supervision of Piet Limburg with technical help of Els Hummel-Tappel.

[3] The diagnosis 'muscle atrophy' is not always easy and if atrophy is present the difference between atrophy by inactivity or by a myogenic or neurogenic origin cannot always be made on clinical grounds or by EMG. Disappearance of subcutaneous fat (weight loss by dysphagia!) may give the impression of the loss of muscle bulk. On the other hand muscle atrophy may be obscured by subcutaneous fat. Real atrophy is accompanied by muscle weakness.

[4] From a clinical point of view the heart function is not affected by MG. Sudden 'unexplained' death in MG patients is usually due to anoxia, caused by respiratory failure. Laryngeal paralysis may be a contributing factor (33). In a series of 108 patients, arrhythmias were found in 16%, of whom 5 died. Three patients with TH showed focal myocarditis at autopsy (34). Focal lymphorrhagic infiltrates or true myocarditis have been reported in autopsy series, particularly in patients with TH (35, 36).

[5] Several problems in the collection of these data should be mentioned:
1. What is the exact definition of an auto-immune disease? If the presence of specific antibodies is an inclusion criterium diseases such as multiple sclerosis, sarcoidosis, hyper- and hypogammaglobulinaemia, hair follicle tricho epithelioma, psoriasis etc. should be omitted. I have followed the general policy used in other publications.
2. Some diseases are more likely to be reported than others: conditions such as vitiligo, psoriasis, polymyalgia rheumatia may have been underreported.
3. Some diseases have a high chance for spontaneous remission, such as sarcoidosis in my MG patients, others are lifelong diseases such as rheumatoid arthritis.
4. The prevalencies found should be interpreted by comparing them with the prevalences in the general population, which are partly unknown. The lifetime prevalence of RA is about 1% in women; of A.I.-thyroid disease about 2%; the prevalence of all-A.I.-diseases depends on inclusion criteria.
5. Thyroid diseases had an A.I. origin in about 70 of patients, but specific antibodies were not always determined.

[6] Using this criteria we had to exclude 12 patients in whom the diagnosis OMG was diagnosed as possible. They all had fluctuating and often periodic symptoms, while other causes were unlikely by the long follow-up. Also from other studies it is known that about 25% of eye muscle pareses remain undiagnosed (37).

[7] The frequent involvement of the extra-ocular and the palpebral levator muscles in MG deserves further explanation (38, 39). The most obvious reason seems to be that

these muscles are continuously active during waking and even during REM-sleep. The clinical detection limit is low since diplopia already occurs if a minimal paresis of one eye muscle develops. Central innervation is symmetrical (Hering's law) which impedes adaption to the asymmetrical pareses.

Eye muscles have a higher innervaton rate than limb muscles and a lower density of AChR's. The blood supply by the internal carotid artery is relatively high which might cause a more abundant exposure to circulating antibodies. Also the higher temperature may influence the safety factor of neuromuscular transmission adversely.

The effect of a small dosis of pure curare is diplopia, which indicates a low safety factor of neuromuscular transmission of the eye muscles.

The antigenic structure of eye muscles is different from that of skeletal muscles: in extraocular muscles the embryonic gamma subunit of the AChR is expressed (40) but the palpebral levator had the common adult epsilon-subunit (41).

AChR-Ab were found that specifically reacted with eye-muscle antigens (42) and even different reactions between single and multiform endplates were demonstrated (43).

8 The first model of flexible lid-crutches was the 'Lundi-loop', developed by Mr R. Lundi BSc described in a Myasthenia gravis companion of the Myasthenia Gravis Association, Great Britain. The device consisted of a double ring of thin wire attached at 2 points of the frame beside the lenses. The crutches shown at the picture are less visible than the Lundi-loop. They also follow more or less the physiological movements of the eyelids. This type was developed on my request by the optician Mr Jonker, Haren. Further information is obtainable from Groeneveld/Jonker Opticians, Raadhuisplein 21, 9751 AP Haren, the Netherlands. Phone 050-5347603, fax 050-5340387.

9 Thymic hypertrophy (medulla > cortex with reaction centres, see fig. 1.7 b) is not specific for MG (review 38). I could confirm this by reviewing a series of 86 thymectomies performed between 1961 and 1966, on indication of a too enthousiastic neurologist. Only 6 patients had MG, the others chronic fatigue syndromes, 5 patients RA. Reaction centres were found in 3 patients with MG but also in 4 out of 5 patients with RA. The thymuses of the other patients showed a variable increase of fat tissue that increased with age.

10 These patients were described in 1955 as cases of congenital MG (44). From their 3 weeks premature birth onwards they had difficult sucking and swallowing which persisted in their first year, but no other signs were noticed. At the age of 13 months both had a crisis coinciding with a chickenpox infection. The twin brother died without diagnosis; no abnormalities were found at autopsy including the central nervous system. The child who survived with neostigmine improved considerably but has always kept MG signs (diplopia, ptosis, some dysphagia) although with periodical fluctuations. In a period of treatment with PR at the age of 25 (which was not indicated to our criteria) he reported a subjective improvement. AChR-Ab were negative. The question later arose whether this was a case of familial infantile MG (congenital) or an

acquired MG. The asymmetrical and fluctuating eye-muscle pareses and ptosis were more indicative for an acquired form, but the history of poor sucking from birth onwards and the same disease in his twin brother pointed more to the congenital form. AChR-Ab were negative but this fact does not differentiate between congenital and early (> 4y) acquired MG. He was previsionally classified as acquired infantile MG.

[11] Osteoporosis is a hot issue in the discussion with patients who are adviced to be treated with prednisone. Since 1990 bone density measurement with the dexa-method can be performed. The measurement values are expressed as standard deviations of the values of normal controls, matched for age and sex. Bone density measurements were performed in the department of nuclear medicine (Dr D.A. Piers) in 31 MG patients who were treated with PR. None of them had clinical signs of osteoporosis. The duration of the PR therapy was 1-3 years in 13 patients, 3-5 years in 4 patients, 6-10 years in 10 patients, 11-15 years in 4 patients. The results are shown in **table 5.20**.

Table 5.20 BONE DENSITY IN 31 MG PATIENTS TREATED WITH PREDNISONE

SD	Lumbar spine	Femur	Radius
> +2	2	1	1
+1/+2	3	1	6
0/+1	6	3	10
0/−1	10	9	11
−1/−2	8	6	2
> −2	2	3	1

The bone density value is expressed as a standard deviation (SD) from the values found in a normal control group matched for age and sex.

Only in 6 patients values of > −2 SD were found. In 9 out of 31 patients the measurements of the lumbar spine and radius were repeated after 1/2-1 year with the same values. This pilot study suggests that in most patients treated with high dosages of PR bone densimetry does not reach unacceptable values. If osteopenia develops it is possibly early during treatment. It is advisable to make bone densimetry measurements before and 3-6 months after treatment, to have a good indication for prophylactic treatment of osteopenia.

6

DIFFERENTIAL DIAGNOSIS OF MG

6.1 False negative and false positive diagnosis

The clinical signs of fully developed MG are highly characteristic so that the experienced neurologist will seldom consider an alternative diagnosis. Problems arise at the onset of the symptoms, particularly if these develop following infections, operations, stress, child birth or if the patient is known to have another disease. It is still not unusual that a patient with MG is submitted to a series of superfluous diagnostic procedures such as CT or MRI of the cerebrum, muscle biopsy, lumbar puncture before the diagnosis is made. Women are more at risk for a delay in diagnosis, partly because of a slower development of symptoms (1) but also because doctors still have a higher suspicion of non-organic disease in this category of patients. A list of confounding factors is given in **table 6.1**.

The most common false negative diagnoses are somatization disorder ('nerves', stress) and modern patients sometimes make this suggestion themselves and prefer 'alternative' treatments. This may be understandable in patients whose signs are confined to the limb muscles, but less so in patients with dysphagia with considerable loss of weight, in whom anorexia nervosa was the diagnosis. In patients who were suspected of having an organic weakness the failure to make the right diagnosis at onset was sometimes the result of undue emphasis on a localized sign. For instance, patients were referred to the ENT specialist for evaluation of their dysarthria without considering their concomitant diplopia. A common occurrence was the diagnosis of incomplete oculomotor (n.III) 'palsy' in patients with multiple eye muscle pareses and ptosis. In the case of limb muscle pareses the omission of tests for exhaustability (2.) could be a reason for missing the diagnosis MG and surmising another neuro-muscular disease. The frequent false positive diagnoses in my patients **(table 6.2)** were ocular problems e.g. ptosis and or diplopia due to other causes and blepharospasm, followed by the chronic fatigue syndrome. An important though minor group consisted of patients with

Table 6.1 CONFOUNDING FACTORS IN THE DELAY OF THE DIAGNOSIS

1. The patient is known to have another disease:
    e.g. acutal infection with high fever, previous carcinoma, recent operation, childbirth, hyperthyroidism, other neuromuscular disease

2. Atypical signs and features:
    1. extreme age "MG is a disease of young women"
    2. spontaneous fluctuations are not noticed or not reported
    3. psychological stress is apparently present at the onset of symptoms
    4. pains or paraesthesias are concomitant or principal complaints
    5. muscle atrophy is present

3. Confirmatory tests are negative:
    1. no reaction to anti-AChE per injection (3.1) or per os
    2. no decerement on repetitive nerve stimulation in one or more muscle groups or abnormalities in SFEMG (3.3)
    3. no AChR-Ab are detectable (3.2)

4. Routine tests, not specific for MG are positive:
    1. Myopathic signs, or denervation in routine EMG (note 3.5)
    2. Muscle biopsies show abnormal findings e.g. lymphorrhagic infiltration, neurogenic lesions (2.2.4)

other diseases of neuromuscular transmission (NMT) i.c. the Lambert-Eaton Myasthenic Syndrome and a 'late onset' congenital Slow Channel Syndrome (2.7). Other NMT syndromes may occur (2) due to intoxication (botulism, viper bites, certain medicaments).

6.2 Diseases and syndromes with ocular signs and symptoms

The most relevant diseases and syndromes to be considered in the presence of ptosis or eye muscle pareses and some distinguishing features are listed in **table 6.3**. Some comments are given, but for more details the reader is referred to neurological and neuro-ophthalmological textbooks.
Ptosis (3) is diagnosed if the upper-eyelid covers more than 2 mm of the cornea and is caused by a weakness of the m.levator palpebrae or the m.tarsalis superior. If no muscle weakness is involved, but an anatomical variation, either physiologic or pathologic (e.g. after orbital trauma, aberrant regeneration after facial nerve lesion), the condition is referred to as pseudoptosis. **(Fig. 6.1)**

Table 6.2 DIAGNOSIS IN PSEUDO-MYASTHENIA

Myasthenic syndromes		11
LEMS	9	
Slow channel syndrome	2	
Neuromuscular diseases		6
Other neurological diseases		10
• Amyotrophic lateral sclerosis (bulbar)	4	
• Multiple sclerosis (diplopia 2, ptosis 1)	3	
• Others (narcolepsy 1, intoxication 1, cerebral gliomatosis 1)	3	
Chronic fatigue syndrome	44	56
Conversion syndrome (1 patient + MG)	12	
Ocular complaints		62
• Ptosis (+ diplopia 4)	29	
• Diplopia (+ ptosis 3)	31	
• Ptosis by d-penicillamine	2	
• Blephrospasm (Meige syndrome 14	20	
other extrapyramidal syndromes 6)		
Other non-neurological diseases		8
		173

If both upper-eyelids are 'drooping' symmetrically it is not always easy to determine whether this is due to muscle paresis. Especially in older people without complaints, the most obvious cause is a displacement of the eyeballs due to the lack of fat tissue. Central innervation may also be deficient in intoxications with sedatives, or in acute large hemisperic lesions, especially of the nondominant side (4).

A diagnostic dendrogram of eyelid drooping is given in **figure 6.2**.

The most frequent cause of senile ptosis is probably a dehiscence or disinsertion of the aponeurosis of the m.levator palpebrae, in a minority a degeneration of this muscle. This affection is slowly progressive, bilateral but often asymmetrical. It develops gradually, without external cause or general disease, occasionally occurring after local trauma including eye operations (6% following cataract operation [5]). It may also be the cause of ptosis in younger patients after a long period of wearing hard contact lenses (6). The main features are ptosis with a good levator function, a raised or absent upper lid skin crease and a thinning of the upper lid above the tarsal plate. A history of

Table 6.3 DISEASES WITH OCULAR SIGNS TO BE CONFUSED WITH MG

Disease	A	B	C	D	E	Remarks
Dysthyroid ophthalmoplegia	2 3 4	3 4	0	1 2	1	D: m.rect.inf, m.rect.med.
Chronic progressive external ophthalmoplegia	**1** 2 3	4 5	2 3	1 2	1	D: no diplopia
Oculopharyngeal myopathy	**3** 4	5	**2** 3 4	1 2	0	also dysphagia
Myotonic dystrophy	1 **2**	5	2 3	1 2	0	D: no diplopia
Botulism	1 2 3 4	1 2	**2** 3 4	1 2	1	autonomic failure
Fisher's syndrome (Guillain-Barré)	1 **2** 3 4	2 3	2 3	1 2	0	ataxia, areflexia
Retro orbital tumor	2 **3** 4	2 3	**1** 3 4	1 2	1	proptosis, n.trig. I
Multiple sclerosis	1 2 3	1 2	1 3	1 2	1	other signs?
Brain stem tumor	2 **3** 4	3 4	1 2 3 4	1 2	1	E: exercise induced
Basilar artery insufficiency	**3** 4	1	1 2 3 4	1 2	2	other signs
Wernicke-Korsakow syndrome	2 **3** 4	1 2	0	1	2	E: thiamine
Intoxication	1 **2** 3 4	2	**2** 3 4	1 2	1	phenytoin, carbamazepine
Conversion spasm	1 2 3 4	2 3	0	1	2	
Meige syndrome	2 **3** 4	3 4	2 4	0	2	other facial dyskinesias
Lambert-Eaton Myasthenic Syndrome	2 **3** 4	3 **4**	(3 4)	0	1	autonomic signs

A. age at onset: **1.** 0-20 years; **2.** 20-40 years; **3.** 40-60 years; **4.** 60-80 years.

B. maximum symptoms: **1.** 0-24 hours; **2.** 1-7 days; **3.** weeks; **4.** months; **5.** years.

C. ptosis: **0.** absent; **1.** one side; **2.** two sides; **3.** partial; **4.** complete.

D. eye muscle paresis: **0.** absent; **1.** horizontal; **2.** vertical.

E. fluctuations: **0.** absent; **1.** minor; **2.** marked.

The bold number indicates the most likely: e.g. mytonic dystrophy A2: age at onset 20-40.

From: Myasthenia gravis, Ed. M de Baets and H J G H Oosterhuis, C R C Press, Boca Raton, 1993.

increasing ptosis at the end of the day is a common finding and may falsely
suggest MG (7). The therapy is surgical correction (8).
Another condition in older people is the presence of excessive skinfolds

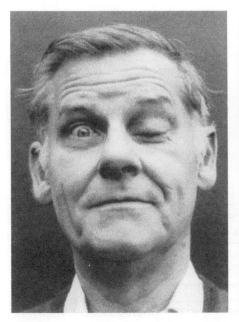 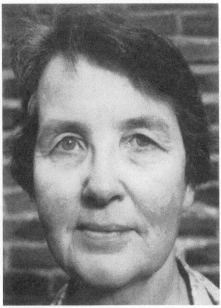

Figure 6.1 M 64. Pseudoptosis due to
diffuse orbital edema (vasculitis).

Figure 6.3 W 64. Mild bilateral
dermatochalazis.

(dermatochalasis), which is most prominent at the lateral eye margin. **(Fig. 6.3)**
A partial unilateral ptosis may be caused by a denervation of the m.tarsalis
superior and relieved by a sympathicomimetic drug (9).
In various myopathies, ptosis is slowly developing over years, bilateral, nearly
symmetrical and rarely the chief complaint of the patient, except in the chronic
progressive external ophthalmoplegia (CPEO).
Confusing is the pseudoptosis in extrapyramidal disorders, especially at the
onset of the Meige syndrome (10). These patients are not aware of active
closure or spasm of the eyelids but report very fluctuating drooping of the
eyelids. This may be influenced by 'tricks', such as laying down, vigorous
chewing, manual work, or changing of environment. Their complaints are
often worse in the course of the day and may react promptly but short-lasting
to a new drug, e.g. pyridostigmine per os or Tensilon, as was my own
experience. Not exceptionally some blepharospasm is also seen in MG patients
with ptosis and the coexistence of MG and Meige has been reported (11).

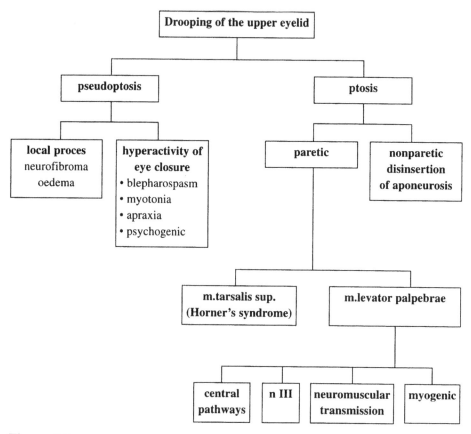

Figure 6.2

Diagnostic dendrogram of upper eyelid drooping (83).

Diplopia due to eye muscle paresis should only be diagnosed if two clearly separated images are reported, one of which disappears after closure of one eye. By intermittent covering of one eye most patients are able to analyze to which eye each image belongs, and how the images change in different directions. In MG the double vision may appear or change if the patient keeps looking in the same direction; this feature is virtually absent in other diseases. If changes in the distance of diplopic images are mentioned in the history, one should try to confirm this by repeated orthoptic tests. It is important to realize that diplopia may occur without visible eye muscle paresis, like in MG, and that slowly developing symmetrical eye muscle pareses usually will not lead to diplopia, like in the chronic external progressive ophthalmoplegias and myotonic dystrophy.

Decompensating heterophoria (latent strabismus) is a common cause of horizontal, but not of vertical diplopia in adults. In these patients, the cover-uncover test will show rapid correcting eye movements and the distance of double images remains more or less equal over a wide range of movement.

Many diseases may cause diplopia or eye muscle pareses, most of which are easily discerned from MG by additional neurological signs and features that are lacking in MG. These include basilar artery insufficiency, Wernicke-Korsakow syndrome, Guillain-Barré and Fisher's syndrome, painful ophthalmoplegia, and acute isolated myositis. The most important conditions that may lead to confusion are listed in **table 6.3**.

A not uncommon cause for diplopia without ptosis in middle age and early senescence is <u>dysthyroid restrictive myopathy</u> (12) or dysthyroid orbitopathy (13) or thyroid ophthalmopathy (14). The full-blown clinical picture with orbital congestion, proptosis, chemosis and upper-eyelid retraction in a patient with thyroid disease is easy to diagnose. Problems may arise at onset if the first sign is diplopia, which is absent on awaking but appears in the course of the day (14). Some patients may have periods of diplopia with spontaneous remissions (14). Diplopia is usually vertical due to an upward restriction of movement. In a later stage, eye movements become restricted in all directions. Lid retraction on one side may give rise to the diagnosis of contralateral ptosis. In a subgroup of patients with thyroid ophthalmopathy, the usual tests for hyperthyroidism (T3, T4) are normal and further tests (TRH stimulation, determination of antibodies against thyroid antigens) are necessary to establish the relation with thyroid disease (14). The diagnosis is made by the demonstration of an enlargement of one or more eye muscles, especially of the m.rectus inferior and the m.rectus internus by CT scanning of the orbit. The shortening and rigidity of the affected eye muscles is demonstrated by the forced abduction test.

A combination of ocular signs of MG and dysthyroid ophthalmoplegia occurred in 6 out of 49 hyperthyroid patients in a total of my 800 myasthenic patients. These patients had also ptosis and anti-AChR antibodies. Treatment with prednisone cured their ptosis but not the eye-muscle paresis, which is a common experience (13).

<u>Chronic progressive external ophthalmoplegy (CPEO)</u> is characterized by a slowly developing symmetrical restriction of eye movements and symmetrical ptosis of variable intensity. Diplopia is uncommon but may occur in the early stage (15). The weakness may be clinically confined to the ocular muscles, or 'descend' to the facial and limb muscles (16, 17) or may be part of a more generalized but variable syndrome with pigmentary retinopathy, deafness, ataxia, dementia, and other signs of central nervous system involvement (16, 18; 'ophthalmoplegia plus'). This syndrome is due to a disturbance of mitochondrial metabolism, which may be localized at different parts of the metabolic chain (16). Muscle biopsies invariably show a typical abnormality (ragged red fibers). The first signs usually appear in the first two decades, but also later (16). The clinical picture may resemble that of MG, since the limb weakness may be induced or exaggerated by exertion (16) and may show

clinical fluctuations (19). Single fiber EMG may show abnormalities. (20).

Oculopharyngeal dystrophy, which usually starts after the age of 50, has a hereditary character in most patients and is characterized by symmetrical or asymmetrical ptosis, rarely accompanied by ophthalmoplegia, and progressive dysphagia (17).

Myotonic dystrophy is a slowly progressive disease with symmetrical ptosis, a restriction of eye movements in part of the patients but without diplopia (21). The facial weakness, the nasal speech, and mild dysphagia are other features in common with MG but are seldom the main complaint of the patient.

Botulism causes ptosis, diplopia, bulbar weakness, and limb muscle weakness especially of the arms but total paralysis in the most severe cases. In addition, symptoms of autonomic disturbance are usually present, including obstipation, urinary retention, dry mouth, and poorly reacting dilated pupils, although the latter signs may be absent (2, 22). Repetitive supramaximal nerve stimulation may show a decrement at 2/s and a marked facilitation at high frequencies, indicating a presynaptic disturbance. Some patients react to edrophonium (23). A problem in the differential diagnosis of MG may appear when either no acute gastrointestinal period precedes the neurologic signs (24), or when the autonomic signs are either not prominent or not recognized.

Poison snake bites are followed in minutes to hours by ptosis, extraocular weakness, later by bulbar and generalized weakness. These symptoms may (2) or may not react to anticholinesterases (25).

Retro-orbital tumors (meningeoma, chondrosarcoma) and aneurysms were reported that caused fluctuating diplopia and ptosis and, in some stages, reacted to edrophonium (26, 27). Also brain stem tumors may initially cause fluctuating, or exercise induced diplopia (28), and may react to edrophonium (29).

Basilar artery insufficiency rarely causes transient diplopia and ptosis as a single sign or transient bulbar weakness. In older patients with fluctuating symptoms of MG, this diagnosis is sometimes made.

Multiple sclerosis starts with diplopia in 5 to 10% of the patients. It is frequently of short duration (weeks) but it lacks the daytime fluctuation characteristic for MG. The sixth nerve function is more commonly affected than that of the third nerve. The failure of the latter is often partial, ptosis and pareses of the elevators being rare (30). Internuclear ophthalmoplegia may be simulated in MG by a nonsymmetrical paresis of the internal rectus of one eye and the external rectus of the other. The nystagmus of the abducting eye is continuous in multiple sclerosis but wears off in MG as the external rectus becomes more paretic.

Drug induced external ophthalmoplegia is reported as an overdosage of amitriptyline, phenytoine (31), and carbamazepine (32), the latter drug may also cause diplopia in normal dosage at the onset of therapy. D-penicillamine induced MG may be mentioned here. I have seen several patients with rheumatoid arthritis or SLE who developed diplopia when treated with chloroquine, which subsided after stopping this drug.

Convergence spasm may cause fluctuating diplopia simulating a bilateral m.rectus externus paresis. It is nearly always of a functional nature and may be seen in patients with the chronic fatigue syndrome but may mimic ocular MG (33). Although it is most frequently seen in unstable individuals, there is a preexistent organic motility disturbance in the majority of cases that centers attention on the eyes and gives rise to complaints of impaired vision (34).

6.3 Diseases with bulbar symptoms and signs

Amyotrophic lateral sclerosis (ALS) with bulbar onset is sometimes diagnosed as MG (35). (Table 6.2) The dysarthria in ALS does not increase at uninterrupted speech (in case of doubt use a tape recorder and ask others to listen). Patients nevertheless have more complaints in the course of the day. A slight reaction to neostigmine may be seen in some patients with ALS, as well as a decremental response at repetitive nerve stimulation (36, 37), but with a low amplitude.

In two patients with juvenile progressive bulbar palsy (ptosis, restricted eye movements, facial weakness, dysarthria), symptoms worsened somewhat during the day. A partial reaction to edrophonium was seen and SFEMG showed increased jitter and blockings (38).

The other most frequent diseases with bulbar weakness are botulism, poliomyelitis, brain stem tumors, basilar artery insufficiency, multiple sclerosis, and dystrophia myotonia. Some patients with isolated complaints and signs of dysarthria have no organic disease. Isolated dysphagia may be due to a mechanical impairment, or to a disturbance in the parasympathetic innervation (achalasia).

6.4 Diseases with weakness of the limb and trunk muscles

Since MG is a disease with muscle weakness of the peripheral type, without sensory or reflex abnormalies, it should be distinguished primarily from the acquired myopathies and motor neuron diseases. Though it is very rare in MG that signs are restricted to the muscles of the limbs and the trunk, they may do so in a certain stage of the disease. Cases of 'limb-girdle' MG have been reported (39, 40, 41) but they are probably extremely rare. If myasthenic weakness is prominent in the leg muscles and not in other muscles the diagnosis Lambert-Eaton Myasthenic Syndrome should be considered (6.5).

Polymyositis may pose the problem of weakness of the girdle, neck, and trunk muscles being associated with dysphagia and very rarely with eye-muscle paresis (42). The weakness is not fluctuating, as in MG, and does not respond to anticholinesterases; no patients are reported with antibodies to AChR or with a positive nerve stimulation test.

The association of MG and polymyositis is described (43) or surmised on ground of round cell infiltrations in muscle, especially in patients with thymoma's.

Endocrinopathies (e.g. hyperthyroidism, hypothyroidism) are frequently associated with abnormal fatigue and proximal weakness, especially of the legs, and sometimes with true MG. The weakness may fluctuate in relation to hypokalemia in hyperaldosteronism, Addison's disease, and hypokalemic periodic paralysis.

In mitochondrial myopathies, weakness of the limbs may be induced or increased by exertion (16, 44), and patients complain about excessive fatiguability and muscle pains after exertion. Other metabolic myopathies such as acid-maltase deficiency and carnitine deficiency may be aggravated by intercurrent infection and starvation.

Prolonged apnoea after narcosis may occur in pseudocholinesterase deficiency, if nondepolarizing muscle relaxants (e.g. succinylcholine) are used. In normal life there is no weakness. Prolonged apnoe may also occur in severely ill patients with multiple organ failure, especially if antibiotics interfering with NMT (e.g. aminoglucosides) are used.

6.5 The Lambert-Eaton Myasthenic Syndrome (LEMS)

In 1957 Eaton and Lambert (45) described 6 patients with weakness and undue fatiguability of the proximal limb muscles, particularly of the legs. In three of them a small cell lung carcinoma (SCLC) was diagnosed and in another two its presence was probable. Their muscle strength was small after a period of rest but increased during repeated voluntary contractions. A similar increase of the initially low muscle action potential occurred after voluntary contractions and also after 20-50/sec nerve stimulation, whereas a decrease was seen at 1-3/sec stimulation. (Fig. 3.6) Muscle stretch reflexes were diminished or absent but could also increase after muscle contractions (46). Some patients complained of paraesthesias in their hands and feet and had muscle aches. These patients showed an equivocal reaction to prostigmin, much less than could be expected in MG, but they had the same increased sensitivity to curare. The first patient of this type was recognized by a prolonged apnoea after narcosis with muscle relaxants (47).

Subsequent reports (46, 48-51) indicated that the ocular and bulbar muscles are affected in most patients but to a much lesser degree than in MG. In a series of 50 patients cranial nerve symptoms, usually mild and transient were experieced by 70% of patients, diplopia and ptosis being the most common. Besides the limb muscle weakness also neck weakness could be found in one third of the patients (46).

Table 6.4 LAMBERT-EATON MYASTHENIC SYNDROME

Symptoms and signs
- •Proximal weakness: legs > arms > neck
- •Oculobulbar signs not prominent or absent
- •Undue fatiguability and exercise intolerance
- •Low or absent muscle strectch reflexes
- •Symptoms decrease by first contractions but increase later
- •Symptoms of parasympathetic dysfunction are common, particularly dry mouth

Diagnosis
EMG: low initial CMAP with decrease at 1-3/sec
nerve stimulation and > 200% increase at 20/sec
Antibodies to VSCC present in 50-80% of patients

Associated diseases
SCLC in 50%, rarely with other malignancies,
LEMS usually preceeds the detection of the tumor
Other A-1 diseases and A-1 antibodies in non-tumor cases

Therapy
a. removal or suppression of tumor activity
b. 3-4 diaminopyridine with pyridostigmine
c. immunosuppressive therapies

A feature that definitely distinguishes LEMS from MG is the loss of parasympathetic functions, causing particularly dry mouth, but also sweating, constipation, sexual impotence, loss of bladder control and orthostatic hypotension have been reported (46).

In later reports it has become clear that LEMS may also occur in patients without carcinoma's; in two larger series there was even a predominance (52) or a 50% incidence (46) of noncarcinoma cases. SCLC was the farmost predominant tumor type, but also other carcinoma's could occur, possibly by chance (46). In two prospective studies the risk for SCLC patients to contract LEMS was 3% (53, 54).

Like other paraneoplastic syndromes LEMS preceded the detection of the tumor by months to years; this risk declines sharply after 2 years and is probbaly not increased after 4-5 years (46). This risk is further decreased if LEMS starts before the age of 40 in a nonsmoker, since SCLS is highly related to excessive smoking.

An increased incidence of (other) autoimmune diseases and autoantibodies was found in non-tumor patients (46, 52). Some patients were reported with a coexistence of MG and LEMS (55-57).

The clinical and electrophysiological features are sufficient to distinguish LEMS from MG, although problems may arise if the first CMAP at nerve stimulation is normal and facilitation after exercise or high rate nerve stimulation is within normal limits (58; one of my patients). A further difference was demonstrated by the increase of secondary clefts and folds of the postsynaptic membrane and signs of reinnervation (59-62). Electrophysiological studies revealed that spontaneous MEPP's have a normal amplitude (in contrast to MG where they are small) and that the degree of depolarization produced by single quanta of ACh is normal (63). These data indicate a primary presynaptic defect to which the morphological changes are an adaptive mechanism. This presynaptic defect was first demonstrated by freeze fracture electromicroscopy showing a paucity of active zones related to synaptic vesicle exocytosis (64), putatively establishing voltage-sensitive calcium channels (VSCC). The hypothesis of an autoimmune aetiology was confirmed by the effect of plasma exchange and immunosuppressive therapy in 3 patients. Injections of the IgG fractions of these patients into mice, produced electrophysiological abnormalities comparable to those of human LEMS (65). IgG from LEMS patients appeared to bind to active zones in the motor nerve terminal and to down regulate the VSCC's (66). The effective mechanism seems to be a cross linking of the active zone particles by the IgG (67). Finally specific antibodies against VSCC were detected.[1]

The natural course of LEMS is a slow progression over months and years leading to a variable degree of disability; in patients with SCLS the poor therapeutic effects determine life expectancy. Remissions of LEMS are reported in patients in whom treatment for SCLC was successful (46, 68).

Symptomatic treatment consist of administration of 3,4-diamino piridine 15-60 mg per day in 4-5 doses, preferably combined with pyridostigmine 5 dd 60-120 mg (69). The effect and dosage adjustment may be controlled by clinical tests and by repetitive nerve stimulation. Side effects are not uncommon but they are usually tolerated and are dosage dependant. They include central effects such as nausea, sleep problems, anxiety, rarely chorea and epileptic fits: peripheral choinergic effects are diarrhoea, blurred vision, bronchal hypersecretion; peripheral adrenergic side effects are palpitations, ventricular extrasystoles peripheral varoconstriction. The most common are perioral and peripheral paraesthesias occurring in a short period after each new dose (69). If this symptomatic therapy is insufficient immunosuppressive therapies in the same regime as in MG may be tried (except thymectomy!). These therapies have a longer mean delay to become affective than in patients with MG (70; own experience). Little is known about adverse side effects of other drugs but calcium antagonists are likely to be contraindicated. One patient was reported who contracted LEMS during treatment with diltiazem, a calcium entry blocker, which disappeared after stopping the drug. This patient did not have a carcinoma nor anti-VSCC-Ab (71).

6.6 The chronic fatigue syndrome

Chronic fatigue is a complaint commonly heard in general practice (72) as well as in the out-patient departments of medical specialists including the neurologist. It may be the chief or single complaint, but more often it is the "background noise" of many other feelings or symptoms of nonwell-being. These patients describe their feelings as "extreme tiredness the whole day long", being "turned-off", or "fed-up", or "sick from fatigue". They tend to lie down a lot but the relief obtained lasts only a short time. Most of them complain that they are already fatigued on awakening, even after a good night's rest. Short lasting muscle activity may decrease rather than increase their tiredness but their endurance in longer lasting work is always diminished, which seems partly due to shortness of breath and palpitations. Their muscle strength is not decreased as far as short action is concerned and they are able to prevent accidents such as sudden falls, which would occur in the case of sudden loss of strength (such as in MG).

The relatively few neurologists who have much experience with MG are consulted by many patients who suffer from excessive, unexplained fatigue and who have no MG, although their referring physicians or they themselves are convinced of this diagnosis (35, 73). The vast majority of these patients are women with many somatic complaints. Their symptoms fluctuate greatly in intensity and may have a variable composition. When they consult the neurologist their symptoms have gradually increased to such an extent as to interfere with their daily duties, and they have usually already consulted other medical specialists who have excluded the main causes of chronic fatigue with reasonable certainty. If their history is taken carefully it appears that their fatigue is not due to weakness. The "double vision" mainly occurs during reading or watching TV and consists of a shadow or vague second contour next to the separate letters and not of two distinct images with (almost) the same brightness. Many patients have the same complaints with monocular vision, which should be routinely examined. Heavy eyelids with a feeling of oppression behind the eyes is another complaint, while no real ptosis is visible. Complaints about the unpleasant feeling of a thick throat "where something is sticking" and the tendency to swallow repeatedly, are often heard. These patients feel unable to hold long conversations, during which their voice becomes weaker although their articulation remains normal and no nasality occurs. Periods of aphonia or hoarseness may suddenly interfere. When examining muscle strength in such patients one often feels that they use antagonistic muscles simultaneously, so that the effect is small. For example, when the biceps is tested and the examiner suddenly releases, the elbow is blocked by the contraction of the triceps. In testing endurance of, for example, the deloid muscles with the outstretched arms test, the patient suddenly fails without the trembling that is typical for the recruitment of all the available muscle power. Moderate exertion, such as 10 to 20 deep knee bends may be accompanied by manifest hyperventilation and sweating, indicating their intolerance to exertion. In a minority of these patients other nonspecific signs are found at the neurological examination, such as sensory loss without organic pattern and some unsteadiness in the tests for ataxia.

The onset of this syndrome is often related to some stressful event: a viral infection (74), a pregnancy or delivery, an operation, illness of their husband or death of parent, although this is not always mentioned in their own story. Some patients have other histories of emotional disturbance or psychiatric illness, but others are described by their partners as stable personalities and hard workers without overt neurotic traits. In those patients who were already diagnosed as having MG, oral anticholinesterases at first seemed to influence their symptoms. A tolerance to rather high dosages, e.g. 900 mg mestinon per day was reported as a remakable feature in these patients (35, 73). In my experience their tolerance is not different from patients with MG, in whom the tolerance may also vary among individuals. It should be emphasized that the reaction to anticholinesterases in these patients had not been tested adequately, i.e., with the use of a placebo, and in most of them only the subjective response was taken into account.

Excessive fatigue may be the first symptom of an organic disease, which must be reasonably excluded before it is attributed to a psychosomatic disorder. In most pseudomyasthenic patients no underlaying somatic disorder can be diagnosed and most of them do not meet the rigid criteria for the tentative diagnosis chronic fatigue syndrome (75). In general, viral infections cannot be traced in their histories. In a study where the complaints of physical and mental fatigue and several parameters of general and psychological health were scored, the patients with chronic fatigue resembled more closely the patients with known psychiatric disorders than those with neuromuscular diseases, including MG (76). It remains to be seen whether recent immunologic findings (reduced suppressor cell activity and increased activation markers) sufficiently explain the clinical symptoms in patients with chronic fatigue syndrome. In fact, these findings could not be related to any known human virus by serology, but they were not detectable in healthy individuals nor in patients with other diseases (77).

Whatever the final outcome of these etiological investigations may be, these patients are not suffering from MG. Modern therapeutic modalities like thymectomy, plasmapheresis, prednisone, and immunosuppressive drugs require a strict diagnostic discipline by which a false positive diagnosis of MG can be avoided.[2]

NOTES

[1] Specific antibodies against Voltage Sensitive Calcium Channels (VSCC) were detected using VSCC-expressing human neuroblastoma cell lines labeled with [125]J-omega-conotoxin (a viper-toxin) which binds specifically to VSCC. This extract was used as antigen for the radioimmuno-assay. Anti-VSCC-Ab were detected in 20 out of 22 patients with clinical LEMS, in 3 out of 7 patients with small lung carcinoma without LEMS, but also in 3 out of 31 controls (78). Using another human neuroblastoma line anti-VSCC-Ab were found in 28% of LEMS patients with SCLC and in 68% of LEMS patients without SCLC and also in 8 of 12 patients with rheumatoid arthritis or systemic lupus erythematosus (79). Antibodies detected by this assay are probably heterogenous and not all are implicated in the cause of LEMS. VSCC complexes could be extracted from SCLC and anti-VSCC-Ab against these complexes were found in 27 out of 52 LEMS patients, but in this study patients with a SCLC had a higher frequency (76%) than those without tumor (30%). These data implicate that tumor associated VSCC are an autoimmunizing stimulus in a subset of patients with LEMS (80). In an assay using another subtype of VSCC derived from cerebellar extracts antibodies were detected in 85% out of 66 LEMS patients and in none of the controls (81).

[2] In 5 patients out of the 180 of my own first series (82) the diagnosis MG had to be rejected later. Four of these patients had a chronic fatigue syndrome, the fifth was suffering from a mild multiple sclerosis causing diplopia and a somatization disorder. In all these patients the reaction to neostigmine was considered to be positive but no placebo had been used.

7

Epilogue

7.1 History

The history of myasthenia gravis reflects that of general medicine. In the last quarter of the 19th century a few German doctors gradually delineated a new disease of which the clinical features did not fit in the diseases known at that time. Apart from the younger age of the patients and the fluctuating course with remissions and exacerbations, the absence of macroscopic or microscopic lesions in the central nervous system was an important argument for the concept of a new disease. The negative argument could be used because many diseases of the central nervous system could be diagnosed at that time by neuro-pathological examination, which was nearly the only way to verify or to refute the clinical diagnosis.

In the patients suffering from the new disease the single abnormalities were tumors of the thymus and lymphorrhagic infiltrates in skeletal muscles which later were also found in other organs (1, 2). A relationship of these abnormalities with the clinical symptoms was far from clear. It was therefore realistic to choose a name that expressed the most striking symptom: muscle weakness (asthenia) although not true paralysis. That this weakness increased by faradic stimulation of the nerve, a therapeutic modality advocated by Duchenne (3), was demonstrated by Jolly (fig. 1.2).

Although it was known by physiologists (Foster 1876) that the propagation velocity of the nerve impulse slows down to about 10% when arriving at the muscle endplates, the notion of discontinuity between nerve and muscle and the existence of a transmitter substance, acetylcholine, emerged only in the 1930's by the discovery of Dale (4). It was in the same period that the effect of physiostigmin in MG was described by Mary Walker (1.4) and the idea of a curarizing substance impeding muscle function at the endplates, revived.

In the first quarter of the 20th century the function of the endocrine glands producing circulating hormones[1] was detected. This gave the impetus for the search of a circulating substance that might cause the muscle weakness in MG.

The main source of this substance was sought in the thymus but experiments never gave convincing results and were abandoned in the late 1950's.

In the 1930's thoracic operations became possible with lesser risks. Since thymic tumors had an unusual high frequency in severe myasthenia patients, a causative role was assumed so that surgical removal was a logical consequence. However the extension of surgery to the non-tumorous thymus was more intuitive than based on firm scientific arguments.

In the 1950's auto-immunity was introduced as a pathophysiological concept. In 1956 Roitt et al (5) demonstrated auto-antibodies against thyroglobulins in patients with Hashimoto's thyroiditis. Burnet (6) proposed a clonal selection theory: in embryonal life immunocompetent lymphocytes are formed which are able to recognize all kind of antigens, but the lymphocytes directed against the body's own proteins are normally deleted. If this elimination mechanism fails, lymphocytes are retained in postembryonal life that may attack the body's own cells by specific antibodies. Later Burnet (7) suggested that the thymus is the site where 'forbidden clones' of immunologically competent cells are destroyed.

Simpson's suggestion that MG was an auto immune disease with an attack on the muscle-endplates, was based on analogous reasoning and clinical intuition. Female preponderance, the fluctuating course of the disease, lymphorrhages in muscles (but not at the endplate), thymic abnormalities (not known then in other diseases) and concomitant occurrence of RA and diseases of the reticulo-endothelial system (of which the cause was unknown) were his main arguments.The proposed antibodies could not been demonstrated.[2]

That the pathophysiological abnormality was caused by a postsynaptic defect was not the prevaling opinion in the 1960's; rather a deficit in ACh-production or a disturbance in ACh- resynthesis was incriminated (8) although some investigators defended a postsynaptic disturbance. (9, 10) This discussion became trivial when in 1973 the loss of AChR was visualized (11). In fact the knowledge of receptor-pathology in general was not yet developed in the 60's. It is now known that ACh-production is increased in MG (12). Increase of transmitters by upregulation is a common event in postsynaptic disturbances.

7.2 Pathophysiology

The pathophysiology of MG has become known in detail by innumerable studies concerning mechanisms of neuromuscular transmission, the immunological breakdown of the AChR, the molecular structure of the AChR, and passively transmitted and antigen induced animal models (reviews 13-16). Acetylcholine receptors are chains of peptides which extend partly outside the membranes of the muscle endplates (fig.1.10). They are in contact with the extra-cellular fluid without a protecting blood-nerve barrier which makes them easily accessible to circulating AChR-antibodies. These play a definite role in the destruction of the AChR by cross-linking (17) following by complement mediated lysis of the postsynaptic membrane (18). In addition a fraction of the antibodies interferes with the site of the AChR molecule where the transmitter (ACh) must bind to initiate the opening of the ion-channel, which is thereby blocked (19). The AChR-Ab are mainly directed to the peptide sequence 67-76 (fig. 1.10) therefore called main immunogenic region. In most patients also antibodies directed to other epitopes can be demonstrated so that antibody production is essentially heterogenous and polyclonal and variable in individual patients.(20) Although T and B cells must be involved in the production of AChR-Ab, they do not seem to play a decisive role in the destruction of the AChR and the postsynaptic membrane. In contrast to the events in the animal model, cellular infiltrates could only be found in 10 intercostal biopsies out of 30 patients; in the positive biopsies no more than 10% of the end-plate zones had cellular infiltrates, and no infiltrate reached the postsynaptic membrane. The membrane attack complex (end product of the complement activation) could be identified in all endplates (21). Endplates that are destructed by focal lysis are internalized in the muscle cell, but new AChR's may develop so that a new balance between pathological destruction and physiological reconstruction is established.

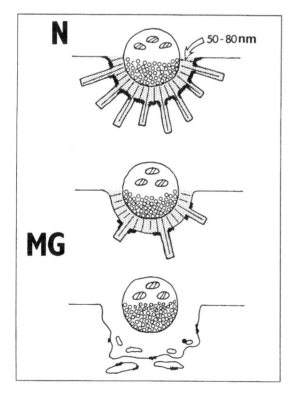

Figure 7.1

Cartoon of the neuromuscular transmission. Nerve ending with three mitochondria and synaptic vesicles containing ACh. AChR are localised at the postsynaptic membrane. (PM) N = normal. MG: mildly and severely affected muscle fibre. In the latter the synaptic cleft is widened, no AChR's are left on the PM but the remnants are visible under the PM. In the severely affected muscle fibre the amount of ACh is increased.

A loss of function at the endplate of a certain muscle fibre will only occur if the receptor density is diminished under a critical level, detectable by blockings in the SFEMG. Since the amount of ACh released may compensate to some extent the loss of functioning AChR's, a physiological increase of ACh by rest and the artificial increase by anti-AChE, will improve the function of fibres that are borderline (SFEMG-jitter).

At the level of the muscle a part of the fibres may still have a normal function, a part is functionally denervated and a part is functioning borderline. The fraction of intact muscle fibres determines the muscle strength that is still left after exhaustion: MG patients 'never' become totally paralysed. The fraction of borderline functioning fibres determines the exhaustibility. In muscle biopsies of MG patients type II fibre atrophy and focal neurogenic lesions with signs of reinnervation (22, 23) (type grouping, increase of innervation ratio) can be observed indicating destruction of muscle fibres and the effect of physiological repair mechanisms. Also at the level of AChR expression in MG muscle biopsies a compensation mechanism was found in severely affected MG patients (24). In some 10% of patients atrophy of large muscle parts occurs, mostly symmetrical but always localized. In observing a large group of patients again the impression arises of a randomized affection of end-plates and muscle fibres. (**Fig. 7.1**)

7.3 Autoimmunity

The cause of this auto-immune proces, of which the effector phase is antibody mediated, is poorly understood. In fact myasthenia gravis shares this ignorance with all other chronic auto-immune diseases (25), whether their effector mechanisms are cellular or humoral. A disturbance in immunomodulation in which T-helper (CD 4+) cells play a major role, (26) is a rather global description of what is probably going on. The mere presence of specific T-cells is not sufficient to cause clinical signs of an antibody mediated autoimmune disease: T-cells that recognize the AChR in in vitro experiments, were also found in the sera of normal controls (27-29) although in a lower percentage than in MG subjects (29). Similarly T cells recognizing myelin basic protein, a candidate antigen for multiple sclerosis, have been recovered from both patients and healthy donors in vitro (30).

These data indicate that antigen specific T-cells are present in the normal immune repertoire and emphasize the role of immune regulation for maintaining a state of tolerance. This state of tolerance is clearly disturbed in patients who have received an allogenic bone marrow transplant, in 40% of whom AChR-Ab were found (31). Some also developed clinical MG (31, 32). A curious experiment of nature is the remission of MG in HIV1 infected patients concomitant with a decrease of their CD4 lymphocytes (33, 34). A further argument for the central role of T-helpers cells was the report of one severely affected MG patient who reacted favourably to a monoclonal antibody against CD4 cells (35).

The question arises again how this disturbance in self-tolerance is triggered[3]. A general medical philosophy states that chronic diseases are probably the result of many stochastic processes including exogenic, endogenic and even psychogenic factors.

Exogenic factors might be viruses, hidden in the body such as the varicella - zoster virus causing herpes zoster with a large interval after infection. Attempts to implicate viruses in the thymus of MG patients had negative results (36), although the possibility was left open that the putative virus could be localized elsewhere in the body or that the techniques used were not sensitive enough. Also in sera of MG patients no significant elevation of antibodies against viruses or other micro-organism could be found (37). The hypothesis of molecular mimicry as a triggering factor has acquired some support in the finding that antibodies of some MG patients bound to a peptide sequence of herpes simplex virus that is homologous to a sequence of the AChR -subunit (39). In general no (viral) infection precedes the onset of MG.

The only exogenic factor known is d-penicillamine that may induce MG in about 1 % of RA patients. (40) In most of these patients the MG disappears after stopping the drug. (5.5.4).[4]

Endogenic factors include a hereditary predisposition. MG is not a hereditary disease in the classic sense but familial acquired MG occurred in 1% (5.1) to 3% of the reported series which is significantly higher than about 7×10^{-5} in the general population. Only about 30% of monozygotic twins are concordant for MG (this partial concordance is also found in other A.I-diseases) so that hereditary disposition cannot be a major factor. In many A.I diseases certain HLA-types associated with the Major Histocompatibility Complex (MHC-II) have a higher frequency than in the general population. Especially the type DR3, DQW2 is increased in young MG patients without thymomas which could make them more "susceptible" for developing MG and also for other A.I diseases, particularly of the thyroid. The higher incidence of rheumatoid arthritis, which is associated with DR4/DR1 cannot be explained by the association with these subtypes in older MG patients. The prevalence of A.I diseases in the MG population is definitely higher than the estimate of 3-4% in the population (25). In general A.I diseases predominate in women, for which a good explanation is still lacking.

The implication of the thymus as a primary factor is contradictory. The thymus has a maximal relative size at birth and early infancy and decreases gradually with age when thymus tissue is replaced by fat. MG has a relative predominance in young females, but not in males and a relatively low prevalence in infancy when the thymus is most active in the development of antibodies against common infections. MG also occurs in older age when the thymus is more or less atrophic. In patients with thymomas no thymus tissue was found at operation in half of my patients (5.6.3).

A possible explanation for the predominance of young women might be a lower safety factor of their neuromuscular transmission expressed as a higher sensitivity to d-tubocurarine. (42) The same difference was also found in rats. (43)

The role of <u>psychogenic factors</u> in the course of MG is evident for most patients and their doctors. Sudden exacerbations may occur in reaction to adverse life events (4.9) or emotions. Again the pathophysiological mechanisms are poorly understood. The exacerbations may be very sudden and transient, so that activation of immunological factors seems unprobable. It might be that catecholamines have a blocking effect on the AChR but experimental evidence is absent and will be difficult to obtain.

7.4 The role of thymus

The role of the thymus in the disturbance of immunomodulation has been the subject of many investigations. A most interesting finding was the presence of myoid cells in the (normal) thymus, that bear surface AChR. These cells were found to be surrounded by antigen presenting cells and T-helpers cells (44), making them particularly vulnerable to immune attack. T-lymphocytes reacting with AChR in vitro were found in all examined thymuses but only in the peripheral blood lymphocytes from 3 out of 10 patients (45, 46). Most thymuses of MG patients also contain B-lymphocytes capable of producing AChR-specific antibodies. This is especially pertinent in hyperplastic thymuses with germinal centres (fig. 1.9.2) which contain cellular complexes formed by AChR-bearing myoid cells and surrounding interdigitating dendritic cells (47). The nature of the cells expressing the intrathymic muscle AChR is unclear. By using a polymerase chain reactions technique it was found that RNA coding for the α-subunit was detectable on thymic epithelial cells in MG thymuses but similarly in thymuses of normal subjects. Also ß and ε-subunits present in the adult AChR were expressed in thymic epithelial cells of MG and control thymuses but not on the thymocytes, while the embryonic subunit (γ) was absent (48). These findings again leave doubt about the specific mechanism of the intrathymic genesis of MG, since the expression of AChR subunits alone is not sufficient to explain the onset of MG.

In thymomas no myoid cells are found and rarely germinal centres. However epitheleal cells of thymomas appear to have AChR epitopes on their surfaces: this was found in 8 MG patients and in 2 out of 6 patients without (yet?) MG. (49). MG in patients with a thymoma may thus be conceived as a paraneoplastic syndrome. The "final common path": destruction of AChR would be the same as in patients without thymoma. Patients with thymoma usually do not improve after thymomectomy and exacerbation of MG in the first year after the operation is not uncommon (5.6.3), with concomitant increase in AChR-Ab levels (50,51). In about 10% of patients undergoing thymomectomy, MG appears at a variable interval after the operation (5.6.2). These data gave rise to the hypothesis that a thymoma has a function in immunoregulation with a predominant inhibitory effect (50).

7.5 Different types of acquired MG and their treatments

7.5.1 Four different types

In the previous chapters a distinction was made between early onset (EO) MG without thymoma, late onset (LO) MG without thymoma, MG with thymoma (TH) and ocular MG (OMG). The age limit of 40 years is somewhat arbitrary and a limit at the age of 50 years may be defended (52, 53).

Table 7.1 GLOBAL COMPARISON OF 4 SUBGROUPS OF MG

	EO	LO	TH	OC
ages (years)	2-39	40-85	20-80	2-80
men : women	1:3	1:1	1:1	2:1
crisis	18%	19%	42%	–
associated A.I. diseases:				
men	17%	6%	13%	5%
women	24%	38%	24%	17%
HLA-B8/DR3	75%	30%	?	?
AChR-Ab	87%	96%	100%	39%
AMA	4%	53%	90%	18%
Effect of thymectomy	++	–	+/–	–
Effect of corticosteroids	+	++	++	++
Effect of azathioprine	+	++	++	(–)
n =	377	182	138	108

HLA-DR-DQ Types are statistically different in EO, LO and TH patients (54-56) and also other features such as sex ratio and antibody production are different. Patients with TH commonly have a more severe MG that is rarely confined to the ocular muscles.

The main reason for distinguishing the 4 groups is the difference in therapeutic approach.

Although the basic symptomatic therapy with anti-AChE is the same, thymectomy is the therapy of choice in EO patients while the second line therapy in older patients is IS therapy. Also patients with TH should be operated because at least one third of the thymomas will grow invasively. Since thymomectomy does not improve their MG, which even may deteriorate, they often need I.S therapy to reach an acceptable clinical condition.

Patients with OMG pose special problems in diagnosis and management.

In OMG the efficacy of thymectomy is controversial. Since anti-AChE have only a partial or no effect in this group, adaptations with mechanical devices are the second line of treatment. Prednisone should be used only if these treatment modalities fail. Azathioprine had no effect in my experience on the ocular signs in patients with generalized MG.

7.5.2 Thymectomy

Although the results of thymectomy in the series operated by Keynes between 1944 and 1956 (57) were convincing in young patients without thymomas, this therapy was not generally accepted in the 1960's. One of the reasons was the risk of postoperative crisis in the severely affected patients, necessitating tracheostomy. On the other hand the natural course of the disease was not always unfavourably, spontaneous improvement and remission could occur, as I could demonstrate in the patients treated in Amsterdam (58). **(Fig. 7.2)**

NATURAL COURSE   MG (n = 73)   **Figure 7.2**
Amsterdam 1926 - '65   Follow up 1985

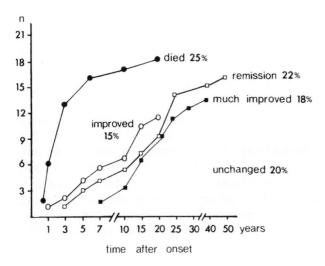

Outcome after long-term follow-up of patients diagnosed in Amsterdam and not treated with thymectomy or I.S therapy.

The improvement of postoperative intensive care in the 1970's and the availability of soft intubation tubes made the operation less risky; the introduction of prednisone in the early 70's and plasmapheresis in the late '70 made intervention in crises possible and could also be used to improve the clinical condition prior to thymectomy. Gradually the indication for thymectomy has been extended to patients with a less severe but generalized signs, who appear to react equally well. Sceptics (59, 60) have stated that the effect of thymectomy is not proved by controlled clinical trials. This may be true but these trials are difficult to organize now even in the categories of older and or of purely ocular patients, where the effect of thymectomy is not established but probably not better than medicamentous treatment (61) (5.4.2). An enquiry among 56 American neurologists revealed that 11 expressed severe reservations about the efficacy of the procedure. They only advocated thymectomy in patients with severe disease or after other (?) modalities had failed. Opinions also differed concerning the age limit, varying from 50-70 years and the indication in purely ocular MG. Other restrictions were as follows: 21 responders reserved thymectomy for those with disabling myasthenia, 14 reserved the procedure for those unresponsive to anti-AChE medication alone (n=10) or those unresponsive to anti-AChE medication and immunosuppressants (n=4) and 12 reserved the procedure for individuals with MG of recent (i.e within 2 to 5 years) onset (62).

I compared the course of the disease in my own thymectomized patients with that of the nonthymectomized EO patients. I found a nearly similar final improvement in both groups (table 5.12a) but the improvement started much sooner in the operated group (fig. 5.10). In most patients of the non-operated group the onset of MG was in an earlier period, and their mean disability score was somewhat lower but otherwise these groups were comparable. This suggests that thymectomy enchanced the natural favourable course of the diseases.

An additional argument for the specific effect of thymectomy was the experience of the inefficacy of partial thymectomy (3 transcervical) in 4 of my patients who improved considerably (2 remissions) after rethymectomy with concomitant decrease of AChR-Ab. In fact these patients had undergone an inadvertant sham-thymectomy! (Fig. 5.11) This experience is shared by many other neurologists (4.4.1).

However the mechanism of action is poorly understood, and a practical problem is that there are non-responders even in maximal thymectomy (63). The advice to undergo thymectomy should always be made with this restriction, but most patients accept this risk. Treating young patients probably life long with immunosuppressive therapy if another riskless treatment modality is possible, seems to be contrary to sound clinical reasoning. Experience with longterm immunosuppressive treatment without thymectomy in early onset patients is apparently scarce and no reports could be found. One of my own patients was treated with prednisone during 3 years, followed by thymectomy.

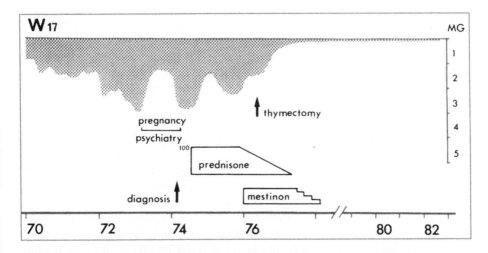

Figure 7.3 W 17. Sudden falls and intermittent arm weakness. Gradual worsening. No diagnosis by 2 neurologists (1974). Improvement in second term of pregnancy when she was under treatment in a psychiatric ward under the diagnosis conversion reaction. Exacerbation after delivery with oculobulbar signs. Diagnosis confirmed by edrophonium test and nerve stimulation test. She improved (DS3 to DS1) by PR 100mg/2 d, which was continued for two years, but she gradually deteriorated again (DS2). She underwent thymectomy which was complicated by an unusual bleeding out of the osteoporotic sternum. Complete remission followed within 1 year after the operation. At the age of 28 she was treated for an A.I.-hyperthyroidism. At the age of 43 she only had some diplopia after looking 10 seconds laterally (DS0).
Comment: In 1974 PR was considered as a "chemical thymectomy" by some
  neurologists so that thymectomy (which had been my initial advice) was
  cancelled. The PR dosage was too long maintained on a high dosage
  without adequate control of the patient. The case suggests the supremacy of
  thymectomy over IS in EO patients.

The indication for thymomectomy is not the MG itself but the risk of invasive growth and the -mainly intrathoracic-metastases. Although it is rare that clinical signs of invasive growth (pain, superior vena cava syndrome, phrenic nerve involvement) are the presenting signs in MG patients, an adherence to or an invasion into pleura and or the pericardium appear to be present at operation in one third of the patients. There is no consensus about the need of postoperative irradiation in those patients in whom resection of the tumor has been complete by macroscopic and microscopic examination (4.4.2). If complete removal cannot be ascertained, postoperative irradiation is generally advised. In this situation there is no consensus about the additional use of chemotherapy. Recurrence of a thymoma may be that of a second tumor which can be removed completely as was the experience in some of my patients. However in patients with an incompletely removed but not irradiated thymoma, recurrence heralds a poor prognosis within 3 to 5 years. In this situation chemotherapy combined or not with irradiation may be tried. Treatment of the thymoma related pancytopenia or aplastic anemia is beyond the skill of a neurologist; some of my patients reacted favourably to high dosage prednisone.

7.5.3 IS therapies

In the period before the use of IS therapies patients had to tolerate the symptoms that were left after thymectomy and an optimal use of anti-AChE. Nowadays doctors seem to have a lower tolerance for their patient's symptoms, knowing that more effective treatments might be employed. The use of IS therapies seemed to be higher in an American study (64) than in our own (53). This was probably not caused by the lesser severity of MG in our patients but due to a more restricted indication. Both doctors and patients make their choices according to their own needs and experiences. In my practice it was not unusual that patients who had been treated effectively with prednisone, nevertheless choose to abandon this therapy. They prefered to have mild or moderate MG symptoms and did not accept actual or possible side effects, even if these seemed minor in their doctor's opinion.

Much clinical experience is needed to estimate the risks of I.S therapies in individual patients. Prednisone has a bad reputation, particularly in women who fear the Cushing face, weight gain and osteoporosis. Although side effects will occur in about one third of the young and in two thirds of the older patients, especially by the high dosage of the initial period, it was relatively rare that prednisone had to be withdrawn.

It is not well possible to predict the risk of side effects in individual patients if no risk factors such as diabetes or hypertension are known from their history. Part of the side effects are dose related and will disappear if the maintenance dosage is reached. Side effects of azathioprine usually appear shortly after the start and often preclude further administration or necessitate an adjustment of the dosage. A problem with the use of azathioprine is the long delay before the effect becomes apparent and again the long delay of the possible reappearance of symptoms if the drug is withdrawn on presumption of the lack of effect.

Exacerbations that are clearly influenced by exogenic or psychological factors are a poor indication for the start of or an increase in dosage of IS therapies.

There is a clear need for more selective therapies, which do not affect the whole antibody productive system. Specific (AChR-reactive) T- and B-cells comprise only about 1‰ of peripheral lymphocytes; they are activated by a continuous antigenic stimulation and therefore more selectively inhibited by IS therapies. But these therapies have unwanted suppressive effects on other cell populations.

On theoretical grounds several possibilities for more selective IS therapies exist, some of which have proved to be effective in animal models (14,65). The main problem in the treatment of human MG is the heterogeneity of the antibody reactivity, which would necessitate the production of CD4+ specific monoclonal antibodies for each individual patient.

7.6 Becoming an expert

My own first confrontation with MG (1959) was in a physiological laboratory in search for the enigmatic circulating substance. Also my experiments failed but my interest in the disease and its patients was raised and I never got rid of it! I had the opportunity to coöperate with Hugo van der Geld and Bert Feltkamp, research fellows in the Central Laboratory of the Blood Transfusion Service in Amsterdam, who were able to determine auto-antibodies with various techniques. The recent report on a circulating IgG fraction that bound to skeletal muscle (66) prompted them to examine the sera of large series of MG patients that I had collected. The finding that this anti-muscle antibody (AMA) also reacted with certain thymic cells (67) confirmed my clinical impression that thymectomy would be of benefit.

For a young clinical neurologist who had to diagnose many untreatable diseases with unknown causes, Myasthenia Gravis was and is an utmost rewarding disease. As in other disciplines of clinical medicine a large experience of patients with a certain disease is a prerequisite to get a good insight into its variability and peculair features. I therefore tried to study patients in other medical centres and could only succeed with the help of many neurologists who gave me access to their patients. Later on they referred their patients in order to get my opinion on the most appropriate way of treatment.

Becoming an "expert" was a gradual process, with the acquirement of "Tacid knowledge" (68), that I tried to explicate in my advices to other neurologists and to my patients. As a matter of fact my personal experience is embedded in that of so many others, who gave me the honour and pleasure of discussing and evaluating my findings and often became good friends in the field of science. I have referred to their work with the best of my knowledge and hope that this book will serve as a frame of reference for our endeavours in the past and for the optimal treatment of Myasthenic Patients.

NOTES

[1] The word "hormone" was first used by Starling in a lecture at the Royal College of Physicians in 1905 (4).

[2] Simpson's fruitful hypothesis was published in a medical journal of minor impact (69) and was not widely citated at the International Congress on Myasthenia Gravis in 1966 (70).

[3] Several mechanisms explaining the development and possible disruption of self tolerance are known (25).
In relation to MG, intrathymic deficits in self-recognition of the body's antigens might be surmised. In later life exogenic factors such as micro-organisms sharing antigens with the host (molecular mimicry) or inducing cell-surface changes that resemble foreign antigens, are considered. Non-deleted self reactive T and B-cells, that are normally present in the body might be activated by bacterial infections. The inactivation of self-reactive lymphocytes would be maintained by idiotypic networks (71) through which antibodies against pathological antibodies are generated. The existence of anti-idiotype antibodies against AChR was reported by some investigators (72-74) but could not be confirmed by others (75) and remains controversial. In general the existence of such networks in A.I. diseases is contested (25). A genetic factor concerns the presence of certain MHC-class II antigens which corresponds with the fact that T-cell-mediated immune responses are MHC-II restricted (76).
The production of multiple diseases non specific antibodies (3.3.5) indicates a more general disturbance in immunomodulation.

[4] D-penicillamine is one of the many drugs that may have the side effect of inducing A.I. responses such as procainamide, hydralazine, gold salts. D-penicilline may also induce other A.I. diseases such as polymyositis, nephrotic syndrome and SLE.

[5] In only one recent study the outcome in a large series of thymectomized and non-thymectomized patients was compared in 3 periods (77). In the period 1940 to 1957 transsternal thymectomy resulted in 20% remissions compared with 10% in the non-operated group (p < 0.02) despite the initially more severe weakness of the operated patients. From 1958 tot 1965 and from 1966 to 1985 the status of thymectomized patients a mean of 17 and 12 years after onset was no better than in patients who were not operated. It is not explicitly stated whether these patients also had received IS therapies. In the last period two thirds of the thymectomies were performed by transcervical approach which may have influenced the results unfavourably.

References

Chapter 1

1. Jolly F 1895 Ueber Myasthenia gravis pseudoparalytica. Berliner Klinische Wochenschrift 32:1-7.
2. Erb W 1879 Zur Casuistik der bulbären Lähmungen. 3 Ueber einen neuen, wahrscheinlich bulbären Symptomencomplex. Archiv fur Psychiatrie und Nervenkrankheiten 9:336-350.
3. Wilks S 1877 On cerebritis, hysteria and bulbar paralysis. Guy's Hospital Reports 22:7-55.
4. Eisenlohr C 1887 Ein Fall von Ophthalmoplegia externa progrssiva und finaler Bulbärparalyse mit negativem Sectionsbefund. Neurologisches Zentralblatt 6:337.
5. Oppenheim H 1887 Ueber einen Fall von chronischer progressiven Bulbärparalyse ohne anatomischer Befund. Virchow's Archiv für pathologische Anatomie und klinische Medizin 108:527.
6. Shaw L E 1890 A case of bulbar paralysis without structural changes in the medulla. Brain 13:96-99.
7. Bernardt M 1890 Zur Lehre von dem nucleären Augenmuskellähmungen and ihren Complicationen. Berliner Klinische Wochenschrift XXVII:981-984.
8. Hoppe H H 1892 Ein Beitrag zur Kenntnis der Bulbärparalyse. Berliner Klinische Wochenschrift 29:332-336.
9. Remak E 1892 Zur Pathologie der Bulbärparalyse. Archiv für Psychiatrie und Nervenkrankheiten 23:919-960.
10. Senator H 1892 Ein Fall von Bulbärlähmung ohne anatomischen Befund. Neurologisches Centrallblatt 168-174.
11. Dreschfeld A 1893 Polioencephalomyelitis without any anatomical lesions. British Medical Journal II: 176-177.
12. Goldflam S 1902 Ueber einen scheinbar heilbaren bulbär paralytischen Symptomencomplex mit Beteiligung der Extremitäten. Deutsches Zeitschrift für Nervenheilkunde 4:312-352.
13. Goldflam S 1902 Weiteres über die asthenische Lähmung nebst einem Obduktionsbefund. Neurologisches Zentralblatt 21:97-107, 154-160, 208-214, 252-258, 303-310, 347-353, 390-397, 447-452, 490-496.
14. Cohn T 1897 Ueber Myasthenia pseudoparalytica gravis. Deutsche Medicinische Wochenschrift 49:785-789.
15. Viets H R 1953 A historical review of myasthenia gravis from 1672 to 1900. Journal of the American Medical Association 153:1273-1280.

16. Campbell H, Bramwell E 1900 Myasthenia gravis. Brain 23:277-336.
17. Starr M A 1912 Myasthenia gravis. Journal of Nervous and Mental Disease 39:721-731.
18. Wayenburg G van 1901 Myasthenia pseudoparalytica gravis. Nederlandsch Tijdschrift voor Geneeskunde 1438-1440.
19. Weigert C 1901 Pathologisch-anatomischer Beitrag zur Erb-schen Krankheit (Myasthenia gravis). Neurologisches Zentralblatt 20:597.
20. Link R 1903 Beitrage zur Kenntnis der Myasthenia gravis mit Befund von Zellherden in zahlreichen Muskeln. Deutsches Zeitschrift für Nervenheilkunde 23:114-124.
21. Buzard E F 1905 The clinical history and postmortem examination of five cases of myasthenia gravis. Brain 28:438-483.
22. Myers Ch S 1902 Myasthenia gravis. Journal of Pathology and Bacteriology 3:306-345.
23. Bell E T 1917 Tumors of the thymus in myasthenia gravis. Journal of Nervous and Mental Disease 45, 130-143.
24. Schumacher C H, Roth P 1912 Thymektomie bei einem Fall von Morbus Basedowi mit Myasthenie. Mitteilungen aus dem Grenzgebieten der Medizin und Chirurgie 25:746-765.
25. Nowell P T, Wilson A 1959 Some effects of foetal whale thymus glands. Quarterly Journal of Experimental Physiology 44:229.
26. Lammers W, Most van Spijk C van de 1954 Unsuccessful attempt to demonstrate a paralytic factor in serum of myasthenia gravis patients. Nature 173:1192-1193
27. Keschner M, Strauss I 1927 Myasthenia gravis. Archives of Neurology and Psychiatry 17:337-376.
28. Thévénard A 1961 Carotid sinus denervation in myasthenia gravis. In: Viets H R (ed) Myasthenia gravis. The second international symposium proceedings. Charles C Thomas, Springfield, 624-633.
29. Mertens H G 1955 Ueber den Verlauf der Myastenie nach Carotissinus-denervierung. Der Nervenarzt 26: 150-154.
30. Edgeworth H 1930 A report of progress on the use of ephedrine in a case of myasthenia gravis. Journal of the American Medical Association.
31. Edgeworth H 1933 The effect of ephedrine in the treatment of myasthenia gravis, second report. Journal of the American Medical Association 100:1401.
32. Walker M B 1934 Treatment of myasthenia gravis with physostigmine. Lancet I: 1200-1201.
33. Walker M B 1935 Case showing the effect of prostigmine on myasthenia gravis. Proceedings of the Royal Society of Medicine 28:33-35.
34. Osserman K E, Kaplan L I 1952 Rapid diagnostic test for myasthenia gravis: increased muscle strength without fasciculations after intravenous administration of edrophonium (Tensilon) chloride. Journal of the American Medical Association 150:265.

35. Osserman K E, Teng P, Kaplan L A 1954 Studies in myasthenia gravis: preliminary report on therapy with mestinon bromide. Journal of the American Medical Association 155:961-966.
36. Schwab R S 1955 WIN 8077 in the treatment of sixty myasthenia gravis patients. American Journal of Medicine 19:734-736.
37. Blalock A, Mason M F, Morgan H J, Riven S S 1939 Myasthenia gravis and tumors of the thymic region. Report of a case in which the tumor was removed. Annals of Surgery 110:544-560.
38. Sloan H E 1943 The thymus in myasthenia gravis. Surgery 13:154-174.
39. Blalock A 1944 Thymectomy in the treatment of myasthenia gravis. Journal of Thoracic Surgery 13:316-339.
40. Keynes G L 1981 The Gates of Memory, Myasthenia gravis. Clarendon Press, Oxford, 276.
41. Keynes 1961 The history of myasthenic gravis. Medical History 5:313-325.
42. Keynes G L 1954 Surgery of the thymus gland. Lancet II: 1197-1208.
43. Simpson J A 1958 Evaluation of thymectomy in myasthenia gravis. Brain 81:112-145.
44. Masaoka A, Monden Y, Nakahara K, Tamioka T 1981 Follow-up study of thymomas with special reference to their clinical stages. Cancer 48:2485-2492.
45. Bennet A E, Cash P T 1942 Curare as a diagnosic test for myasthenia gravis. Curarization an etiologic clue in the disease. Transactions of the American Neurological Association 68:102-106.
46. Bernard Cl 1966 Introduction à l'étude de la médecine expérimentale. Garmer-Flammarion, Paris.
47. Harvey A M, Masland R L 1941 The electromyogram in myasthenia gravis. Bulletin of the John Hopkins Hospital 69:1-13.
48. Grob D, Johns R J 1961 Further studies on the mechanism of the defect in neuromuscular transmission, with particular reference to the acetylcholine-insensitive block. In: Viets H R (ed) Myasthenia gravis. The second international symposium proceedings. Charles C Thomas, Springfield, 127-149.
49. Desmedt J E 1958 Myasthenic-like features of neuromuscular transmission after administration of an inhibitor of acetylcholine synthesis. Nature 182:1673-1674.
50. Zacks S I, Bauer W C, Blumberg J M 1962 The fine structure of the myasthenic neuromuscular junction. Journal of Neuropathology and Experimental Neurology 21:335-347.
51. Zacks S I, Shields D R, Steinberg S A 1966 A myasthenic syndrome in the dog: a case report with electron microscopic observations on motor end-plates and comparisons with the fine structure of end-plates in myasthenia gravis. Annals of the New York Academy of Sciences 135:79-97.
52. Engel A G, Santa T 1971 Histometric analysis of the ultrastructure of the neuromuscular junction in myasthenia gravis and in the myasthenic syndrome. Annals of the New York Academy of Sciences 183:46-63.
53. Fambrough D M, Drachman D B, Satyamurti S 1973 Neuromuscular junction in myasthenia gravis: decreased acetylcholine receptors. Science 182:293-295.

54. Roitt I M, Doniach D, Campbell P N, Hudson R V 1956 Auto antibodies in Hashimoto's disease (lymphadenoid goitre). Lancet II: 820.

55. Burnet M F 1959 Clonal selection theory of acquired immunity. Vanderbilt and Cambridge University Presses.

56. Burnet M F 1962 The role of the thymus and related organs in immunity. British Medical Journal 265:807.

57. Smithers S W 1959 Tumors of the thyroid gland in relation to some general concepts as neoplasia. Journal of the Faculty of Radiologists 10:3-16.

58. Simpson J A 1960 Myasthenia gravis, a new hypothesis. Scottish Medical Journal 5:419-436.

59. Nastuk W L, Strauss A J L, Osserman K E 1959 Search for a neuromuscular blocking agent in the blood of patients with myasthenia gravis. American Journal of Medicine 26:394-409.

60. Miller J F A P 1961 Immunologic function of the thymus. Lancet II: 748.

61. Strickroot F L, Schaeffer R L, Bergo H E 1942 Myasthenia gravis occurring in an infant born of a myasthenic mother. Journal of the American Medical Association 120:1207-1209.

62. Nastuk W L, Plescia O J, Osserman K E 1960 Changes in serum complement activity in patients with myasthenia gravis. Proceedings of the Society for Experimental Biology and Medicine 105:177-184.

63. Strauss A J L, Seegal B C, Hsu K C, Burkholder P M, Nastuk W L, Osserman K E 1960 Immunofluorescence demonstration of a muscle binding, complement fixing serum globulin fraction in myasthenia gravis. Proceedings of the Society of Experimental Biological Medicine 105:184-191.

64. Geld H van der, Oosterhuis H J G H 1963 Muscle and thymus antibodies in myasthenia gravis. Vox sanguinis 8:196-204.

65. Velde R L van de, Friedman N B 1966 The thymic "myoidzellen" and myasthenia gravis. Journal of the American Medical Association 198:287-288.

66. Oosterhuis H J G H, Feltkamp T E W, Geld H W R van der 1967 Studies in myasthenia gravis, part II. The relations of some clinical and immunological data. Journal of the Neurological Sciences 4:417-434.

67. Geld H van der, Feltkamp T E W, Loghem J J van, Oosterhuis H J G H, Biemond A 1963 Multiple antibody production in myasthenia gravis. Lancet II: 373-375.

68. Millikan C H, Eaton L M 1951 Clinical evaluation of ACTH in myasthenia gravis. Neurology 1:145-152.

69. Reis G von, Liljestrand A, Matell G 1966 Treatment of severe myasthenia gravis with large doses of ACTH. Annals of the New York Academy of Sciences 135:409-416.

70. Delwaide P J, Salmon J, Van Cauwenberger H 1967 Premiers essais de traitement de la myasthénie par azathioprine. Acta Neurologica Belgica 67:701-712.

71. Mertens H G, Balzereit F, Leipert M 1969 The treatment of severe myasthenia gravis with immunosuppressive agents. European Neurology 2:321-339.

72. Warmolts J R, Engel W K 1971 Benefit from alternate-day prednisone in myasthenia gravis. Neurology 21:412.

73. Stricker E, Thölen H, Massini M, Staub H 1960 The effect of haemodialysis in myasthenia gravis. Journal of Neurology, Neurosurgery and Psychiatry 23:291.

74. Hedger R W, Davis F A, Schwartz F D, Ing T S 1971 Improvement of myasthenia gravis by hemodialysis in a patient with chronic rental failure. Annals of Internal Medicine 75:749-752.

75. Bergström K, Franksson C, Matell G, Von Reis G 1973 The effect of thoracic duct lymph drainage on myasthenia gravis. European Neurology 9:157-167.

76. Lindström J M, Seybold M E , Lennon B A, Whittingham S, Duane D D 1976 Antibody to acetylcholine receptor in myasthenia gravis. Neurology 26:1054-1059.

77. Patrick J, Lindstrom J 1973 Autoimmune response to acetylcholine receptor. Science 180:871-872.

77a. Almon R R, Andrew C G, Appel S H 1974 Serum globulin in myasthenia gravis: Inhibition of alpha-bungarotoxin binding to acetylcholine receptors. Science 186:55-57.

78. Fambrough D M, Drachman D B, Sayamurti S 1973 Neuromuscular junction in myasthenia gravis: decreased acetylcholine receptors. Science 182:293-295.

79. Drachman D B, Angus R N, Adams R N, Michelson J D, Hoffmann G J 1978 Myasthenic antibodies cross-link acetylcholine receptors to accelerate degradation. New England Journal of Medicine 298:1116-1122.

80. Engel A G, Arakata K 1987 The membrane attack complex complement at the endplate in myasthenia gravis. Annals of the N.Y. Academy of Sciences 505:326-332.

81. Toyka K V, Drachman D B, Pestronk A, Kao I 1975 Myasthenia gravis: passive transfer from man to mouse. Science 109:397-399.

82. Lindstrom J 1980 Experimental autoimmune myasthenia gravis. Journal of Neurology, Neurosurgery and Psychiatry 43:568-576.

83. Wekerle H, Müller-Hermelink H K 1986 The thymus in myasthenia gravis. In: Müller-Hermelink H K Ed. The human thymus. Springer Verlag, Berlin, 179-206.

84. Melms A, Schalke B C, Kirchner T, Müller-Hermelink H K, Albert E, Wekerle H 1988 Thymus in myasthenia gravis. Isolation of T-lymphocyte lines specific for the nicotinic acetylcholine receptor from thymusses of myasthenic patients. Journal of Clinical Investigation 81:902-908.

85. Kuks J B M, Oosterhuis H J G H, Limburg P C , The T H 1991 Anti-acetylcholine receptor antibodies decrease after thymectomy in patients with myasthenia gravis. Clinical correlations. Journal of Autoimmunity 4:197-211.

86. Kirchner T, Hoppe F, Müller-Hermelink H K 1987 Acetylcholine receptor epitopes on epithelial cells of thymoma in myasthenia gravis. Lancet I: 218.

87. Müller-Hermelink H K, Marx A, Gender K, Kirchner T H 1993 The pathological basis of thymoma associated myasthenia gravis. New York Academy of Sciences 681:56-65.

88. Molenaar P C 1993 Physiology, biochemistry and pathology of neuromuscular transmission. In: DeBaets M, Oosterhuis H J G H Eds. Myasthenia gravis. C.R.C. Press, Boca Raton, 44-97.

89. Beeson D, Brydson M, Wood H, Vincent A, Newsom-Davis J 1989 Human muscle acetylcholine receptor: cloning and expression in Escherichia coli of c DNA for the alpha-subunit Biochemical Society Transactions 17:219-20.

89a. Conti-Tronconi B, McLane K E, Raftery M A, Grando S A, Protti M P 1994 The structure of the acetylcholine receptor: structure and autoimmune pathology. Critical Reviews in Biochemistry and Molecular Biology 29, 69-123.

90. Lindstrom J 1977 An essay for antibodies to human acetylcholine receptor in serum from patients with myasthenia gravis. Clinical Immunology and Immunopathology 7:36-43.

91. Vincent A, Newsom Davis J 1980 Anti-acetylcholine receptor antibodies. Journal of Neurology, Neurosurgery and Psychiatry 43:590-600.

92. Vincent A, Whiting P J, Schluep M, Heidenreich F, Lang B, Roberts A, Willcox N, Newsom-Davis J 1987 Antibody heterogeneity and specificity in Myasthenia gravis. New York Academy of Sciences 505:106-120.

93. Pinching A J, Peters D K, Newsom-Davis J 1976 Remission of myasthenia gravis following plasma exchange. Lancet II: 1373-1376.

93a. Drachman D B 1994 Myasthenia gravis. The New England Journal of Medicine 330:1797-1810.

94. Engel A G, Lambert E H, Gomez M R 1977 A new myasthenic syndrome with end-plate acetylcholin-esterase deficiency, small nerve terminals and reduced acetylcholine release. Annals of Neurology 1:315-330.

95. Engel A G 1993 The investigation of congenital myasthenic syndromes. Annals of the New York Academy of Sciences 682:425-434.

96. Aoki T, Drachman D B, Asher D M, Gibbs C J, Bahmanyar S, Wolinski J S 1985 Attempts to implicate viruses in myasthenia gravis. Neurology 35:185-192.

97. Bucknal R C, Dixon A S J, Glick E N, Woodland J, Zutshi D W 1975 Myasthenia gravis associated with penicillamine treatment for rheumatoid arthritis. British Medical Journal 1:600-602.

98. Oosterhuis H J G H 1993 Clinical aspects. In DeBaets M, Oosterhuis H J G H Eds. Myasthenia gravis. C.R.C. Press, Boca Raton 33.

99. Feltkamp T E W, Berg-Loonen P M van der, Nijenhuis L E, Engelfriet C P, Loghem J J van, Rossum A L van, Oosterhuis H J G H 1974 Myasthenia gravis auto antibodies and HLA antigens. British Medical Journal I:131-133.

100. Oppenheim H 1901 Die Myasthenische Paralyse (Bulbärparalyse ohne anatomischen Befund). Berlin, S Karger.

101. Collins J 1897 Asthenic bulbar paralysis. Internal Medicin Magazin 5:203.

102. Guthrie L G 1903 Myasthenia gravis in the seventeenth century. Lancet I: 330-331.

103. Pordage S 1683 Two discourses concerning the soul of brutes. Translation of de Anima Brutorum. Willis T 1672, 431-432.

104. Hérard M 1868 De la paralysie glosso-labio-laryngée. Société Médecine des Hopitaux 44-46.

105. Charcot J M, Guinon G, Parmentier E 1890 De l'ophthalmoplégie externe. Nouvelle iconographie de la salpètrière, Lecroisnier et Babé (eds) Paris, 305-306.

106. Charcot J M, Guinon G 1892 Cinq cas d'ophtalmoplégie externe (paralysie bulbaire supérieure) combinée soit à la paralysie labio-glosso-laryngie (paralysie bulbaire totale) soit à l'atrophie musculaire généralisée (polioencéphalomyelite) Diagnostic. In: Clinique des maladies du système nerveux Tome I, XI, 208-242.
107. Murri A 1896 Sur un cas de maladie d'Erb. Archives Italiennes de Biologie (Pisa) 25:64-92.
108. Remen L 1932 Zur Pathogenese und Therapie der Myasthenia gravis pseudoparalytica. Deutsches Zeitschrift für Nervenheilkunde 128:66-78.
109. Grob D 1958 Myasthenia gravis: current status of pathogenesis, clinical manifestations and management. Journal of Chronic Diseases 8:536-566.
110. Walker M B 1938 A case in which fatigue of the forearm muscles could induce paralysis of the extraocular muscles. Proceedings of the Royal Society of Medicine 31:722.
111. Wilson A, Stoner B H 1944 Myasthenia gravis: a consideration of its causation in a study of 14 cases. The Quarterly Journal of Medicine 37:1-18.
112. Grosse-Brockhoff F, Welte E 1950 Ueber selten beobachtete Ermüdungserscheinungen bei Myasthenia Gravis Pseudoparalytica. Deutsche Medizinische Wochenschrift 75:698-700.
113. Strüppler A 1955 Experimentelle Untersuchungen zur Pathogenese der Myasthenie. Zeitschrift für die gesammte experimentelle Medizin 125:244.
114. Tsukiyama K, Nakai A, Mine R, Kitani T 1959 Studies on a myasthenic substance present in the serum of patients with myasthenia gravis. Medical Journal of Osaka University 10(2).
115. Most-van Spijk D van de, Lammers W 1955 Unsuccessful attempt to demonstrate a paralytic factor in the serum of myasthenia gravis patients. Acta physiologica et pharmacologica neerlandica IV, 591-594.
116. Desmedt J E 1956 Contribution à la physiopathologie de la myasthénie. Thèse Bruxelles (BRU 464) p 46-48.

Chapter 2

1. Harvey A McG 1948 Some preliminary observations in the clinical course of myasthenia gravis before and after thymectomy. Bulletin of the New York Academy of Medicine 24: 505-522.
2. Kennedy F S, Moersch F P 1937 Myasthenia gravis. A clinical review of 87 cases observed between 1915 and the early part of 1932. Canadian Medical Association Journal 37:216-223.
3. Oosterhuis H J G H 1964 Studies in myasthenia gravis. Journal of the Neurological Sciences 1:512-546.
4. Osserman K E 1958 Myasthenia gravis. Grune & Stratton, New York
5. Osserman K E 1967 Ocular myasthenia gravis. Investigative Ophthalmology 6:277-287.

6. Simpson J A 1981 Myasthenia gravis and myasthenic syndromes. In: Walton J (ed) Disorders of voluntary muscle, 4th edn. Churchill Livingstone, Edinburgh p 585-624.

7. Oppenheim H 1901 Die Myasthenische Paralyse (Bulbärparalyse ohne anatomischen Befund). Berlin, S Karger.

8. Cogan D G 1965 Myasthenia gravis. A review of the disease and a description of lid twitch as a characteristic sign. Archives of Ophthalmology 74:217-221.

9. Glaser J S 1978 Neuro-ophthalmology, Harper & Row Publishers, Hagerstown, p 273-275.

10. Osher R H, Griggs R C 1979 Orbicularis fatigue. The 'Peek' sign of myasthenia gravis. Archives of Ophthalmology 97:677-679.

11. Fontaine M 1952 Les symptômes oculaires de la myasthénie. Archives d'Ophthalmologie (Paris) 12:157-169.

12. Walsh F B, Hoyt W F 1969 Clinical neuro-ophthalmology, 3rd edn, Williams & Wilkins Company, Baltimore Vol II: 1283.

13. Spector R H, Daroff R B 1976 Edrophonium infra-red optokinetic nystagmography in the dignosis of myasthenia gravis. Annals of the New York Academy of Sciences 274:642-651.

14. Retzlaff J A, Kearns Th P, Howard F M, Cronin M L 1969 Lancester red-green test in evaluation of edrophonium effect in myasthenia gravis. American Journal of Ophthalmology 67:13-21.

15. Glaser J S 1966 Myasthenic pseudo-internuclear ophthalmoplegia. Archives of Ophthalmology 75:363-366.

16. Cogan D G, Yee R D, Gittinger J 1976 Rapid eye movements in myasthenia gravis. I. Clinical observations. Archives of Ophthalmology 94:1083-1085.

17. Pucklin J E, Sacks J G, Boshes B 1976 Transient eye lid retraction in myasthenia gravis. Journal of Neurology, Neurosurgery and Psychiatry 39:44-47.

18. Simpson J A 1960 Myasthenia gravis, a new hypothesis. Scottish Medical Journal 5:419-436.

19. Alajouanine Th, Castaigne P, Nick J, Contamin F, Lhermitte F 1957 Sur l'existence de signes sensitifs et sensoriels au cours de la myasthénie. Revue Neurologique 96:242-248.

20. Gowers W R 1902 Remarks on Myasthenia and ophthalmoplegia. British Medical Journal 1253-1256.

21. Sneddon J 1980 Myasthenia gravis: the difficult diagnosis. British Journal of Psychiatry 136:92-93.

22. Blom S, Ringqvist I 1971 Neurophysiological findings in myasthenia gravis. Electroencephalography and Clinical Neurophysiology 30:477-487.

23. Stålberg E 1980 Clinical electrophysiology in myasthenia gravis. Journal of Neurology, Neurosurgery and Psychiatry 43: 622-633.

24. Osserman K E 1958 Myasthenia gravis. Grune & Stratton, New York p 73.

25. Ploeg R J O van der, Oosterhuis H J G H, Reuvekamp J 1984 Measuring muscle strength. Journal of Neurology 231:200.

26. Ploeg R J O van der, Fidler V, Oosterhuis H J G H 1991 Hand-held myometry: reference values. Journal of Neurology, Neurosurgery and Psychiatry 54:244-247.

27. Berger W, Kunze K 1977 Lungenfunktion. In: Hertel G u. A (Ed) Myasthenia gravis. G Thieme, Berlin 183-190.

28. Magyar P, Szathamary I, Szobor A 1979 Myasthenia gravis: lung function studies without and with edrophonium chloride. European Neurology 18:59-65.

29. Reuther P, Hertel G, Ricker K, Bürkner R 1978 Lungenfunktionsdiagnostik bei myasthenia gravis. Verhandlungen der Deutsche Gesellschaft für Innere Medizin 84:1579-1582.

30. Ringqvist I, Ringqvist T 1971 Respiratory mechanisms in untreated myasthenia gravis with special reference to the respiratory forces. Acta Medica Scandinavica 190:499-508.

31. Szathmary I, Magyar P, Szobor A 1981 Maximaler respiratorischer Druck bei Einatmung von krisengefährdeten und nicht gefährdeten myasthenischen Kranken. Aktuelle Neurologie 8:76-79.

32. Campbell H, Bramwell E 1900 Myasthenia gravis. Brain 23: 277-336.

33. Alajouanine T, Lemair A, Bourgignon A 1954 Sur un syndrome myasthénique et myalgique réalisant une pseudomyopathie à évolution périodique. Revue Neurologique 90:3-12.

34. Struppler A 1955 Experimentelle Untersuchungen zur Pathogenese der Myasthenie. Zeitschrift für die gesammte Experimentelle Medizin 125:244-273.

35. Steidl R M, Oswald A J, Kottke F J 1962 Myasthenic syndrome with associated neuropathy. Archives of Neurology 6:451-459.

36. Jesel M, Stoebner P, Zenglein J P, Isch F 1969 Syndrome myasthéniforme et polymyosite. Correlations cliniques, electromyographiques et ultrastructurales dans deux cas. Revue Oto-Neuro-Ophthalmologia 41:175-183.

37. Bonduelle M, Bouygues P, Puech H 1956 Ophthalmoplégie d'emblée permanente et insensible à la prostigmine, ayant précédé de six mois un syndrome myasthénique périphérique. Revue Neurologique 94:246-249.

38. Griffin S G, Natrass F J, Posk E A 1956 Thymectomy during respiratory failure in a case of myopathy with myasthenia gravis. Lancet II: 704-708.

39. Hausmanowa-Petrusewicz I, Falkiewiczowa S, Jedrzejewska H, Kamieniecka Z, Fidiauska A 1965 Descending dystrophy or advanced myasthenia. Schweizer Archiv für Neurologie, Neurochirurgie und Psychiatrie 95:233-244.

40. Hosotte A 1951 Myasthénie avec atrophies de type myopathique. Presse Médicale 59:1146.

41. Garcin R, Fardeau M, Godet-Guillain M 1965 A clinical and pathological study of a case of alternating and recurrent external ophthalmoplegia with amyotrophy of the limbs observed for forty-five years: discussion of the relationship of this condition with myasthenia gravis. Brain 88:739-752.

42. Hopf H C, Ludin H P 1968 Neurogene Muskelatrophien, aufgetreten im Verlauf einer vornehmlich oculären Myasthenia gravis. Der Nervenarzt 39:416-422.

43. Lapresle J, Fardeau, M 1965 Diagnostic histologique des atrophies et hypertrophies musculaire. Proceedings of the 8th International Congress of Neurology, Vienna 1965 Neuromuscular diseases p 47-66.

44. Kinoshita M, Nakazato H, Wakata N, Satoyoshi E 1982 Myasthenic neuromyopathy. European Neurology 21:5-58.

45. Oosterhuis H J G H, Bethlem J 1973 Neurogenic muscle involvement in myasthenia gravis. Journal of Neurology, Neurosurgery and Psychiatry 36:244-254.

46. Schimrigk K, Samland O 1977 Muskelatrophien bei Myasthenia gravis. Der Nervenarzt 48:65-68.

47. Simpson J A 1958 Evaluation of thymectomy in myasthenia gravis. Brain 81:112-145.

48. Uono M, Tanabe H, Nakao K 1970 Clinicopathological studies of myasthenia gravis with muscle atrophy. Advances in Neurological Science, Tokyo 14:485-491.

49. Kinnier Wilson S A 1940 Neurology, vol II, London, Edward Arnolds Co 1598.

50. Osserman K E, Genkins G 1971 Studies in myasthenia gravis: review of a twenty year experience in over 1200 patients. Mt. Sinai Journal of Medicine 38:497.

51. Besinger U A, Toyka K V, Heininger K, Fateh-Mogadam A, Schumm F, Sandel P, Birnberger K L 1981 Long-term correlation of clinical course and acetylcholine receptor antibody in patients with myasthenia gravis. Annuals of the New York Academy of Sciences 377, 812.

52. Mann J D, Johns T R, Campa J F 1976 Long-term administration of corticosteroids in myasthenia gravis. Neurology 26:729.

53. Gajdos Ph, Simon N, Rohan-Chabot P de, Rafael J C, Goulon M 1983 Effets à longterm des échanges plasmatiques au cours de la myasthénie. Presse Médicale 12:939.

54. Szobor A 1990 Myasthenia gravis. Akadémiai Kiadó, Budapest 147.

55. Oosterhuis H J G H 1984 Myasthenia gravis. Churchill Livingstone, Edinburgh.

56. Schumm F, Wiethölter H, Fateh-Moghadam A, Dichgans J 1985 Thymectomy in myasthenia gravis with pure ocular symptoms, Journal of Neurology, Neurosurgery and Psychiatry 48:332.

57. Oosterhuis H J G H 1981 Myasthenia gravis. A review. Clinical Neurology and Neurosurgery 83:105-135.

58. Grob D, Brunner N G, Namba T 1981 The natual course of myasthenia gravis and the effect of various therapeutic measures. Annals of the New York Academy of Sciences 377:652-669.

59. Oosterhuis H J G H 1977 Epidemiologie der Myasthenie in Amsterdam. In: Hertel G u A (ed) Myasthenia gravis, G Thieme, Berlin 103-108.

60. Oosterhuis H J G H 1981 Observations of the natural history of myasthenia gravis and the effect of thymectomy. Annals of the New York Academy of Sciences 377:678-689.

61. Kennedy F S, Moersch F P 1937 Myasthenia gravis. A clinical review of 87 cases observed between 1915 and the early part of 1932. Canadian Medical Association Journal 37:216-223.
62. Schwab R S, Leland C 1953 Sex and age in myasthenia gravis as critical factors in incidence and remission. Journal of the American Medical Association 153:1270-1273.
63. Osserman K E, Kornfeld P, Cohen E, Genkins G, Mendelow H, Goldberg H, Windsley H, Kaplan L I 1958 Studies in myasthenia gravis. A M A Archives of Internal medicine 102:72-81.
64. Plauché W C 1979 Myasthenia gravis in pregnancy: an up date. American Journal of Obstetrics and Gynaecology 135:691-697.
65. Pirskanen R 1981 Discussion to Oosterhuis H J G H: the natural history of myasthenia gravis. In: Satoyoshi E (ed) Myasthenia gravis, University of Tokyo Press, Tokyo 371.
66. Borenstein S, Demedt J E 1974 Temperature and weather correlates of myasthenia fatigue. Lancet II: 63-66.
67. Goldflam S 1893 Ueber einen scheinbar heilbaren bulbär paralytischen Symptomencomplex mit Beteiligung der Extremitäten. Deutsches Zeitschrift für Nervenheilkunde 4:312-352.
68. Guttman L 1980 Heat-induced myasthenic crises. Archives of Neurology 37:671-672.
69. Storm Mathisen A 1984 Epidemiology of myasthenia gravis in Norway. Acta Neurologica Scandinavica 70, 274.
70. Pirskanen R 1977 Genetic aspects in myasthenia gravis, a family study of 264 Finnish patients. Acta Neurologica Scandinavica 56:365.
71. Araki S, Uchino M, Kumamoto T 1987 Prevalence studies of multiple sclerosis, myasthenia gravis and myopathies in Kumamotodistrict, Japan, Neuroepidemiology 6:120.
72. Oosterhuis H J G H 1989 The natural course of myasthenia gravis: a longterm follow-up study. Journal of Neurology, Neurosurgery and Psychiatry 52:1121.
73. Skallebaek D, Kuks J B M, Oosterhuis H J G H 1997 Epidemiological investigation of myasthenia gravis in the three Northern Provinces of the Netherlands.
74. Giagheddu M, Puggioni G, Sanna G, Tamburini G, Marrosu F, Rachele M G, Murgia B, Rosati G 1989 Epidemiological study of myasthenia gravis in Sardinia, Italy. Acta Neurologica Scandinavica 79:326.
75. D'Alessandro R, Granieri E, Benassi G, Tola M R, Casmiro M, Mazzanti B, Gamberini G, Caniatti L 1991 Comparative study on the prevalence of myasthenia gravis in the provinces of Bologna and Ferrara, Italy. Acta Neurologica Scandinavica 2:83.
76. Somnier F E, Keiding N, Paulson 0 B 1991 Epidemiology of myasthenia gravis in Denmark, A longitudinal and comprehensive population survey. Archives of Neurology 48:733.

77. Sorensen T T, Holm E B 1989 Myasthenia gravis in the county of Viborg, Denmark. European Neurology 29:177.

78. Phillips L H, Torner J C, Anderson M S, Cox G M 1992 The epidemiology of myasthenia gravis in central and western Virginia, Neurology 42:1888-93.

79. Cohen M S 1987 Epidemiology of myasthenia gravis. Monographs in Allergy 21:246.

80. Mantegazza R, Beghi E, Pareyson D, Antozzi C, Peluchetti D, Sghirlanzoni A, Cosi V, Lombardi M, Piccolo G, Tonali P et al 1990 A multicentre follow-up study of 1152 patients with myasthenia gravis in Italy. Journal of Neurological Sciences 237, 339.

81. Grob D, Arsura E L, Brunner N G, Namba T 1987 The course of myasthenia gravis and therapies affecting outcome. Annals of the New York Academy of Sciences 505:472.

82. Fukuyama Y, Hirayama Y, Osawa M, 1981 Epidemiological and clinical features of childhood myasthenia gravis in Japan, in Myasthenia gravis. Japan Medical Research Foundation University of Tokyo Press, Tokyo p 19.

83. Hawkins B R, Yu Y L, Wong V, Woo E, Ip M S, Dawkins R L 1989 Possible evidence of a variant of myasthenia gravis based on HLA and acetylcholine receptor antibody in Chinese patients. Quarterly Journal of Medicine 70:235.

84. Thorlacius S, Aarli J A, Riise T, Matre R, Johnsen H J, 1989 Associated disorders in myasthenia gravis: autoimmune diseases and their relation to thymectomy. Acta Neurologica Scandinavica 80:290.

85. Beekman R, Kuks J B M, Oosterhuis H J G H 1997 Myasthenia gravis: diagnosis and follow-up of 100 consecutive patients. Journal of the Neurological Sciences 244:112-118.

86. Cohen M S, Younger D, 1981 Aspects of the natural history of myasthenia gravis: crisis and death. Annals of the New York Academy of Sciences 377:670.

87. Oosterhuis H J G H 1988 Longterm effects of treatment in 374 patients with myasthenia gravis. Monographs in Allergy 25, 75.

88. Wolf S M, Rowland L P, Schotland D L, McKinney A S, Hoefer P F A, Aranow H 1966 Myasthenia as an autoimmune disease; clinical aspects. Annals of the New York Academy of Sciences 135, 517.

89. Papatestas A E, Genkins G, Kornfeld P, Eisenkraft J B, Fagerstrom R P, Pozner, J, Aufses Jr A H 1987 Effects of thymectomy in myasthenia gravis. Annals of Surgery 206:79.

90. Keynes G 1955 Investigations into thymic disease and tumour formation. British Journal of Surgery XLII: 449.

91. Mulder D G, Herrmann Chr, Keesey J, Edwards H 1983 Thymectomy for myasthenia gravis. American Journal of Surgery 146:61.

92. Maggi G, Casadio C, Cavallo A, Cianci R, Molinatti M, Ruffini E 1989 Thymectomy in myasthenia gravis, Results of 662 cases operated upon in 15 years. European Journal of Cardiothoracic Surgery 3:504.

93. Evoli A, Batocchi A P, Provenzano C, Ricci E, Tonali P 1988 Thymectomy in the treatment of myasthenia gravis: report of 247 patients. Journal of the Neurological Sciences 235, 272.

94. Namba T, Brunner N G, Grob D 1978 Myasthenia gravis in patients with thymoma with particular reference to onset after thymectomy. Medicine 57:411.

95. Monden Y, Uyama T, Taniki T, Hashimoto J, Fujii Y, Nakahara K, Kawashima Y, Masaoka A 1988 The characteristics of thymoma with myasthenia gravis: a 28-year experience. Journal of Surgical Oncology 38:151.

96. Levasseur P, Menestrier M, Gaud C, Dartevelle P, Julia P, Rojas-Miranda A, Navajas M, Le Brigand H, Merlier M, 1988 Thymomes et maladies associées, A propos d'une serie de 255 thymomes operées. Revue Maladies de Respiration 5:178.

97. Slater G, Papatestas A E, Genkins G, Kornfeld P, Horowitz S H, Bender A 1978 Thymomas in patients with myasthenia gravis. Annals of Surgery 188:171.

98. Monden Y, Uyama T, Kimura S, Taniki T 1991 Extrathymic malignancy in patients with myasthenia gravis. European Journal on Cancer 27:745.

99. Simpson J A 1966 Myasthenia gravis as an autoimmune disease: clinical aspects,. Annals of the New York Academy of Sciences 135:506.

100. Downes J M, Greenwood B M, Wray S H, 1966 Autoimmune aspects of myasthenia gravis. Quarterly Journal of Medicine, New Series 35:85.

101. Hertel G, Ricker K, Schumm F, Fuchs P 1977 Begleitskrankheiten der Myasthenie. In: Myasthenia Gravis, Hertel G, Mertens H G, Ricker K, Schimrigk K, Eds. George Thieme Verlag, Stuttgart 127.

102. Goulon M, Gadjos P, Estournet B, Andre C, Tulliez M 1980 Myasthénie et maladies associées: étude d'une serie de 145 cas. Annales de Medicine Interne 131:9.

103. Scherbaum W A, Schumm F, Maisch B, Müller C, Fateh-Moghadam A, Flüchter S H, Seif F J, Bottazzo G F, Berg P A, 1983 Myasthenia gravis: overlap with "polyendocrine autoimmunity". Klinisches Wochenschrift 61:509.

104. Thorlacius S, Aarli J A, Riise T, Matre R, Johnsen H J 1989 Associated disorders in myasthenia gravis: autoimmune diseases and their relation to thymectomy. Acta Neurologica Scandivica 80:290.

105. Monden Y, Uyama T, Nakahara K, Fujii Y, Hashimoto J, Ohno K, Masaoka A, Kawashima Y 1986 Clinical characteristics and prognosis of myasthenia gravis with other autoimmune diseases. Annals of Thoracic Surgery 41:189.

106. Christensen P B, Jensen T S, Tsiropoulos I, Sørensen T, Kjaer M, Højer-Pedersen E, Rasmussen M J K, Lehfeldt E 1995 Associated autoimmune diseases in myasthenia gravis. Acta Neurologica Scandinavica 91:192-195.

107. Tola M R, Caniatti L M, Casetta I et al 1994 Immunogenic heterogeneity and associated autoimmune disorders in myasthenia gravis: a population-based survey in the province of Ferrara, Northern Italy. Acta Neurologica Scandinavica 90:318-323.

108. Furszyfer J, Kurland L T, McConahey W M, Elveback L R 1970 Grave's disease in Olmsted county, Minnesota, 1935 through 1967. Proceedings of the Mayo Clinics 45:636.

109. Nyström E, Bengtsson C, Lindquist O, Lundberg S, Lindstedt G, Lundberg P A, 1984 Serum triiodothyronine and hyperthyroidism in a population sample of women. Clinical Endocrinology 20, 31.

110. Ohno M, Hamada N, Yamakawa J, Noh J, Morii H, Ito K 1987 Myasthenia gravis associated with Grave's disease in Japan, Japanese Journal of Medicine 26:2.

111. Bucknall R C, Dixon A S J, Glick E N, Woodland J, Zutshi D W 1975 Myasthenia gravis associated with penicillamine treatment for rheumatoid arthritis. British Medical Journal 1:600.

112. Albers J W, Hodach R J, Kimmel D W, Tracy W L 1980 Penicillamine associated myasthenia gravis. Neurology 30:1246.

113. Dawkins R L, Christiansen F T, Garlepp M J 1981 Autoantibodies and HLA antigens in ocular, generalised and penicillamine-induced myasthenia gravis. Annals of the New York Academy of Sciences 377, 372.

114. Seitz D, Fischer K, Hopf H C, Janzen R W C, Meyer W 1977 D-penicillamine-induzierte Myasthenie bei chronischer Polyarthritis, in Myasthenia Gravis. Hertel, G., Mertens, H. G., Ricker K., and Schimrigk, K., Eds, George Thieme Verlag, Stuttgart 162.

115. Mizon J P, Morcamp D, Lefebre P, Froissart M, Guidicelli C P, Goasguen J, 1979 Les associations myasthénie-lupus erythémateux disséminé, A propos de deux observations avec revue complète de la literature. Annales de Médicine Interne 130:489.

116. Turner J W, 1974 Myasthenia gravis, Proc. R. Soc. Med. 67:763.

117. Martin R W, Shah A 1991 Myasthenia gravis coexistent with Crohn's disease. J. Clinical Gastroenterology 13:112.

118. Noguchi S, Nishitani H 1976 Immunologic studies of a case of myasthenia gravis associated with pemphigus vulgaris after thymectomy. Neurology 26:1075.

119. Dumas P, Archambeaud-Mouveroux F, Vallat J M, Barussaud D, Hugon J, Dumas M 1985 Myasthenia gravis associated with adrenocortical insufficiency, report of two cases. Journal of the Neurological Sciences 232:354.

120. Bosch E P, Reith P E, Cranner D K 1977 Myasthenia gravis and Schmidt Syndrome. Neurology 27:1179.

121. Jansen P H, Renier W O, Vaan de G, Reekers P, Vingerhoets D M, Gabreels F. J, 1987 Effect of thymectomy on myasthenia gravis and autoimmune thrombocytopenic purpura in a 13-year-old girl. European Journal of Pediatry 146:587.

122. Veenhoven W A, Oosterhuis H J G H, Schans G S van der 1979 Myasthenia gravis and Werlhof's disease. Acta Medica Scandinavica 206:131-135.

123. Kuki S, Morgan R L, Tucci J R 1981 Myasthenia gravis and premature ovarian failure. Archives of Internal Medicine 141:1230.

124. Bayne L 1990 Primary ovarian failure: a rare autoimmune presentation of myasthenia gravis, Neurology, Suppl. 1: 349.

125. Oh S J, Dwyer D S, Bradley R J 1987 Overlap myasthenic syndrome: combined myasthenia gravis and Eaton-Lambert syndrome. Neurology 37:1411.
126. Taphoorn M J, Van Duijn H, Wolters E C 1988 A neuromuscular transmission disorder: combined myasthenia gravis and Lambert-Eaton syndrome in one patient, Journal of Neurology, Neurosurgery and Psychiatry 51:880.
127. Brenna A, Curzo N, d'Urso D, d'Avanzo F, 1989 A neuromuscular transmission disorder: combined myasthenia gravis and Lambert-Eaton syndrome in one patient. Journal of Neurology, Neurosurgery and Psychiatry 52:684.
128. Spalek P, Orolin D, Lisy L 1989 Immunosuppressive drug treatment in overlap myasthenic syndrome: combined myasthenia gravis and Lambert-Eaton myasthenic syndrome. In: Neurology in Europe I, Bartko D, Gerstenbrand F, Turcani P, Eds. John Libbey & Co 603.
129. Newsom-Davis J, Leys K, Vincent A, Ferguson I, Modi G, Mills K 1991 Immunological evidence for the co-existence of the Lambert-Eaton myasthenic syndrome and myasthenia gravis in two patients. Journal of Neurology, Neurosurgery and Psychiatry 54:452.
130. Brown A C, Crounse R G, Winkelmann R K 1969 Generalised hair-follicle hamartoma associated with alopecia, aminoaciduria and myasthenia gravis, Archives of Dermatology 99:478.
131. Ridley C M, Smith N 1981 Generalized hair-follicle hamartoma associated with alopecia and myasthenia gravis; report of a second case, Clinical Experimental Dermatology 6:283.
132. Starink Th M, Lane E B, Meyer Ch J L M, 1986 Generalized trichoepitheliomas with alopecia and myasthenia gravis: clinicopathologic immunohistochemical study and comparison with classic and desmoplastic trichoepithelioma. Journal of the American Academy on Dermatology 15:1104.
133. Satoyoshi E, Kinoshita M, Nakazato H, Saku A 1975 Combination of myasthenia gravis and multiple sclerosis, Rinsho Shinheigaku (Clinical Neurology) 15:888.
134. Somer H, Mueller K, Kinnunen E 1989 Myasthenia gravis associated with multiple sclerosis. Epidemiological survey and immunological findings. Journal of the Neurological Sciences 89:37.
135. Namba T, Brunner N G, Brown S B, Muguruma M Grob D 1971 Familial myasthenia gravis. Archives of Neurology 25, 49.
136. Szobor A 1989 Myasthenia gravis: familial occurrence, a study of 1100 myasthenia gravis patients, Acta Medica Hungarica 46:13.
137. Behan P O 1980 Immune disease and HLA association with myasthenia gravis. Journal of Neurology, Neurosurgery and Psychiatry 43:611.
138. Strickroot F L, Schaeffer R L, Bergo H E 1942 Myasthenia gravis occurring in an infant born of a myasthenic mother. Journal of the American Medical Association 120:1207-1209.
139. Namba T, Brown S B, Grob D 1970 Neonatal myasthenia gravis: report of two cases and review of the literature. Pediatrics 45:488-504.
140. Branch C E, Swift Th R, Dijken P R 1978 Prolonged neonatal myasthenia gravis: electrophysiological studies. Annals of Neurology 3:416-418.

141. Teng P, Osserman K E 1956 Neonatal and juvenile type. Report of 21 cases and a review of 188 cases. Journal of the Mount Sinai Hospital 23:711-727.

142. Oosterhuis H J G H, Feltkamp T E W, Geld H W R van der 1966 Muscle antibodies in myasthenic mothers and their babies. Lancet II: 1226-1227.

143. Vollmer A C, Landolt R F, Kristaly S Z, Grob P J 1971 Myasthenia gravis neonatorum transitoria mit Nachweis muskelspezifischer Antikörper. Schweizerische Medizinische Wochenschrift 101:1052-1054.

144. Donaldson J O, Penn A S, Lisak R P, Abramsky O, Brenner T, Schotland D L 1981 Antiacetylcholine receptor antibody in neonatal myasthenia gravis. American Journal of Diseases of Children 135:222-226.

145. Keesey J, Lindstrom J M, Cokely H, Herrmann C 1977 Antiacetylcholine receptor antibody in neonatal myasthenia gravis. New England Journal of Medicine 296:55.

146. Lindstrom J M, Seybold M E, Lennon V A, Whittingham S, Duane D D 1976 Antibody to acetylcholine receptor in myasthenia gravis. Neurology 26:1054-1059.

147. Eymard B, Vernet-der Garabedian B, Berrih-Aknin S, Pannier C, Bach J F, Morel E, 1991 Anti-acetylcholine receptor antibodies in neonatal myasthenia gravis: heterogeneity and pathogenic significance. Journal Autoimmunity 4:185-95.

148. Ohta M, Matsubara P, Hayashi K, Nakao K, Nishitani H 1981 Acetylcholine receptor antibodies in infants of mothers with myasthenia gravis. Neurology 31:1019-1022.

149. Brenner T, Beyth Y, Abramsky O 1980 Inhibitory effect of alpha-fetoprotein on the binding of myasthenia gravis antibody to acetylcholine receptor. Proceedings of the National Academy of Sciences of the USA 77:3635-3639.

150. Lefvert A K, Osterman P O 1982 Newborn infants to myasthenic mothers: a clinical study and an investigation of acetylcholine receptor antibodies in 17 children. Annals of Neurology 33:133-138.

151. Vernet-der Garabedian B, Lacokova M, Eymard B, Morel E, Faltin M, Zajac J, Sadovsky O, Dommergues M, Tripon P, Back J-F 1994 Association of neonatal myasthenia gravis with antibodies against fetal acetylcholine receptor. Journal of Clinical Investigation 94:555-559.

152. Bowman J R 1948 Myasthenia gravis in young children. Pediatrics, I, 472-7.

153. Engel A G 1994 Congenital Myasthenic Syndromes, Neurologic Clinics of North America 12:401-437.

154. Mora M, Lambert E H, Engel A G 1987 Synaptic vesicle abnormality in familial infantile myasthenia. Neurology 37:206.

155. Engel A G, Lambert E H, Mulder D M et al 1982 A newly recognised congenital myasthenic syndrome attributed to a prolonged open time of the acetylcholine-induced ion channel. Annuals of Neurology, 11:53.

156. Oosterhuis H J G H, Newsom-Davis J, Wokke J H J Molenaar P C, Weerden T van, Oen B S, Jennekens F G I, Veldman H, Vincent A, Wray D W, Prior C, Murray N M F 1987 The slow channel syndrome: Two new cases. Brain 110:1061.

157. Chauplannas G, Bady B 1994 Syndromes myasthéniques héréditaires à révélation tardive. Revue Neurologique (Paris) 150:142-148.
158. Smit L M E, Barth P G 1980 Arthrogryposis multiplex congenita due to congenital myasthenia. Developmental Medicine and Child Neurology 22:371-374.
159. Smit L M E, Hageman G, Veldman H, Molenaar P C, Oen B S, Jennekens F G I 1988 A myasthenic syndrome with congenital paucity of synaptic clefts: CPSC syndrome. Muscle Nerve 11:337-348.
160. Conomy J P, Levinsohn M, Fanaroff A 1975 Familial infantile myasthenia gravis, a case of sudden death in young children. Journal of Pediatrics 87:428-429.
161. Hart Z, Sahashi K, Lambert E H, Engel A G, Lindstrom J M 1979 A congenital familial myasthenic syndrome caused by a presynaptic defect of transmitter resynthesis or mobilization. Neurology 29:556-557.
162. Robertson W C, Chun R W M, Kornguth S E 1980 Familial infantile myasthenia. Archives of Neurology 37:117-119.
163. Seybold M E, Lindstrom J M 1981 Myasthenia gravis in infancy. Neurology 31:476-480.
164. Walls T J, Engel A G, Nagel A S Harper C M, Trastek V F 1993 Congenital myasthenic syndrome associated with paucity of synaptic vesicles and reduced quantal release. Annals of the New York Academy of Sciences 681:461.
165. Bady B, Chauplannaz G, Carrier H 1987 Congenital Lambert-Eaton myasthenic syndrome. Journal of Neurology, Neurosurgery and Psychiatry 50:476.
166. Vincent A, Newson-Davis J, Wray D, Shillito P, Harrison J, Betty M, Beeson D, Mills K, Palace J, Molenaar P C, Murray N 1993 Clinical and experimental observations in patients with congenital myasthenic syndromes. Annals of the New York Academy of Sciences, 681:451-460.
167. Engel A G, Lambert E H, Gomex M R 1977 A new myasthenic syndrome with end-plate acetylcholinesterase deficiency, small nerve terminals, and reduced acetylcholine release. Annals of Neurology 1:315.
168. Hutchinson D O, Engel A G, Walls T J, Nakano S, Camp S, Taylor P, Harper C M, Brengman J M 1993 The spectrum of congenital end-plate acetylcholinesterase deficiency. Annals of the New York Academy of Sciences 681:469-486.
169. Jennekens F G I, Hesselmans F G M, Veldman H, Jansen E N H, Spaans F, Molenaar P C 1992 Deficiency of acetylcholine receptors in a case of end-plate acetylcholinesterase deficiency: a histochemical investigation. Muscle Nerve 15:63-72.
170. Wokke J H J, Jennekens F G I, Molenaar P C, Oord C J M van den, Oen B S, Busch H F M 1989 Congenital paucity of secondary synaptic clefts (CPSC) syndrome in 2 adult sibs. Neurology 39:648-654.
171. Engel A G, Hutchinson D O, Nakano S, Murphy L, Griggs R C, Gu Y, Hall Z W, Lindstrom J 1993 Myasthenic syndromes attributed to mutation affecting the epsilon subunit of the acetylcholine receptor. Annals of the New York Academy of Sciences 681:497-508.

172. Nagel A, Engel A G, Walls T J, Harper C M, Waisburg H A 1993 Congenital end-plate acetylcholine receptor deficiency and short channel open time. Annals of the New York Academy of Sciences 681:509-14.

173. Engel A G, Uchitel O, Walls T J, Nagel A, Harper C M, Bodensteiner J, 1993 Newly recognized congenital myasthenic syndrome associated with high conductance and fast closure of the acetylcholine receptor channel. Annals of Neurology 34:38-47.

174. Uchitel O, Engel A G, Walls T J et al 1993 Congenital myasthenic syndromes: II. A syndrome attributed to abnormal interaction of acetylcholine with its receptor. Muscle Nerve 16:1293.

175. McQuillen M P 1966 Familial limb-girdle myasthenia. Brain 89:121.

176. Goldhammer Y, Blatt I, Sadeh M 1990 Congenital myasthenia associated with facial malformations in Iraqi and Iranian Jews. Brain 113:1291-1306.

177. Palace J, Wiles C M, Newsom-Davis J 1991 Diaminopyridine in the treatment of congenital (hereditary) myasthenia. Journal of Neurology, Neurosurgery and Psychiatry 54:1069-1072.

178. Gomez Ch, Maselli R, Gammack J, Lasalde J, Tamamizu S, Cornblath D R, Lehar M, McNamee M, Kuncl R W 1996 A beta-subunit mutation in the acetylcholine receptor channel gate causes severe Slow-Channel syndrome. Annals of Neurology 39:712-23.

179. Millichap J G, Dodge Ph R 1960 Diagnosis and treatment of myasthenia gravis in infancy, childhood and adolescence: a study of 51 patients. Neurology 10:1007-1014.

180. Szobor A, Mattyus A, Molnar J, 1988-89 Myasthenia gravis in childhood and adolescence. Report on 209 patients and review of the literature. Acta Paediatrica Hungarica 29:299-312.

181. Batocchi A P, Evoli A, Palmisani M T, Lo Monaco M, Bartoccioni M, Tonali P 1990 Early-onset myasthenia gravis: clinical characteristics and response to therapy. European Journal of Pediatrics 150:66-68.

182. Wong V, Hawkins B R, Yu Y L 1992 Myasthenia gravis in Hong Kong Chinese. Acta Neurologica Scandinavica 86:68-72.

183. Bastedo D L A 1950 Acute fulminating myasthenia gravis in children. Canadian Medical Association Journal 63:388-389.

184. Biemond A, Trotsenburg L V 1955 Over congenitale en infantiele myasthenie. Maandschrift voor Kindergeneeskunde 23:155-164.

185. Andrews P I, Massey J M, Sanders D B 1993 Acetylcholine receptor antibodies in juvenile myasthenia gravis. Neurology 43:977-982.

186. Alvarez G 1980 Bell's phenomenon in normal adults and in Parkinson's disease. Acta Neurologica Scandinavica 62:127-131.

187. Baptista A G, Silva E, Souza H 1961 Pupillary abnormalities in myasthenia gravis. Neurology 11:210-213.

188. Herishami Y, Lavy S 1971 Internal ophthalmoplegia in myasthenia gravis. Ophthalmologica 163:302-305.

189. Lepore F E, Sanborn G E, Slevin J 1979 Pupillary dysfunction in myasthenia gravis. Annals of Neurology 6:29-33.
190. Yamazaki A, Ishikawa S 1976 Abnormal pupillary responses in myasthenia gravis. British Journal of Ophthalmology 60:575-580.
191. Molbech S, Johansen S H 1969 Endurance time in static work during partial curarization. Journal of Applied Physiology 27:44-48.
192. Campbell E J M, Edwards R H T, Hill D K, Jones D A, Sykes M K 1977 Perception of effort during partial curarization. Journal of Physiology 263:186-187.
193. Zwarts M J, Van Weerden T W, Haenen H T M 1987 Relationship between average muscle fibre conduction velocity and EMG power spectra during isometric contraction, recovery and applied ischemia. European Journal of Applied Physiology 56:212-216.

Chapter 3

1. Jankovic J, Patten B M 1987 Blepharospasm and autoimmune diseases. Movement Disorders 2:159-63.
2. Beekman R, Kuks J B M, Oosterhuis H J G H, 1997 Myasthenia gravis: diagnosis and follow-up of 100 consecutive patients. Journal of Neurology, 244:112-118.
3. Oh S J, Kurioglu R 1992 Chronic limb girdle myasthenia gravis. Neurology 42:1153.
4. Azulay J Ph, Pouget J, Figarella-Branger D, Colamarino R, Pellissier J-F, Serratrice G 1994 Faiblaisse musculaire proximale isolé révélatrice d'un syndrome myasthénique. Revue Neurologique (Paris) 150:377-381.
5. Ploeg R J O van der, Oosterhuis H J G H, Reuvekamp J 1984 Measuring muscle strength. Journal of Neurology 231:200.
6. Nicklin J, Karni Y, and Wiles C M 1987 Shoulder abduction fatiguability, Journal of Neurology, Neurosurgery and Psychiatry 50:423.
7. Ploeg R J O van der, Fidler V, Oosterhuis H J G H 1991 Hand-held myometry: reference values, Journal of Neurology, Neurosurgery and Psychiatry 54:244.
8. Viets H R, Schwab R S 1935 Prostigmin in the diagnosis of myasthenia gravis. New English Journal of Medicine 213:1280.
9. Viets H R, Schwab R S 1955 Problems in the diagnosis of myasthenia gravis, a 20 year report of the neostigmine test. Trans. Am. Neurol. Assoc. 80:36.
10. Osserman K E, Kaplan L I 1952 Rapid diagnostic test for myasthenia gravis: increased muscle strength without fasciculations after intravenous administration of edrophonium (Tensilon) chloride. Journal of the American Medical Association 150:265.
11. Osserman K E, Genkins G 1966 Critical reappraisal of the use of edrophonium (Tensilon) chloride tests in myasthenia gravis and significance of clinical classification. Annals of the New York Academy of Sciences 135:312.

12. Magyar P, Szathamary I, Szobor A 1979 Myasthenia gravis: lung function studies without and with edrophonium chloride. Eur. Neurol. 18:59.

13. Dijk J L van, Florence L 1980 The tensilon-test: a safe office procedure. Ophthalmology 87:210.

14. Nicholson G A, Mcleod J G, Griffiths L R 1983 Comparison of diagnostic tests in myasthenia gravis. Clinical and Experimental Neurology 19:45.

15. Oosterhuis H J G H, Kuks J B M 1991 The diagnosis of myasthenia gravis. A mathematical approach. Journal of Autoimmunity 4, XX.

16. Philips L H 2nd, Melnick P A 1990 Diagnosis of myasthenia gravis in the 1990s. Seminars in Neurology 10:62.

17. Evoli A, Tonali P, Bartoccioni E, Lo Monaco M 1988 Ocular myasthenia: diagnostic and therapeutic problems. Acta Neurologica Scandinavica 77:31.

18. Schwab R S, Perlo V P 1966 Syndromes simulating myasthenia gravis. Annals of the New York Academy of Sciences 135:350.

19. Mulder D W, Lambert E H, Eaton L M 1959 Myasthenic syndrome in patients with amyotrophic lateral sclerosis. Neurology 9:627.

20. Cherington M 1974 Botulism. Ten-year experience. Archives of Neurology 30:432.

21. Oh S J, Cho H K 1990 Edrophonium responsiveness not necessarily diagnostic of myasthenia gravis. Muscle Nerve 13:187.

22. O'Neill J H, Murray N M, Newsom-Davis J 1988 The Lambert-Eaton myasthenic syndrome. A review of 50 cases. Brain 111:577.

23. Dirr L Y, Donofrio P D, Patton J F, Troost B T 1989 A false-positive edrophonium test in a patient with a brainstem glioma. Neurology 39:865.

24. Moorthy G, Behrens M M, Drachman D B, Kirkham T H, Knox D L, Miller N R, Slamovitz T L, Zinreich S J 1989 Ocular pseudomyasthenia or ocular myasthenia 'plus': a warning to clinicians. Neurology 39:1150.

25. Lindstrom J 1977 An essay for antibodies to human acetylcholine receptor in serum from patients with myasthenia gravis. Clinical Immunology Immunopathology 7:36.

26. Le Forrestier N, Gherardi R K, Meyrignac C, Annane D, Marsac C, Gray F, Gajdos P 1995 Myasthenic symptoms in patients with mitochondrial myopathies. Muscle Nerve 18, 1338-1340.

27. Miller N R, Morris J E, Maquire M 1982 Combined use of neostigmine and ocular motility in the diagnosis of myasthenia gravis. Ophthalmology 100:761-763.

28. Lindstrom J M, Seybold M E, Lennon B A, Whittingham S, Duane D D 1976 Antibody to acetylcholine receptor in myasthenia gravis. Neurology 26:1054.

29. Lefvert A K, Bergström K, Matell G, Osterman P O, Pirskanen R 1978 Determination of acetylcholine receptor in myasthenia gravis: clinical usefulness and pathogenetic implication. Journal of Neurology, Neurosurgery and Psychiatry 41:394.

30. Limburg P C, The H, Hummel-Tappel E, Oosterhuis H J G H 1983 Anti-acetylcholine receptor antibodies in myasthenia gravis. Their relation to the clinical state and the effect of therapy. Journal of the Neurological Sciences 58:357.

31. Toyka K V, Heiniger K 1986 Acetylcholin-Rezeptor-Antikörper in der Diagnostik der Myasthenia gravis. Deutsches Medisches Wochenschrift 111:1435.

32. Vincent A, Newsom-Davis J 1985 Acetylcholine receptor antibody as a diagnostic test for myasthenia gravis: results in 153 validated cases and 2967 diagnostic essays. Journal of Neurology, Neurosurgery and Psychiatry 48:246.

33. Somnier F E 1993 Clinical implementation of anti-acetylcholine receptor antibodies. Journal of Neurology, Neurosurgery and Psychiatry 56: 496-504.

34. Soliven B C, Lange D J, Penn A S, Younger D, Jaretzki 3rd A, Lovelace R E, Rowland L P 1988 Seronegative myasthenia gravis. Neurology 38:514.

35. Massey J M, Sanders D B, Howard J F 1990 Sensitivity of diagnostic tests in myasthenia gravis. Neurology 40:348.

36. Newsom-Davis J, Willcox N, Schluep M, Harcourt G, Vincent A, Mossman S, Wray D, Burges J 1987 Immunological heterogeneity and cellular mechanisms in myasthenia gravis. Annals of the New York Academy of Sciences 505:12.

37. Evoli A, Bartoccioni E, Batocchi A P, Scuderi F, Tonali P 1989 Anti-AChR-negative myasthenia gravis: clinical and immunological features. Clin. Invest. Med. 12:104.

38. Oosterhuis H J G H, Limburg P C, Hummel-Tappel E, The T H 1983 Anti-acetylcholine receptor antibodies in myasthenia gravis: clinical and serological follow-up of individual patients. Journal of the Neurological Sciences 58:371.

39. Vincent A, Newsom-Davis J, Newton P, Beck N 1983 Acetylcholine receptor antibody and clinical response to thymectomy in myasthenia gravis. Neurology, 33:1276.

40. Hohlfield R, Toyka K V, Besinger U A, Gerhold B, Heiniger K 1985 Myasthenia gravis: reactivation of clinical disease and of autoimmune factors after discontinuation of long-term azathioprine. Annals of Neurology 17:238.

41. Drachman D B, Adams R N, Josifek L F 1982 Functional activities of auto-antibodies to acetylcholine receptors and the clinical severity of myasthenia gravis. New English Journal of Medicine 307:769.

42. Besinger U A, Toyka K V, Hömberg M, Heiniger K, Hohlfeld R, Fateh-Moghadam A 1983 Myasthenia gravis: long-term correlation of binding and bungarotoxin blocking antibodies against acetylcholine receptors with changes in disease severity. Neurology 33:1316.

43. Howard F M Jr, Lennon V A, Finley J, Matsumoto J, Elveback L R 1987 Clinical correlations of antibodies that bind, block, or modulate human acetylcholinereceptors in myasthenia gravis. Annals of the New York Academy of Sciences 505, 526.

43a. Morel E, Vernet-der Garabedian B, Eymard B, Raimond F, Bustarret F A, Bach J F 1988 Binding and blocking antibodies to the human acetylcholine receptor: are they selected in various myasthenia gravis forms? Immunological Research 7:212-7.

44. Eymard B, Vernet-der Garabedian B, Berrih-Aknin S 1991 Anti-acetylcholine receptor antibodies in neonatal myasthenia gravis: heterogeneity and pathogenic significance. Journal of Autoimmunity 4:185.

45. Oda K, Shibasaki H 1988 Antigenic difference of acetylcholine receptor between single and multiple form endplates of human extraocular muscle. Brain Research 449:337.

46. Garlepp M J, Dawkins F L, Christiansen F T 1983 HLA-antigens and acetylcholine receptor antibodies in penicillamine induced myasthenia gravis. British Medical Journal 286, 338.

47. Sundewall A C, Lefvert A K, Olsson R 1984 Antibodies against the acetylcholine receptor in primary biliary cirrhosis. Acta Neurologica Scandinavica 69:202.

48. Ohta M, Ohta K, Mori F, Itoh N, Nashitani H, Hayashi K 1990 Improved radio assay of anti-acetylcholine receptor antibody: application for the detection of extremely low titers in sera from patients with myasthenia gravis. Clinical Chemistry 36:911-913.

49. Garlepp M J, Kay P H, Dawkins R L 1982 The diagnostic significance of auto-antibodies to the acetylcholine receptor. Journal of Neuroimmunology 3:337.

50. Lefvert A K, Bjoerkholm M 1987 Antibodies against the acetylcholine receptor in hematologic disorders: implications for the development of myasthenia gravis after bone marrow grafting. New English Journal of Medicine 317:170.

51. Tanaka M, Miyatake T 1983 Anti-acetylcholine receptor antibody in aged individuals and in patients with Down's Syndrome. J. Immunol. 4:17.

52. Robb S A, Vincent A, McGregor M A, McGregor A M, Newsom-Davis J M 1985 Acetylcholine receptor antibodies in the elderly and in Down Syndrome. Journal of Neuroimmunology 9:139.

53. Lieberman J A, Bradley R J, Rubinstein M, Kane J M 1984 Antibodies to acetylcholine receptors in tardive dyskinesia. Lancet 1, 1066.

54. Pirskanen R, Lefvert A K, Matell G, Nilsson B Y, Smith C I E, Svanborg E 1984 Muscle function, SFEMG, receptor antibodies and HLA in relatives of myasthenia gravis patients. Acta Neurologica Scandinavica 69:214.

55. Pascuzzi R M, Phillips L H, John T R, Lennon B A 1988 The prevalence of electrophysiology and serologic abnormalities in asymptomatic relatives of patients with myasthenia gravis. Neurology 38:125.

56. Hara H, Hayachi K, Ohta K, Itoh N, Nishitani H, Ohta M 1993 Detection and characterization of blocking-type anti-acetylcholine receptor antibodies in sera from patients with myasthenia gravis. Clinical Chemistry 39:2053-2057.

57. Desmedt J E, Borenstein S 1976 Diagnosis of myasthenia gravis by nerve stimulation. Annals of the New York Academy of Sciences 274:174.

58. Ozdemir C, Young R R 1976 The results to be expected from electrical testing in the diagnosis of myasthenia gravis. Annals of the New York Academy of Sciences 274:203.

59. Stalberg E 1980 Clinical electrophysiology in myasthenia gravis. Journal of Neurology, Neurosurgery and Psychiatry 43:622.

60. Keesey J C 1989 Electrodiagnostic approach to defects of neuromuscular transmission. Muscle Nerve 12:613.

61. Borenstein S, Desmedt J E 1975 Local cooling in myasthenia: improvement of neuromuscular failure. Archives of Neurology 32:152.

62. Ricker K, Hertel G, Stodieck S 1977 Influence of temperature on neuromuscular transmission in myasthenia gravis. Journal of the Neurological Sciences 216, 273.

63. Desmedt J E, Borenstein S 1977 Double step nerve stimulation test for myasthenic block: sensitization of postactivation exhaustion by ischemia. Annals of Neurology 1:55.

64. Gilchrist J M, Sanders D B 1987 Double-step repetitive stimulation in myasthenia gravis. Muscle Nerve 10:233.

65. Botello S Y, Deaterly Ch, Comroe J H 1952 EMG from orbicularis oculi in normal persons and in patients with myasthenia gravis. American Medical Association Archives of Neurology and Psychiatry 67:348.

66. Schumm F, Stöhr M 1984 Accessory nerve stimulation in the assessment of myasthenia gravis. Muscle Nerve 7:147.

67. Mier A, Brophy C, Moxham J, Green M 1992 Repetitive stimulation of phrenic nerves in myasthenia gravis. Thorax 47:640-644.

68. Scopetta C, Casali C, d'Agostini S, La Cesa I, Parisi L 1990 Repetitive stimulation in myasthenia gravis: decrementing response revealed by anticholinesterase drugs. Electroencephalographic Clinical Neurophysiology 75:122.

69. Bernstein L P, Antel J P 1981 Motor neuron disease: decremental responses to repetitive nerve stimulation. Neurology 31:202.

70. Denijs E H, Forbes F H 1979 Amyotrophic lateral sclerosis: impairment of neuromuscular transmission. Archives of Neurology 36:202.

71. Aminoff M J, Layzu R B, Satya-Murti S, Faden A I 1977 The declining electrical response of muscle to repetitive nerve stimulation in myotonia. Neurology, 27:812.

72. Eaton L M, Lambert E L 1957 Electromyography and electric stimulation of nerves in diseases of the motor unit: Observations on myasthenic syndrome associated with malignant tumors. Journal of the American Medical Association 162:1117.

73. Lambert E H, Rooke E D, Eaton L M, Hodgson C H 1961 Myasthenic syndrome occasionally associated with bronchial neoplasm: neurophysiological studies. In: Myasthenia Gravis, Viets H R, Ed, Charlie C Thomas, Springfield, 362.

74. Ekstedt J 1964 Human single muscle fiber action potentials. Acta Physiologica Scandinavica 226:61.

75. Stålberg E, Trontelj J V 1994 Single fibre electromyography, 2nd Edition. Raven Press New York, 158-177.
76. Trontelj J V, Khuraibet A, Mihelin M 1988 The jitter in stimulated orbicularis oculi muscle: technique and normal values. Journal of Neurology, Neurosurgery and Psychiatry 51:814.
77. Sanders D B, Howard J F Jr 1986 Single-fiber electromyography in myasthenia gravis. Muscle Nerve 9:809.
78. Jabre J F, Chirico-Post J, Weiner M 1989 Stimulation SFEMG in myasthenia gravis. Muscle Nerve 12:38.
79. Emeryk B, Rowinska-Marcinska K, Nowak-Michalska T 1990 Pseudoselectivity of the neuromuscular block in ocular myasthenia: a SFEMG study. Electromyographic Clinical Neurophysiology 30, 53.
80. Oey P L, Wieneke G H, Hoogenraad T U, Huffelen A C van 1993 Ocular myasthenia gravis: the diagnostic yield of repetitive nerve stimulation and stimulated single fibre EMG of orbicularis oculi muscle and infrared reflection oculography. Muscle Nerve 16:142-149.
81. Thiele B, Stalberg E 1975 Single fiber EMG findings in polyneuropathies of different aetiology. Journal of Neurology, Neurosurgery and Psychiatry 38:881.
82. Komishi T, Nishitani H, Motomura S 1982 Single fiber electromyography in chronic renal failure. Muscle Nerve 5:458.
83. Thurston S E, Phillips L H II 1984 Disorder of neuromuscular transmission in a peripheral neuropathy. Muscle Nerve 7:495.
84. Krendel D A, Sanders D B, Massey J M 1985 Single fiber electromyography in chronic progressive external ophthalmoplegia. Muscle Nerve 8:624.
85. Weir S, Hansen S, Ballantyne J P 1979 Single Fibre Electromyographic jitter in multiple sclerosis. Journal of Neurology, Neurosurgery and Psychiatry 42:1146.
86. Jamal G A, Hansen S 1985 Electrophysiological studies in the post-viral fatigue syndrome. Journal of Neurology, Neurosurgery and Psychiatry 48:691.
87. Stålberg E, Trontelj J, Schwartz M 1976 Single fibre recording of the jitter phenomenon in patients with myasthenia gravis and in members of their families. Annals of the New York Academy of Sciences 274:189.
88. Pirskanen R, Bergström K, Hammerström L, Knuttson E, Lefvert A K, Matell G, Nilsson B Y, Smith C I E 1981 Neuromuscular safety margin: genetical, immunological and electrophysiological determinants in relatives of myasthenic patients. Annals of the New York Academy of Sciences 377:606.
89. Geld H van der, Feltkamp T E W, Oosterhuis H J G H 1964 Reactivity of myasthenia gravis serum - globulin with skeletal muscle and thymus demonstrated by immunofluorescence. Proceedings of the Society for Experimental Biology 115:782-785.
90. Feltkamp T E W, Berg-Loonen P M van der, Nijenhuis L E, Engelfriet C P, Loghem J J van, Rossum A L van, Oosterhuis H J G H 1974 Myasthenia gravis, auto antibodies and HLA antigens. British Medical Journal I: 131-133.

91. Oosterhuis H J G H, Feltkamp T E W, Geld H W R van der 1967 Studies in myasthenia gravis, part II. The relations of some clinical and immunological data. Journal of the Neurological Sciences 4:417-434.

92. Limburg P C, The H, Hummel-Tappel E, Oosterhuis H J G H 1983 Anti acetylcholine receptor antibodies in myasthenia gravis. I. Their relation to the clinical state and the effect of therapy. Journal of the Neurological Sciences 58:357-370.

93. Kuks J B M, Limburg P C, Horst G, Oosterhuis H J G H 1993 Antibodies to skeletal muscle in myasthenia gravis, part 3. Relation with clinical course and therapy. Journal of the Neurological Sciences 120:168-173.

94. Ohta M, Itoh M, Hara H, Itoh N, Nishitani H, Hayashi K, Ohta K 1991 Anti-skeletal muscle and anti-acetylcholine receptor antibodies in patients with thymoma without myasthenia gravis: relation to the onset of myasthenia gravis. Clin. Chim. Acta 201:201-205.

95. Peers J, McDonald B L, Dawkins R L 1977 The reactivity of the antistriational antibodies associated with thymoma and myasthenia gravis. Clinical and Experimental Immunology 27:66-73.

96. Gilhus N E, Aarli J A, Matre R 1984 Myasthenia gravis, difference between thymoma associated antibodies and cross-striational skeletal muscle antibodies. Neurology 34:246-249.

97. Kuks J B M, Limburg P C, Horst G, Dijksterhuis J, Oosterhuis H J G H 1993 Antibodies to skeletal muscle in myasthenia gravis, part 1. Diagnostic value for the detection of thymoma. Journal of the Neurological Sciences 119:183-188.

98. Kuks J B M, Limburg P C, Horst G, Oosterhuis H J G H 1993 Antibodies to skeletal muscle in myasthenia gravis, part 2. Prevalence in non-thymoma patients. Journal of the Neurological Sciences 120:78-81.

99. Komiyama A, Kamo I, Furukawa S, Akazawa S, Hirayama K, Satoyoshi E 1988 Antibodies against saline-soluble components of skeletal muscle in myasthenia gravis. Journal of Neurology 235:207-213.

100. Gautel M, Lakey A, Barlow D P, Zolmes Z, Scales S, Leonard K, Labeit S, Mygland A, Gilhus N E, Aarli J A 1993 Titin antibodies in myasthenia gravis. Neurology 43:1581-1585.

101. Skeie O, Mygland A, Aarli J A, Gilhus N E 1995 Titin antibodies in patients with late onset myasthenia gravis: Clinical correlations. Autoimmunity 20:99-104.

102. Gilhus N E, Matre H, Aarli J A, Hofstad H, Thunold S 1986 Thymic lymphoepitheliomas and skeletal muscle expressing common antigen(s). Acta Neurologica Scandinavica 73:428-433.

103. Geld H van der, Feltkamp T E W, Loghem J J van, Oosterhuis H J G H, Biemond A 1963 Multiple antibody production in myasthenia gravis. Lancet 2, 373-375.

104. Simpson J A 1966 Myasthenia gravis as an auto immune disease: clinical aspects. Annals of the New York Academy of Sciences 135:506-516.

105. Comston D A S, Vincent A, Newsom-Davis J, Batchelor J R 1980 Clinical, pathological, HLA antigen and immunological evidence for disease heterogeneity in myasthenia gravis. Brain 103:579-601.

106. Kiessling W R, Pflughaupt K W, Ricker K, Haubitz I, Meertens H G 1981 Thyroid function and circulating antibodies in myasthenia gravis. Neurology 31:771-774.

107. Kornfeld P 1964 Serum proteins in myasthenia gravis. Journal of the American Medical Association 190:463.

108. Aach R, Kissane J 1968 The unusual association of myasthenia gravis and hypergammaglobulinemia. American Journal of Medicine 45:451-459.

109. Oosterhuis H J G H, Geld H W R van der, Feltkamp T E W, Peetoom F 1964 Myasthenia gravis with hypergammaglobulinaemia and antibodies. Journal of Neurology, Neurosurgery and Psychiatry 27:345-350.

110. Rowland L P, Osserman E F, Scharfman W B, Balsam R F, Ball S 1969 Myasthenia gravis with a myeloma-type gamma-(IgG) immunoglobulin abnormality. American Journal of Medicine 46:599-605.

111. Yamamoto T, Sato T, Sugita H 1987 Antifilamin, antivinculin, and antitropomyosin antibodies in myasthenia gravis. Neurology 37, 1329-1333.

112. Hoogenraad T U, Gmelig Meyling F H 1987 Putative role of antireticulin antibody in antiacetylcholine-receptor-antibody-negative myasthenia gravis. Archives of Neurology 44:536-538.

113. Ohta M, Ohta K, Itoh N, Kurobe M, Hayashi K, Nishitani H, 1990 Anti-skeletal muscle antibodies in the sera from myasthenic patients with thymoma: identification of anti-myosin, actomyosin, actin, and alpha-actinin antibodies by a solid-phase radioimmunoassay and a Western blotting analysis. Clin. Chim. Acta 187:255-264.

114. Muller K M 1989 Anti-neuroblastoma antibodies in myasthenia gravis: clinical and immunological correlations. Journal of Neurological Sciences 93:263-275.

115. Michaelson D M, Korczyn A D, Sokolovsky M 1982 Antibodies to muscarinic acetylcholine receptors in myasthenia gravis. Biochemical and Biophysical Research Communications 104:52-57.

116. Lu C Z, Link H, Mo X A, Xiao B G, Zhang Y L, Qin Z 1991 Anti-presynaptic membrane receptor antibodies in myasthenia gravis. Journal of Neurological Sciences 102:39-45.

117. Pirskanen R 1976 Genetic association between myasthenia gravis and the HLA system. Journal of Neurology, Neurosurgery and Psychiatry 39:23-33.

118. Fritze D, Herrmann C, Naiem F, Smith G S, Waldford R L 1974 HLA antigens in myasthenia gravis. Lancet 1, 240-242.

119. Naiem F 1978 Association of HLA-B8, DRw3 and anti-acetylcholine receptor antibodies in myasthenia gravis. Tissue Antigens 12:381-386.

120. Szobor D, Gyodi E 1980 HLA-Antigene und geschlechtsbedingte genetische Factoren bei Myasthenia gravis. Aktuelle Neurologie 7:19-26.

121. Keesey J, Naiem F, Lindstrom J, Roe D 1982 Acetylcholine receptor antibody titer and HLA B8 antigen in myasthenia gravis. Archives of Neurology 39:73-77.

122. Berg-Loonen E M van der, Nijenhuis L E, Engelfriet C P, Feltkamp T E W, Rossum A L van, Oosterhuis H J G H 1977 Segregation of HLA haplotypes in 100 families with a myasthenia gravis patient. Journal of Immunogenetics 4:331-340.

123. Bell J, Rassenti L, Smoot S, Smith K, Newby C, Hohlfeld R, Toyka K, McDevitt H, Steinman L 1986 HLA-DQ beta-chain polymorphism linked to myasthenia gravis. Lancet 1, 1058-1060.

124. Kuks J B, Lems S P, Oosterhuis H J G H 1992 HLA type is not indicative for the effect of thymectomy in myasthenia gravis. Neuroimmunology 36:217-224.

125. Pirskanen R, Lefvert A K, Matell G, Osterman P O, Satoyoshi E, Tsuchiya M, Tsuchimoto K 1981 HLA, receptor antibodies and clinical state in Japanese, Finnish and Swedish myasthenia gravis. In: Satoyoshi E (ed) Symposium on myasthenia gravis. University of Tokyo Press, Tokyo, 233-248.

126. Kida K, Hayashi M, Yamada I, Matsuda H, Yoshinaga J, Takami S, Yashiki S, Sonoda S 1987 Heterogeneity in myasthenia gravis: HLA phenotypes and autoantibody responses in ocular and generalized types, Annals of Neurology 274-278.

127. Kayashi M, Kida K, Yamada I, Matsuda H, Sonoda S, Inoue H, Shiga S 1988 Involvement of HLA in clinical courses of myasthenia gravis. Journal of Neuroimmunology 171-179.

128. Hawkins B R, Ip M S, Lam K S, Ma J T, Wy C L, Yeung R T, Dawkins R L 1986 HLA antigens and acetylcholine receptor antibody in the subclassification of myasthenia gravis in Hong Kong Chinese. Journal of Neurology, Neurosurgery and Psychiatry 49:316-319.

129. Hawkins B R, Yu Y L, Wong V, Woo E, Ip M S, Dawkins R L 1989 Possible evidence for a variant of myasthenia gravis based on HLA and acetylcholine receptor antibody in Chinese patients. Quarterly Journal of Medicine 70:235-241.

130. Hare W S C, Mackay I R 1963 Radiological assessment of thymic size in myasthenia gravis and systemic lupus erythematosus. Lancet 1, 746.

131. Ellis K, Austin J H, Jartzki A 1988 III, Radiologic detection of thymoma in patients with myasthenia gravis. American Journal of Radiology 151, 873.

132. Keesey J, Bein M, Mink J 1980 Detection of thymoma in myasthenia gravis. Neurology 30:233.

133. Janssen R S, Kaye A D, Lisak R P, Schatz N J, Arger P A, Savino P J 1983 Radiologic evaluation of the mediastinum in myasthenia gravis. Neurology 33:534.

134. Juliani G 1990 Radiological diagnosis of thymoma in myasthenia gravis. Review of a series of 523 surgically controlled cases. Clin. Imagin. 14:48.

135. Moore A V, Korobkin M, Powers B, Olanow W, Ravin C E, Pufman C E, Breiman R S, Ram P C 1982 Thymoma detection by mediastinal CT; patients with myasthenia gravis. American Journal of Roentgenology 138, 217.

136. Fon G F, Bein M E, Mancuso A A, Keesey J C, Lupetin A R, Wong W S 1982 Computed tomography of the anterior mediastinum in myasthenia gravis. Radiology 142, 135.

137. Glate S, Neufang K F R, Haupt F W 1989 Was leistet die radiologische Thymus diagnostik bei der Myasthenia gravis? Röntgen Blätter 42:455-461.

138. Baron R L, Lee J K T, Sagel S S, Levitt R G 1982 Computed tomography of the abnormal thymus. Radiology 142:127.

139. Batra P, Herrmann C Jr, Mulder D 1987 Mediastinal imaging in myasthenia gravis: correlation of chest radiography, CT, MR, and surgical findings. American Journal of Radiology 148, 515.

140. Emskoetter T, Trampe H, Lachenmayer L 1988 Kernspintomographie bei Myasthenia gravis. Eine Alternative zur mediastinalen Computertomographie?, Deutsches Medisches Wochenschrift 113:1508.

141. Wright R B, Glantz R G, Turner D A, Siegel I M 1988 Mediastinal computed tomography (CT) and magnetic resonance imaging in myasthenia gravis: preliminary results and considerations. Neurology 38, 108.

142. Sabbagh S N, Garza J S, Patten B 1995 Thoracoscopic thymectomy in patients with myasthenia gravis. Muscle and Nerve 18:1475-1477.

143. Kornfeld P, Merav A, Fox S, Maier K 1993 How reliable are imaging procedures in detecting residual thymus after previous thymectomy? Annals of the New York Academy of Sciences 681:575-576.

144. Miller R G, Milner-Brown H S, Dan P C 1981 Antibody-negative acquired myasthenia gravis: successful therapy with plasma exchange. Muscle and Nerve 4:255.

145. Vincent A, Li Z, Hart A, Barret-Jolly R, Yamamoto T, Burges J, Wray D, Byrne N, Molenaar P C, Newsom-Davis J 1993 Seronegative myasthenia gravis: evidence for plasma factor(s) interfering with acetylcholine receptor function. Annals of the New York Academy of Sciences 681:529.

146. Gou T, Motamura M, Matsua H 1993 Effect of myasthenic IgG on degradation of junctional acetylcholine receptor. Muscle Nerve 16:840-848.

147. Martino G, DuPont B L, Wollmann R L 1993 The human-severe combined immunodeficiency myasthenic mouse model: a new approach for the study of myasthenia gravis. Annals of Neurology 34:48-56.

148. Oosterhuis H J G H, Hootsmans W J M, Veenhuizen H B, Zadelhoff I van 1972 The mean duration of motor unit action potentials in myasthenia gravis. Electroencephalography and Clinical Neurophysiology 32:697-700.

149. Huber A 1989 Ocular myography Bulletin Société Belge d'Ophthalmologie 237, 425.

150. Rivero A, Crovetto L, Lopez L, Maselli R, Nogues M 1995 Single fibre electromyography of extraocular muscles: a sensitive method for the diagnosis of ocular myasthenia gravis. Muscle Nerve 18:943-947.

151. Somnier F E 1994 Anti-acetylcholine receptor (AChR) antibodies measurement in myasthenia gravis: the use of cell line TE 671 as a souce of AChR antigen. Journal Neuroimmunology 51:63-68.

152. Beeson D, Amar M, Bermudez I, Vincent A, Newsom-Davis J 1996 Stable functional expression of the adult subtype of human muscle acetylcholine receptor following transfection of the human rhabdomyosarcoma cell line TE 671 with cDNA encoding the epsilon subunit. Neuroscience Letters 207:57-60.

Chapter 4

1. Sneddon J 1980 Myasthenia gravis: a study of social, medical and emotional problems in 26 patients. Lancet I:526-528.

2. D J Shale, D L Lane, Chr J F Davis 1983 Air flow limitation in myasthenia gravis. American Review of Respiratory diseases 128:618-621.

2a. Beekman R, Kuks J B M, Oosterhuis H J G H 1997 Myasthenia gravis: diagnosis and follow-up of 100 consecutive patients. Journal of Neurology 244:112-118.

3. Lambert D 1981 Myasthenia gravis. Lancet I:937.

4. Hardell L I, Lindström B, Lünnerholm G, Osterman P O 1982 Pyridostigmine in human breast milk. British Journal Clinical Pharmacology 14:565-567.

5. Schwab R S 1955 WIN 8077 in the treatment of sixty myasthenia gravis patients. American Journal of Medicine 19:734-736.

6. Westerberg M R 1956 Clinical evalution of Ambenonium (Mysuran) chloride. Archives of Neurology and Psychiatry 75:91.

7. Szobor A 1970 Crises in Myasthenia gravis. Akadémiai Kiadó Budapest.

8. Hoefer P F A, Aranow H, Rowland L P 1961 Long-acting compounds, especially BC-51 in the treatment of myasthenia gravis. In: Viets H R (ed) Myasthenia gravis. The second international symposium proceedings. Charles C Thomas, Springfield, p 303-308.

9. Bingle J P, Rutherford J D, Woodrow D 1979 Continuous subcutaneous neostigmine in the management of severe Myasthenia gravis. British Medical Journal I:1050.

10. Dooley J M, Goulden K J, Gatien J G, Gibson E J, Brown B St J 1986 Topical therapy for oropharyngeal symptoms of myasthenia gravis. Annals of Neurology 19:192-194.

11. Ricciardi R, Rossi B, Nicora M, Sghirlanzoni A, Muratorio A J 1991 Acute treatment of Myasthenia Gravis with intranasal neostigmine;clinical and electromyographic evalution. Journal of Neurology Neurosurgery Psychiatry 54:12:1061-1062.

12. Black J T, Braint K A, DeJesus V, Harner N, Rowland L P 1973 Myasthenia gravis lacking response to cholinergic drugs. Neurology 23:851-853.

13. Rowland L P 1955 Prostigmin-responsiviness and the diagnosis of myasthenia gravis. Neurology 5:612-624.

14. Argov Z, Mastaglia F L 1979 Disorders of neuromuscular transmission caused by drugs. New England Journal of Medicine 301:409-413.

15. Kaeser H E 1984 Drug-induced myasthenic syndromes. Acta Neurologica Scandinavica 70 (suppl 100):39-47.

16. Howard J F 1990 Adverse drug effects on neuromuscular transmission. Seminars in Neurology 10:89-102.
17. Schumm F, Wiethoelter H, Fateh-Moghadam A 1981 Myasthenie-Syndrome unter Chloroquin Therapie. Deutsches Medizinische Wochenschrift 106:1745-1747.
18. Robberecht W, Bednarik J, Bourgeois P, Hees J van, Carton H 1989 Myasthenic syndrome caused by direct effect of chloroquine or neuromuscular function. Archives of Neurology 46:464-468.
19. Drachman D A, Skom J H 1965 Procainamide - a hazard in myasthenia gravis. Archives of Neurology 13:316-320.
20. Kornfeld P, Horowitz S H, Genkins G, Papatestas A E 1976 Myasthenia gravis unmasked by anti-arhythmic agents. The Mount Sinai Journal of Medicine 43:10-14.
21. Oosterhuis H J G H 1964 Studies in myasthenia gravis. Journal of the Neurological Sciences I:512-546.
22. Bescausa E, Nicolas M, Aguado C, Toledano M, Vitrals M 1991 Myasthenia gravis aggravated by pyrantel pamoate. Journal of Neurology, Neurosurgery and Psychiatry 54:563.
23. Hokkanen E 1964 The aggravating effect of some antibiotics on the neuromuscular blockade in myasthenia gravis. Acta Neurologica Scandinavica 40:346-352.
24. McQuillen M P, Canter H E, O'Rourke J R 1968 Myasthenic syndrome associated with antibiotics. Archives of Neurology 18:402-415.
25. Wright E A, McQuillen M P 1971 Antibiotic-induced neuromuscular blockade. Annals of the New York Academy of Sciences 183:358-368.
26. Martins E I F, Ansink B J J 1979 A Myasthenia-like syndrome and polyneuropathy, complications of gentamycin therapy. Clinical Neurology and Neurosurgery 81:241-246.
27. Pauker S G, Kopelman R I 1993 Weak reasoning: diagnosis by drug reaction. New England Journal of Medicine 328:336-9.
28. Swift Th R 1981 Disorders of neuromuscular transmission other than myasthenia gravis. Muscle and Nerve 4:334-353.
29. Durand J M, Prince-Zucchelli M A, Galland M C, Pouget J, Harle J R, Weiller P J, Mongin M 1986 Syndrome myasthénique et doxycycline. Revue de Medecine Interne 7:68-9.
30. Mumford C J, Ginsberg L 1990 Ciprofloxacin and myasthenia gravis. British Medical Journal 301 (6755):818.
31. Rauser E H, Ariano R E, Anderson B A 1990 Exacerbation of myasthenia gravis by norfloxacin. DICP, the annals of Pharmacotherapy 24:207-208.
32. Argov Z, Brenner T, Abramsky O 1986 Ampicillin may aggravate clinical and experimental myasthenia gravis. Archives of Neurology 43:255-256.
33. Sonawalla A B, Lance J W 1989 Relapse of myasthenia gravis after amoxycillin therapy. Journal of Pakistan Medical Association 39:18-9.

34. Leys D, Pasquier F, Vermersch P, Gosset D, Michiels H, Kassiotis P, Petit H 1987 Possible revelation of latent myasthenia gravis by labetalol chlorhydrate. Acta Clinica Belgica 42:475-6.

35. Hermann Jr Chr 1961 Crisis in myasthenia gravis. In: Viets H R (ed) Myasthenia gravis. Charles C Thomas, Springfield, p 637-652.

36. Shaivitz S A 1974 Timolol and Myasthenia Gravis. J.A.M.A. 242:1611-1612.

37. Coppeto J R 1984 Timolol-associated myasthenia gravis (letter). American Journal Ophthalmology 98:244-245.

38. Verkyk A 1985 Worsening of myasthenia gravis with Timolol maleate eyedrops. Annals Neurology 17:211-212.

39. Confavreux C, Charles N, Aimard G 1990 Fulminant myasthenia gravis soon after initiation of acebutolol therapy. European Neurology 30:279-81.

40. Swash M, Ingram D 1992 Adverse effect of verapamil in myasthenia gravis. Muscle Nerve 15:396-398.

41. Lecky B R, Weir D, Chong E 1991 Exacerbation of myasthenia by propafenone. Neurology Neurosurgery Psychiatry 54:377.

42. McQuillen M P, Gross M, Johns R J 1963 Chlorpromazine-induced weakness in myasthenia gravis. Archives of Neurology 8:286-290.

43. Neil J F, Himmelhoch J M, Licata S M 1976 Emergence of myasthenia gravis during treatment with lithium carbonate. Archives of General Psychiatry 33:1090-1092.

44. Lipton I D 1987 Myasthenia gravis unmasked by lithium carbonate. Journal Clinical Psychopharmacology 7:57.

45. Norris F H, Colella J, McFarlin D 1964 Effect of diphenylhydantion on neuromuscular synapse. Neurology 14:869-876.

46. Regli F, Guggenheim P 1965 Myasthenisches Syndrom als seltene Komplikation unter Hydantoin Behandlung. Nervenarzt 36:315-318.

47. Brumlik J, Jacobs R S 1974 Myasthenia gravis associated with diphenylhydantoin therapy for epilepsy. Canadian Journal Science 1:127-129.

48. Milonas J, Kountouris D, Scheer E 1983 Myasthenisches Syndrom nach langzeitiger Diphenylhydantoin-Therapie. Nervenartz 54:437-8.

49. Peterson H 1966 Association of trimethadione therapy and myasthenia gravis. New English Journal of Medicine 274:506-7.

50. Booker H E, Chun R W M, Sanguino M 1970 Myasthenia gravis syndrome associated with trimethadione. JAMA 212:2262-2263.

51. Ueno S, Takahashi M, Kajiyama K, Okahisa N, Hazama T, Yorifuji S, Tarui S 1987 Parkinson's disease and myasthenia gravis: adverse effect of trihexyphenidyl on neuromuscular transmission. Neurology 37:832-3.

52. Canal N, Franceschi M 1983 Myasthenic crisis precipitated by iothalamic acid. Lancet I:1288.

53. Chagnac Y, Hadani M, Goldhammer Y 1985 Myasthenic crisis after intravenous administration of iodinated contrast agent. Neurology 35:1219-1220.

54. Frank J H, Cooper G W, Black W C, Phillips L H 2d 1987 Iodinated contrast agents in myasthenia gravis. Neurology 37:1400-2.

55. Bonmarchand G, Weiss P, Clavier E, Lerebours-Pigeonniere G, Massari P, Leroy J 1987 Myasthenic crisis following the injection of an iodinated contrast medium. Intensive Care Medicine 13:365.

56. Mosbaek Nordenbo A, Sommier F E 1992 Acute deterioration of myasthenia gravis after intravenous administration of gadolinium-DTPA. Lancet 340:1168.

57. Jonkers L, Swerup Ch, Pirskanen R, Bjelak S, Matell G 1996 Acute effects of intravenous injection of beta-adrenoreceptor and calcium antagonists in myasthenia gravis. Muscle Nerve 19:959-965.

58. Milonas I, Kountouris D, Müller E 1981 Das Jitter-Phänomen bei Myasthenia gravis und die Wirkung von Diazepam: eine Studie zur Einzelfaser Elektromyographie. Zeitschrift für Elektroenzephalographie, Elektromyographie und verwandte Gebiete 12:183-184.

59. Oosterhuis H J G H 1984 Myasthenia Gravis. Churchill Livingstone Edingburgh p.62-67.

60. Otto T J, Strugalska H 1987 Surgical treatment for myasthenia gravis. Thorax 42:199-204.

61. Papatestas A E, Genkins G, Kornfeld P, Eisenkraft J B, Fagerstrom P, Pozner J, Aufses E H 1987 Effects of thymectomy in myasthenia gravis. Annals of Surgery 206:79-88.

62. Evoli A, Batocchi A P, Provenzano C, Ricci E, Tonali P 1988 Thymectomy in the treatment of myasthenia gravis: report of 247 patients. Journal of Neurology 235:272-6.

63. Maggi G, Casadio C, Cavallo A, Cianci R, Molinatti M, Ruffini E 1989 Thymectomy in myasthenia gravis. Results of 662 cases operated upon in 15 years. European Journal Cardiothoracic Surgery 3:504-9.

64. B eghi E, Autozzi C, Batocchi A P, Cornelio F, Cosi V, Evoli A, Lombardi M, Mantegazza R, Monticelli M L, Piccolo G, Tonali P, Trevisan D, Zarrelli M 1991 Prognosis of myasthenia gravis: a multicentre follow up study of 844 patients. Journal of the Neurological Sciences 106:213-220.

65. Durelli L, Maggi G, Casadio C, Ferri R, Rendine S, Bergamini L 1991 Actuarial analysis of the occurrence of remissions following thymectomy for myasthenia gravis in 400 patients. Journal of Neurology Neurosurgery and Psychiatry 54:406-11.

65a. Kuks J B M 1993 The thymus and myasthenia gravis. Thesis Groningen, Ch II B. Thymectomy for myasthenia gravis. A 16-year experience with 100 patients p 37-51.

66. Jaretzki III A, Penn A S, Younger D S, Wolff M, Olarte M R, Lovelace R E, Rowland L P 1988 "Maximal" thymectomy for myasthenia gravis. The Journal of Thoracic and Cardiovascular sugery 95:747-57.

67. Mulder D G Discussion to Jaretzki (66).

68. Mulder D G, Graves N, Hermann C 1989 Thymectomy for myasthenia gravis: recent observations and comparisons with past experience. Annals of Thoracic Surgery 48:551-5.

69. Matell G, Bjelak S, Björnsen L, Brögger Christensen P 1994 Effect of thymectomy after the age of 40 in myasthenia gravis. EuroMyasthenia IV Versailles 245.

70. Evoli A, Batocchi A P, Tonali P, Palmisani M T, Lino M 1996 Thymectomy for Late-Onset Myasthenia Gravis. Neurology 46:A310.

71. Schumm F, Wiethölter H, Fateh-Moghadam A, Dichgans J 1985 Thymectomy in myasthenia gravis with pure ocular symptoms. Journal of Neurology Neurosurgery Psychiatry 48:332-337.

72. Rosenberg M, Jáuregui W O, DeVega M E, Herrera M R, Roncoroni A J 1983 Recurrence of thymic hyperplasia after thymectomy in myasthenia gravis. The American Journal of Medicine 74:78-82.

73. Pirskanen R, Matell G, Henze A 1987 Results following transsternal thymectomy after failing transcervical "thymectomy". Annals of the New York Academy of Sciences 505:866-867.

74. Miller R G, Filler-Katz A, Kiprov D, Roan R 1991 Repeat thymectomy in chronic refractory myasthenia gravis. Neurology 41:923-4.

74a. Ashour M1995 Prevalence of ectopic thymic tissue in myasthenia gravis and its clinical significance. Journal of Thoracic Cardiovascular Surgery 109:632-635.

75. Jaretzki A 3d, Wolff M 1988 "Maximal" thymectomy for myasthenia gravis. Surgical anatomy and operative technique. Journal of Thoracic Cardiovascular Surgery 96:711-6.

76. Fukai I, Funato Y, Mizuno T, Hashimoto T, Masaoka A 1991 Distribution of thymic tissue in the mediastinal adipose tissue. Journal of Thoracic and Cardiovascular Surgery 101:1099-102.

77. Oosterhuis H J G H, Limburg P C, Hummel-Tappel E, Van den Burg W, The TH 1985 Anti-acetylcholine receptor antibodies in myasthenia gravis. Part 3. The effect of thymectomy. Journal of the Neurological Sciences 69:335-43.

78. Kuks J B M, Oosterhuis H J G H, Limburg P C, the TH 1991 Anti-acetycholine receptor antibodies decrease after thymectomy in patients with myasthenia gravis: Clinical correlations. Journal of Autoimmunity 4:197-211.

79. Fuji N, Itoyama Y, Machi M, Goto I 1991 Analysis of prognostic factors in thymectomized patients with myasthenia gravis: correlation between thymic lymphoid cell subsets and postoperative clinical course. Journal of Neurology Science 105:143-9.

80. Melms A, Malcherek G, Gern U, Sommer N, Weissert R, Wiethölter H, Bühring H J 1993 Thymectomy and asathioprine have no effect on phenotype of CD4 T lymphocyte subsets in myasthenia gravis. Journal of Neurology Neurosurgery and Psychiatry 56:46-51.

81. Sabbach S N, Garza J S, Patten B 1995 Thoracoscopic thymectomy in patients with myasthenia gravis. Muscle Nerve 18:1475-1477.

82. Oosterhuis H J G H 1984 Myasthenia gravis. Churchill Livingstone Edingburgh p 68-73.

83. Maggi G, Casadio C, Cavallo A, Cianci R, Molinatti M, Ruffini E 1991 Thymoma: results of 241 operated cases. Annals of Thorac Surgery 51:152-6.

84. Somnier F E, 1994 Exacerbation of myasthenia gravis after removal of thymomas. Acta Neurologica Scandinavica 90:56-66.

85. Monden Y, Nakahara K, Nanjo S, Fuji Y, Matsumura A, Masaoka A, Kawashima Y 1984 Invasive thymoma with myasthenia gravis. Cancer 54:2513-2518.

86. Palmisani M T, Evoli A, Batocchi A P, Provenzano C, Tonali P 1993 Myasthenia gravis associated with thymoma: clinical characteristics and long-term out-come. European Neurology 34:78-82.

87. Masaoka A, Monden Y, Nakahara K, Tamoika T 1981 Follow-up study of thymomas with special reference to their clinical stages. Cancer 48:2485-2492.

88. Pescarmona E, Rendina E A, Venuta F, D'Arcangelo E, Pagani M, Ricci C, Ruco L P, Baroni C D 1990 Analysis of prognostic factors and clinicopathological staging of thymoma. Annals of Thoracic Surgery 50:534-8.

89. Müller-Hermelink H K, Marino M, Palestro G 1986 Pathology of thymic epithelial tumors. Müller-Hermelink H K Ed The Human Thymus, Springer Berlin p 207.

90. Nakahara K, Ohno K, Hashimoto J 1988 Thymoma: results with complete resection and adjuvant postoperative irradiation in 141 consecutive patients. Journal of Thoracic and Cardiovascular Surgery 95:1041-1047.

91. Kirschner P A 1990 Reoperation for thymoma: report of 23 cases. Annals of Thoracic Surgery 49:550-555.

92. Ohmi M, Ohuchi M 1990 Recurrent thymoma in patients with myasthenia gravis. Annals of Thoracic Surgery 50:243-7.

93. Loehrer P J, Chen M, Kun K, Aisner S C, Einhorn L H, Livingston R, Johnson D 1996 Cisplatin, doxorubicin and cyclosphamide plus thoracic radiation therapy for limited stage, unresectable thymoma: an intergroup trial. Journal of clinical oncology submitted.

94. Hu E, Levine J 1986 Chemotherapy of malignant thymoma. Cancer 57:1101-1104.

95. Schumm F, Brinkmann A, Fateh-Moghadam A 1984 Antikörperkontrollierte zytostatische Therapie des Malignen Thymoms bei begleitender Myasthenia gravis. Deutsches Medizinische Wochenschrift 109:1244-46.

96. Giaccone G, Ardizzoni A, Kickpatrick A, Clerico M, Sahmoud T, Zandwijk N van 1996 Cisplatin and etoposide combination chemotherapy: for locally advanced or metastatic thymoma. Journal of Clinical Oncology 14:814-820.

97. Warmolts J R, Engel W K, Whitaker J N 1970 Alternate day prednisone in a patient with myasthenia gravis. Lancet II:1198-1199.

98. Oosterhuis H J G H 1977 Erfahrungen mit Glykocorticoïden bei Patiënten mit Myasthenia gravis. In: Hertel G uA (eds) Myasthenia gravis, Thieme Verlag, Stuttgart:246-251.

99. Sghirlanzoni A, Peluchetti D, Fiacchio F, Mantegazza R, Cornelio F 1983 Myasthenia gravis: long term treatment with steroïds. Neurology 33.

100. Pascuzzi R M, Coslett H B, Johns T R 1984 Long term corticosteroïd treatment of myasthenia gravis; report of 116 patients. Annals of Neurology 15:291-298.

101. Seybold M E, Drachman D B 1974 Gradually increasing doses of prednisone in myasthenia gravis. New England Journal of Medicine 290:81-84.
102. Oosterhuis H J G H 1984 Myasthenia gravis. Churchill Livingstone Edingburgh: 197.
103. Arsura E L, Brunner N G, Namba T, Grob D 1985 High-dose intravenous methylprednisolone in myasthenia gravis. Archives of Neurology 42:1149-1153.
104. Oosterhuis H J G H 1984 ibid. p. 193.
105. Mertens H G, Balzereit F, Leipert M 1969 The treatment of severe myasthenia gravis with immunosuppressive agents. European Neurology 2:321-339.
106. Mertens H G, Hertel G, Reuther P, Ricker K 1981 Effect of immunosuppressive drug (azathioprine). Annals of the New York Academy of Sciences 377:691-699.
107. Matell G 1987 Immunosuppressive drugs: azathioprine in the treatment of myasthenia gravis. Annals of the New York Academy of Sciences 505:588-594.
108. Scherpbier H J, Oosterhuis H J G H 1987 Factors influencing the relapse risk at steroid dose reduction in myasthenia gravis. Clinical Neurology Neurosurgery 89:145-50.
109. Gajdos P and Myasthenia gravis clinical study group 1993 A randomised clinical trial comparing prednisone and azathioprine in myasthenia gravis. Results of the second interim analysis. Journal of Neurology, Neurosurgery and Psychiatry 56:1157-1163.
110. Palace J, Newsom-Davis J, Lecky B and the Myasthenia Study Group Oxford U.K. 1996 A multicentre, randomized, double blind trial of prednisolone plus azathioprine versus prednisolone plus placebo in myasthenia gravis. Neurology 46:A332.
111. Mantegazza R, Antozzi C, Peluchetti D, Sghirlanzoni A, Cornelio F 1988 Azathioprine as a single drug or in combination with steroïds in the treatment of myasthenia gravis. Journal of Neurology 235:449-53.
112. Oosterhuis H J G H 1988 Long-term effects of treatment in 374 patients with myasthenia gravis. Monographs in Allergy 25:75-85.
113. Valli G, Jann S, Premoselli S, Scarlato G 1987 Myasthenia gravis treatment: twelve years experience on 110 patients. Italian Journal of Neurology Sciences 8:593-601.
114. Kuks J B M, Djojoatmodjo S, Oosterhuis H J G H 1991 Azathioprine in myasthenia gravis: observations in 41 patients and a review of the literature. Neuromuscular disorders 1:423-431.
115. Oosterhuis H J G H 1981 Myasthenia gravis. A review. Clinical Neurology and Neurosurgery 83:105-135.
116. Hohlfeld R, Michels M, Heininger K, Besinger U, Toyka K V 1988 Azathioprine toxicity during long-term immunosuppression of generalized myasthenia gravis. Neurology 38:258-61.
117. Kissel J T, Levy R J, Mendell J R, Griggs R C 1986 Azathioprine toxicity in neuromuscular disease. Neurology 36:35-39.
118. Berlit P, Gretz N 1993 Azathiprin (Imurek). Internist 34:788-793.

119. Donaldson D H, Ansher M, Horan S, Rutherford R B, Ringel S P 1990 The relationship of age to outcome in myasthenia gravis. Neurology 40:786-90.

120. Panegyres P K, Squier M, Mills K P, Newsom-Davis J 1993 Acute myopathy associated with large parenteral dose of corticosteroid in myasthenia gravis. Journal of Neurology, Neurosurgery and Psychiatry 56:702-704.

120a.Vallet B, Fourrier F, Hurtevent J F, Parent M, Chopin C 1993 Myasthenia gravis and steroid induced myopathy of respiratory muscles. Intensive Care Medicine 18:424-426.

121. Kaplan J G, Barasch E, Hirschfeld A, Ross L, Einberg K, Gordon M 1989 Spinal epidural lipomatosis: a serious complication of iatrogenic Cushing'ssyndrome. Neurology 39:1031-1034.

122. Fonseca V, Havard C W 1988 Portal hypertension secondary to azathioprine in myasthenia gravis. Postgraduate Medical Journal 64:950-52.

123. Mertens H G, Hertel G, Reuther P, Ricker K 1981 Effect of immunosuppressive drugs (azathioprine). Annals of the New York Academy of Sciences 377:691-699.

124. Kornfeld P, Ambinder E P, Matta R, Bender A, Papatestas A E, Gross H, Genkins G 1985 Azathioprine experience in severe, generalized, recalcitrant myasthenia gravis. Mount Sinai Journal of Medicine (NY) 52:347-52.

125. Fischer B von, Gigon U, Sidiropoulos D, Montandona C 1981 Pregnancy and immunosuppressives. Gynäkologische Rundschau 21:141-158.

126. Rasmussen P, Fasth A, Ahimen J, Brynger H, Iwarson S, Kiellmer I 1981 Children of female renal transplant recipients. Acta Paediatrica Scandinavica 70:869-874.

127. Waltzer W C, Coulain C B, Zincke H, Sterioff S, Frohnert P P 1980 Pregnancy in renal transplantation. Transplantation Proceedings 12:221-226.

128. Pinching A J, Peters D K, Newsom Davis J 1976 Remission of myasthenia gravis following plasma exchange. Lancet II:1373-1376.

129. Dau P C 1980 Plasmapheresis therapy in myasthenia gravis. Muscle and Nerve 3:468-482.

130. Cumming W J K, Hudgson P 1986 The role of plasmaphoresis in preparing patients with myasthenia gravis for thymectomy. Procedings Intern Congress for Neuromuscular diseases, Marseille 25:3.

131. Antozzi C, Gemma M, Regi B, Berta E, Confalonieri P, Peluchetti D, Mantegazza R, Baggi F, Marconi M, Fiacchino F 1991 A short plasma exchange protocol is effective in severe myasthenia gravis. Journal of Neurology 238:103-7.

132. Reuter P, Wiebecke D, Fateh-Moghadan A, Besinger K, Mertens H G 1981 The role of plasma exchange in the treatment of myasthenia gravis. Plasma Exchange Therapy:Borberg H, Reuter P (Ed) George Thieme Verlag Stuttgart186-193.

133. Newsom-Davis J, Wilson S G, Vincent A, Ward C D 1979 Long term effects of repeated plasma exchange in myasthenia gravis. Lancet I:464-468.

134. Gajdos Ph, Surron N, Rohan-Chabot P de, Rafael J C, Goulon M 1983 Effets à long term des échanges plasmatiques au cours de la myasthènie. La Presse Médicale 12:939-942.

135. Fornasari P M, Riva G, Piccolo G, Cosi V, Lombardi M 1985 Short and long-term clinical effects of plasma-exchange in 33 cases of myasthenia gravis. International Journal Artificial Organs 8:159-62.

136. Kornfeld P, Ambinder E P, Mittag Th, Bender A N, Papatestas A E, Goldberg J, Genkins G 1981 Plasma pheresis in refractory generalized myasthenia gravis. Archives of Neurology 38:478-481.

137. Thorlacius S, Aarli J A, Jacobsen H, Halvorsen K 1985 Plasma exchange in myasthenia gravis: clinical effect. Acta Neurologica Scandinavica 72:464-8.

138. Howard Jr J F 1982 Treatment of myasthenia gravis with plasma exchange. Seminars in neurology 2:273-279.

139. Cohen M S, Younger D 1981 Aspects of the natural history of myasthenia gravis: crisis and death. Annals of the New York Academy of sciences 377:670-677.

140. Patten B M 1980 Discussion on plasma exchange. Annals of the New York Academy of Sciences 377:742.

141. Thorlacius S, Mollnes T E, Garred P, Aarli J A, Matre R, Toender O, Halvorsen K 1988 Plasma exchange in myasthenia gravis: changes in serum complement and immunoglobulins. Acta Neurologica Scandinavica 78:221-7.

142. Evoli A, Batocchi A P, Lo Monaco M, Servidei S, Padua L, Majolini L, Tonali P 1996 Clinical heterogeneity of seronegative myasthenia gravis. Neuromuscular disorders 6:155-161.

143. Miller R G, Milner-Brown H S, Dau P C 1981 Antibody negative acguired myasthenia gravis: successful therapy with plasma exchange. (Letter) Muscle nerve 4:255.

144. Sato T, Nishimiya J, Amai K, Anno M, Yamawaki N, Koroda T, Inagaki K 1983 Selective removal of anti-acetylcholine receptor antibodies in sera from patients with myasthenia gravis in vitro with a new adsorbent. Therapeutic plasmapheresis III:565-568.

145. Heininger K, Hartung H P, Toyka K V, Gaczkowski A, Borberg H 1987 Therapeutic plasma exchange in myasthenia gravis: semiselective adsorption of anti-AchR autoantibodies with tryptophane-linked polyvinylalcohol gels. Annals of the New York Academy of Sciences 505:898-900.

146. Sato T, Ishigahi Y, Komiya T, Tsuda H 1988 Therapeutic immuno adsorption of acetylcholine receptor antibody in MG. Annals of the New York Academy of Science 540:554-556.

147. Grob D, Simpson D, Mitsumoto H, Hoch B, Mokhtarain F, Bender A, Greenberg M, Koo A, Nakayama S 1995 Treatment of myasthenia gravis by immunoadsorption of plasma. Neurology 45:338-344.

148. Shibuya N, Sato T, Osame M, Takegami T, Doi S, Kawanami S 1994 Immunoadsorption therapy for myasthenia gravis. Journal of Neurology Neurosurgery Psychiatry 57:578-81.

149. Somnier F E, Langvad E 1989 Plasma exchange with selective immunoadsorption of anti-acetylcholine receptor antibodies. Journal Neuroimmunology 22:123-7.

150. Antonini G, Bove R, Filippine C, Millefiorini M 1990 Results of an open trial of cyclosporine in a group of steroïdo-dependant myasthenic subjects. Clinical Neurology Neurosurgery 92:317-322.

151. Goulon M, Elkharrat D, Gajdos P 1989 Traitement de la myasthenia grave par la ciclosporine. Etude ouverte de 12 mois. Presse Med 18:341-6.

152. Nyberg-Hansen R, Gjerstad L 1988 Myasthenia gravis treated with ciclosporin. Acta Neurology Scandinavica 77:307-13.

153. Schalke B C G, Kappos L, Rohrbach E, Melms A, Kalies I, Dommasch D, Mertens H G 1988 Ciclosporin A vs Azathioprine in the Treatment of Myasthenia Gravis: Final Results of a Randomized, Controlled Double-blind Clinical Trial. Neurology 38(suppl):135.

154. Tindall R S A, Phillips Th, Rollins J, Wells L, Hall K 1993 A clinical therapeutic trial of cyclosporine in myasthenia gravis. Annals of the New York Academy of Sciences 681:539-551.

155. Smith J L, Wilkinson A H, Hunsicker L G, Tobacman J , Kapelanski D P, Johnson M, Wright F H, Behrendt D M, Corry R J 1989 Transplantation Proceedings 21:3199-3200.

156. Perez M C, Buot W L, Mercado-Danguilan C, Bagabaldo Z G, Renales L D 1981 Stable remission in myasthenia gravis. Neurology 31:32-37.

157. Maza M de la, Duke H, Patten B M 1980 Cytotoxic drugs for myasthenia gravis. Neurology 30:389.

158. Niakan E, Harati Y, Rolak L A 1986 Immunosuppressive drug therapy in myasthenia gravis. Archives of Neurology 43:155-156.

159. Kinlen L J, Peto J, Doll R, Sheil A G R 1981 Cancer in patients treated with immunosuppressive drugs. British Medical Journal 282:474.

160. Leövey A, Szobor A, Szegedi G, Szathmary I, Petranyi 1975 Myasthenia gravis: ALG treatment of seriously ill patients. European Neurology 13:422-432.

161. Pirofski B, Reid R H, Basdana E J, Baker R L 1979 Myasthenia gravis treated with purified anti-thymocyte antiserum. Neurology 29:112-116.

162. Ahlberg R, Yi Q, Pirskanen R, Matell G, Swerup C, Rieber E H, Riethmüller G, Holm G, Lefvert A K 1994 Treatment of myasthenia gravis with anti - CD4 antibody. Neurology 44:1732-1737

163. Engel W K, Lichter A S, Dalakas M C 1981 Splenic and total body irradiation treatment of myasthenia gravis. Annals of the New York Academy of Sciences 377:744-754.

164. Durelli L, Ferrio M F, Urgesi A, Poccardi G, Ferrero B, Bergamini L 1993 Total body irradiation for myasthenia gravis: a long term follow-up. Neurology 43:2215-2221.

165. Zweiman B 1989 Theoretical mechanisms by which immunoglobulin therapy might benefit myasthenia gravis. Clinical Immunology Immunopathology 53:983-91.

166. Dwyer J M 1992 Manipulating the immune system with immune globulin. New England Journal of Medicine 326:107-106.

167. Fateh-Moghadam A, Besinger U, Geursen R G 1982 Ein klinisches Modell zur Regulation der humoralen Immunantwort: Infusion Therapie. Beitr Infusionther Klin Ernahr 9:69-72.

168. Arsura E L, Bick A, Brunner N G, Grob D 1988 Effects of repeated doses of intravenous immunoglobulin in myasthenia gravis. The American Journal of Medical Science 295:438-443.

169. Ferrero B, Durelli L, Cavallo R et al 1993 Therapies for exacerbation of myasthenia gravis. The mechanism of action of intravenous high-dose immunoglobulin G. Annals of the New York Academy of Sciences 681:563-569.

170. Evoli A, Palmisani M T, Bartoccioni E, Padua L, Tonali P 1993 High-dose intravenous immunoglobulin in myasthenia gravis. Italian Journal Neurology Science 14:233-237.

171. Meché F G A van der, Doorn P A van 1997 The current place of high-dose immunoglobulins in the treatment of neuromuscular disorders. Muscle Nerve 20:136-147.

172. Ippoliti G, Cosi V, Piccolo G, Lombardi M, Mantegary R 1984 High-dose intravenous gamma globulin for myasthenia gravis. Lancet II:809.

173. Cosi V, Lombardi M, Piccolo G, Erbetta A 1991 Treatment of myasthenia gravis with high-dose intravenous immunoglobulin. Acta Neurologica Scandinavica 84:81-84.

174. Besinger U, Fateh-Moghadam A, Knorr-Held S, Wick M, Kissel H, Albitz M 1987 Immunomodulation in myasthenia gravis by high-dose 7S-intravenous gammaglobulins. Annals of the New York Academy of Sciences 505:828-31.

175. Cook L, Howard J F, Folds T D 1988 Immediate effect of intravenous IgG administration on peripheral blood band T-cells and polymorphonuclear cells in patients with myasthenia gravis. Journal of Clinical Immunology 8:23-31.

176. Kolmolvarin N, Hemachudka T, Ongpipattanakul et al 1989 Plasma C3c changes in myasthenia gravis patients receiving high-dose intravenous immunoglobulin during crisis. Acta Neurologica Scandinavica 80:324-326.

177. Gajdos Ph, Outin H D, Morel E et al 1987 High dose intravenous gammaglobulin for myasthenia gravis: an alternative to plasma exchange? Annals of the New York Academy of Sciences 505:842-44.

178. Stricker R B, Kwiatkowska B J, Habis J A, Kiprov D D 1993 Myasthenic crisis. Response to plasmapheresis following failure of intravenous gamma-Globulin. Archives of Neurology 50:837-840.

179. Thornton Ch. A, Ballow M 1993 Safety of intravenous immunoglobulin. Editoral. Neurology 50:135-136.

180. Arsura E 1989 Experience with intravenous immunoglobulin in myasthenia gravis. Clinical Immunology and Immunopathology 53:170-179.

181. Lohi E-L, Lindberg Ch, Andersen O 1993 Physical training effects in myasthenia gravis. Archives of Physical Medicine and Rehabilitation 74:1178-1180.

182. Brolley M, Hollander M H 1955 Psychological problems of patients with myasthenia gravis. Journal of Nervous and Mental Disease 122:178-184.

183. Chafetz M E 1966 Psychological disturbances in myasthenia gravis. Annals of the New York Academy of Sciences 135:424-427.

184. Martin R D, Flegenheimer W von 1971 Psychiatric aspects of the management of the myasthenic patient. Mount Sinai Journal of Medicine 38:594-601.

185. Oosterhuis H J G H, Wilde G J S 1964 Psychiatric aspects of myasthenia gravis. Psychiatra, Neurologia et Neurochirurgia 67:484-496.

186. Szobor A 1967 Die bei Myasthenia gravis vorkommenden psychischen Zustände und psychopathologischen Phänomene. Psychiatrica et Neurologica 153:63-72.

187. MacKenzie K R, Martin M J, Howard F M 1969 Myasthenia gravis: psychiatric concomitants. Canadian Medical Association Journal 100:988-991.

188. Perlman B, Hogben G, Rosenthal J, Wolf-Dorlester B 1976 Myasthenia gravis and psychological illness in an adolescent: a case report. Mount Sinai Journal of Medicine 43:578-580.

189. Schwartz M L, Cahill R 1971 Psychopathology associated with Myasthenia gravis and its treatment by psychotherapeutically oriented group counseling. Journal Chronical Disease 24:543-552.

190. Nicholson G A, Wilby J, Tennant Ch 1986 Myasthenia gravis: the problem of a "psychiatric" diagnosis. The Medical Journal of Australia 144:632-638.

191. Magni G, Micaglio G F, Lalli R, Bejato L, Candeago M R, Merskey H, Angelini C 1988 Psychiatric disturbances associated with myasthenia gravis. Acta Psychiatrica Scandinavica 77:443-5.

192. Bartel P R, Lotz B P 1995 Neuropsychological test performance and affect in myasthenia gravis. Acta Neurologica Scandinavica 91:266-270.

193. Doering S, Heuze T, Schüssler G 1993 Coping with myasthenia gravis and implications for psychotherapy. Archives of Neurology 50:617-620.

194. Luetzenkirchen J, Bomhard M von, Lurati M 1977 Psychosomatische Aspekte. In: Hertel G (ed) Myasthenia gravis. Springer Verlag, Stuttgart: 153-156.

195. Tucker D M, Roeltgen D P, Wann Ph D Wertheimer R I 1988 Memory dysfunction in myasthenia gravis: evidence for central cholinergic effects. Neurology 38:1173-1177.

196. Lewis S W, Ron M A, Newsom-Davis J 1989 Absence of central functional cholinergic deficits in myasthenia gravis. Journal of Neurology, Neurosurgery and Psychiatry 52:258.

197. Hoefer P F A, Aranow H, Rowland L P 1958 Myasthenia gravis and epilepsy.A.M.A. Archives of Neurology and Psychiatry 80:10.

198. Hokkanen E 1969 Myasthenia gravis. A clinical analysis of the total material from Finland with special references to endocrinological and neurological disorders. Annals of Clinical Research 1:94-108.

199. Storm Mathisen A 1984 Epidemiology of myasthenia gravis in Norway. Acta Neurologica Scandinavica 70:274.

200. Simpson J A 1960 Myasthenia gravis, a new hypothesis. Scottish Medical Journal 5:419-436.

201. Hokkanen E, Toivakka E 1969 Electroencephalographic findings in myasthenia gravis. Acta Neurologica Scandinavica 45:556.

202. Papazian O 1976 Rapid eye movement sleep alteration in myasthenia gravis. Neurology 26:311.

203. Bergonzi P, Mazza S, Mennuni G, Morante M, Sollazo D, Scopetta C 1981 Central nervous system involvement in myasthenia gravis. Annals of the New York Academy of Sciences 377:810.

204. Shintani S, Shizawa Z, Shindo K, Matsui T, Tsunoda S 1989 Sleep apnea in wellcontrolled myasthenia gravis. Rinsho Shinkeigaku 29:547.

205. Whiting P J, Cooper J, Lindstrom J M 1987 Antibodies in sera from patients with myasthenia gravis do not nicotinic acetylcholine receptors from human brain. Journal of Neuroimmunologica 16:205.

206. Magni G, Micaglio G, Ceccato M B, Lalli R, Bejato L, Angelini C 1989 The role of life events in the myasthenia gravis outcome: a one-year longitudinal study. Acta Neurologica Scandinavica 79:288-291.

207. Rohr W 1992 Myasthenia gravis in the frontier of psychiatric diagnosis. Psychiatric Praxis 19:157-63.

208. Martin R D, Flegenheimer W von 1971 Psychiatric aspects of the management of the myasthenic patient. Mount Sinai Journal of Medicine 38:594-601.

209. Wainwright A P, Brodrick P M 1987 Suxamethonium in myasthenia gravis. Anaesthesia 42:950-7.

210. Ramsay F M, Smith G D 1985 Clinical use of atracurium in myasthenia gravis: a case report. Canadian Anaesthesia Soc J 32:642-5.

211. Hunter J M, Bell C F, Florence A M, Jones R S, Utting J E 1985 Vecuronium in the myasthenic patient. Anaesthesia 40:848-53.

212. Nilsson E, Meretoja O A 1990 Vecuronium dose-response and maintenance requirements in patients with myasthenia gravis. Anesthesiology 73:28-32.

213. Nilsson E, Muller K 1990 Neuromuscular effects of isoflurane in patients with myasthenia gravis. Acta Anaesthesiologica Scandinavica 34:126-31.

214. Schumm F, Gaertner H J, Wiatr G, Dichgans J 1985 Serumspiegel von Pyridostigmin bei Myasthenia gravis: Methoden und Klinische Bedeutung. Fortschr Neurol Psychiatr 53:201-11.

215. Aquilonius S M, Eckernäs S A, Hartvig P, Lindström P O, Osterman P O 1980 Pharmacokinetics and oral bio-availability of pyridostigmine in man. European Journal of Pharmacology 18:423-428.

216. Calvey T N, Chan K 1976 Plasma pyridostigmine levels in patients with myasthenia gravis. Clinical Pharmacology and Therapeutics 21:184-193.

217. Breyer-Pfaff U, Schmezer A, Maier U, Brinkmann A, Schumm F 1990 Neuromuscular function and plasma drug levels in pyridostigmine treatment of myasthenia gravis. Journal of Neurology, Neurosurgery Psychiatry 53:502-6

218. White M C, Silva P de, Harvard C W H 1981 Plasma pyridostigmine levels in myasthenia gravis. Neurology 31:145-150.

219. Rothenberg D M, Berns A S, Barkin R, Glantz R H 1990 Bromide intoxication secondary to pyridostigmine bromide therapy. Journal of American Medical Association 268:1121-2.

220. Jacobs R, Karczmar A G, Brumlick J 1973 Theophylline compounds and myasthenia gravis. Clinical Pharmalogical Therapy 14:374-379.
221. Molenaar P C, Biewenga J E, Van Kempen G Th, De Priester J A 1993 Effect of ephedrine in muscle weakness in a model of myasthenia gravis in rats. Neuropharmacology 32:373-6.
222. Laflin M J 1977 Interaction of pancuronium and corticosteroïds. Anesthesiology 47:471-472.
223. Fuchs S, Bartfeld D, Eshhar Z, Fetngold C, Moshly-Rosen D, Novick D, Schwarts M, Tarrab-Hazdai R 1980 Immune regulation of experimental Myasthenia. Journal of Neurology, Neurosurgery and Psychiatry 43:634-643.
224. Komar J, Szalay M, Szel I 1987 Myasthenische Episode nach Einnahme grosser Mengen Betablocker. Fortschr Neurol Psychiatr 55:201-2.
225. Molgo J, del Ponzo E, Bahos J E, Anqaut-Petit D 1991 Changes of quantal transmitter releae caused by gadolinium ions at the frog neuromuscular function. British Journal of Pharmacology 104:133-138.
226. Kirjner M, Lebourges J, Caums J P 1980 Myasthénie induite par pyrithioxine au cours du traitement d'une polyarthrite rhumatoide. La Nouv. Presse Médicale 41:3098.
227. Swash M, Ingram D A 1992 Adverse effect of Verapamil in myasthenia gravis. Muscle Nerve 15:396-398.
228. Pestronk A, Drachman D B 1980 Lithium reduces the number of acetylcholine receptors in skeletal muscle. Science 210:342-343.
229. Glaser G H 1966 Crises, precrises and drug resistance in myasthenia gravis. Annals of the New York Academy of Sciences 135(I):335-349.
230. Osserman K E 1958 Myasthenia gravis. Grune & Stratton New York and London.
231. Tether J E 1955 Management of myasthenic and cholinergic crisis. American Journal of Medicin 19:740-742.
232. Szobor A 1970 Crises in myasthenic gravis. Akadémiai Kiadó, Budapest.
233. Jongste M J L de, Oosterhuis H J G H, Lie K I 1986 Intractable ventricular tachycardia in a patient with giant cell myocarditis, thymoma and myasthenia gravis. International Journal of cardiology 13:374-378.
234. Hermann Jr Chr 1961 Crisis in myasthenia gravis. In Viets H R (Ed) Myasthenia gravis Charles C Thomas Springfield 637-652.
235. Ferguson I T, Murplug R P, Lascelles R G 1982 Ventilatory failure in myasthenia gravis. Journal of Neurology, Neurosurgery, Psychiatry 45:217-222.
236. Hohlfeld R, Toyka K V, De Baets M H, Oosterhuis H J G H 1993 Myasthenia gravis. CRC Press Boca Raton 254-255.

Chapter 5

1. Geld H v d 1963 ch 1.64.
2. Geld H v d 1963 ch 1.67.

3. Feltkamp T E W, Van der Geld H, Oosterhuis H J G H 1963 Studies on sera from cases of Myasthenia Gravis using the Fluorescent Antibody Technique. Vox Sang. 8:317-327.

4. Feltkamp T E W, Van der Geld H, Kruyff K, Oosterhuis H J G H 1963 Antinuclear factor in myasthenia gravis. Lancet I/7282 667.

5. Geld H v d 1964 ch 3.89.

6. Oosterhuis H J G H 1966 ch 2.142.

7. Oosterhuis H J G H 1967 ch 3.91.

8. Oosterhuis H J G H 1981 ch 2.60.

9. Oosterhuis H J G H 1988 ch 2.87.

10. Oosterhuis H J G H 1989 ch 2.78.

11. Beekman R 1997 ch 2.85.

12. Limburg P C 1983 ch 3.30.

13. Oosterhuis H J G H, Limburg P C, Hummel-Tappel E, The T H 1983 Anti-acetylcholine receptor antibodies in myasthenia gravis. Part. 2 clinical and serological follow-up of individual patients. Journal of the Neurological Sciences 58:371-385.

14. Kuks J B M, Limburg P C, Oosterhuis H J G H, The H 1992 Antibodies to acetylcholine receptors in myasthenia gravis. In vitro synthesis by peripheral blood lymphocytes before and after thymectomy. Clinical and Experimental Immunology 87:246-250.

15. Garcin R, Fardeau M, Godet-Guillain M 1965 A clinical and pathological study of a case of alternating and recurrent external ophthalmoplegia with amyotrophy of the limbs observed for forty-five years: discussion of the relationship of this condition with myasthenia gravis. Brain 88 (IV):739-752.

16. Oosterhuis H J G H 1973 ch 2.45.

17. Veenhoven W A 1979 ch 2.122.

18. Oosterhuis H J G H, Van der Geld H, Feltkamp T E, Peetoom F 1964 Myasthenia gravis with hypergammaglobulinaemia and antibodies. Journal of Neurology, Neurosurgery, Psychiatry 27/4:345-350.

19. Starink Th 1986 ch 2.132.

20. Kuks J B M 1991 ch 4.114.

21. Oosterhuis H J G H 1964 ch 4.185.

22. Feltkamp T E W 1974 ch 3.90.

23. Kuks J B M 1992 ch 3.124.

24. Oosterhuis H J G H 1975 The relation between the histopathology of the thymus gland and the effect of thymectomy in myasthenia gravis. In: Recent Advances in myology Ed. W.G. Bradley et al. 517-521. Excerpta Medica Intern Congr Series no 360.

25. Kuks J B M 1992 The thymus and myasthenia gravis. Academic Thesis Groningen:137-151.

26. Blom R J, Kuks J B M, Westerterp-Maas A, Oosterhuis H J G H 1997 Gunstige resultaten van plasma ferese bij ernstige myasthenia gravis. Nederlands Tijdschrift voor Geneeskunde 141:381-384.

27. Oosterhuis H J G H, Kuks J B M 1997 Myasthenia gravis with thymoma. Marx A, Müller-Hermelink H K Ed. Epithelial tumors of the thymus: Pathology, Biology, Treatment. Plenum N.Y.

28. Oosterhuis H J G H, Slooten P J van der 1973 The effect of Aldactone-A on intracellular potassium in patients with myasthenia gravis. Journal of the Neurological Sciences 19:453-460.

29. Oosterhuis H J G H 1987 ch 2.156.

30. Croxen R, Newland C, Beeson D, Oosterhuis H, Chanplannaz G, Vincent A, Newsom-Davis J 1997 Mutations in different functional domains of the human muscle acetylcholine receptor -subunit in patients with the slow channel congenital myasthenic syndrome. Human molecular genetics, May.

31. Sieb J P, Milone M, Engel A G 1994 Effects of Quinine and Quinidine on neuromuscular transmission. Neurology 44 (suppl 2) A289.

32. Wokke J H J 1989 ch 2.170.

33. Hermann Chr 1961 ch 4.234.

34. Hofstad H, Ohm O J, Mörk S J, Aarli J A 1984 The heart in myasthenia gravis. Acta Neurologica Scandinavica 70:176.

35. Ashok P P, Ahuja G K, Manchanda S C, Jalal S 1983 Cardiac involvement in myasthenia gravis. Acta Neurologica Scandinavica 68:113-120.

36. Gibson T C 1975 The heart in myasthenia gravis. American Heart Journal 90:389-396.

37. Richards B W, Jones F R, Younge B R 1992 Causes of paralysis of the oculomotor, trochlear and abducens cranial nerves. American Journal Ophthalmology 113:489-96.

38. Oosterhuis H J G H 1984 Myasthenia gravis. Churchill Livingstone Edinburgh:101-102.

39. Kaminski H J, Maas E, Spiegel P, Ruff R L 1990 Why are eye muscles frequently involved in myasthenia gravis? Neurology 40:1663-69.

40. Horton R M, Manfredi A A, Conti-Tronconi B M 1993 The 'embryonic' gamma subunit of the nicotinic acetylcholine receptor is expressed in adult extra ocular muscle. Neurology 43:983-6.

41. Kaminski H J, Kusner L L, Nash K V, Ruff R L 1995 The -subunit of the acetylcholine receptor is not expressed in the levator palpebrae superiors. Neurology 45:516-518.

42. Vincent A, Newsom-Davis J 1980 Anti-acetylcholine receptor antibodies. Journal of Neurology, Neurosurgery, Psychiatry 43:590-600.

43. Oda K, Shibasaki H 1988 Antigenic difference of acetylcholine receptor between single and multiple form endplates of human extraocular muscle. Brain Res 449 (1-2) 337-40.

44. Biemond A ch 2.184.

Chapter 6

1. Beekman R, Kuks J B M, Oosterhuis H J G H 1997. Myasthenia gravis: diagnosis and follow-up of 100 consecutive patients. Journal of Neurology 244:112-118.
2. Swift Th R 1981 Disorders of neuromuscular transmission other than myasthenia gravis. Muscle Nerve 4:334.
3. Sturzenegger M 1989 Ptose-klinische Differential Diagnose. Schweizerische Medizinische Wochenschrift 119:1386.
4. Lepore F E 1986 Bilateral Cerebral Ptosis. Neurology 36:251.
5. Feibel R M, Custer P L, Gordoz M O 1993 Postcataract ptosis. A randomized double masked comparison of peribulbar and retrobulbar anaesthesia. Ophthalmiology 100:660-665.
6. Bosch W van der, Lemy H G 1992 Blepharoptosis induced by prolonged hard contact lens wear. Ophthalmology 99:1759-1765.
7. Deady J P, Morrell A J, Sutton G A 1989 Recognising aponeurotic ptosis. Journal of Neurology, Neurosurgery, Psychiatry 52:996.
8. Jones L T, Quickert M H, Wobig J L 1975 The cure of ptosis by aponeurotic repair. Archives of Ophthalmology 93:629-634.
9. Conrad B, Meinck H M, Beneke R, Mühlendyck H 1984 Zur Differentialdiagnose der isolierten Ptosis. Nervenarzt 55:432.
10. Jankovic J, Ford J 1983 Blepharospasm and orofacial-cervical dystonia: Clinical and pharmacological findings in 100 patients. Annals of Neurology 13:402.
11. Kurlan R, Jankovic J, Rubin A, Patten B, Griggs R, Shoulson I 1987 Coexistent Meige's syndrome and myasthenia gravis. A relationship between blinking and extra-ocular muscle fatigue? Archives of Neurology 44:1057.
12. Glaser J S 1978 Neuro-ophthalmology. Harper & Pow Publishers, Hagerstown:273.
13. Dresner S C, Kennerdell J S 1985 Dysthyroid orbitopathy. Neurology 35:1628.
14. Spector R H, Carlisle J A 1987 Minimal thyroid ophthalmopathy. Neurology 37:1803.
15. Bastiaensen L A K Chronic progressive external ophthalmoplegia. Thesis Nijmegen, Koninklijke Drukkerij G J Thieme B V.
16. Petty R K H, Harding A E, Morgan-Hughes J A 1986 The clinical features of mitochondrial myopathy. Brain 109:915.
17. Serratrice G, Pellissier J F 1987 Myopathies oculaires. La Presse Médicale 16:1969.
18. Drachman D A 1968 Ophthalmoplegia plus. The neuro degenerative disorders associated with progressive external ophthalmoplegia. Archives of Neurology 18:654.
19. Matsuda Y, Sakata C, Sunohara N, Nonaka I, Satoyoshi E 1989 Two cases of mitochondrial myopathy, long-term follow-up on a diagnosis of ocular type myasthenia gravis. Rinsko Shinkeigaku 29:1180.
20. Weir S, Hansen S, Ballantyne J P 1979 Single fibre electromyographic jitter in multiple sclerosis. Journal of Neurology, Neurosurgery, Psychiatry 42:1146.

21. Harper P S 1979 Myotonic Dystrophy. W B Saunders, Philadelphia p 165.

22. Cherington M 1974 Botulism. Ten-year experience. Archives of Neurology 30:432.

23. Rapoport S, Warkins P B 1984 Descending paralysis resulting from occult wound botulism. Annals of Neurology 16:359.

24. Tyler H R 1963 Botulism;physiological observations in human botulism. Archives of Neurology 9:652.

25. Pettigrew L C, Glass J P 1985 Neurologic complications of a coral snake bite. Neurology 35:589.

26. Moorthy G, Behrens M M, Drachman D B, Kirkman T H, Knox D L, Miller N R, Slamovitz T L, Zinreich S J 1989 Ocular pseudomyasthenia or ocular myasthenia 'plus': a warning to clinicians. Neurology 39:1150.

27. Lindstrom J 1977 An essay for antibodies to human acetylcholine receptor in serum from patients with myasthenia gravis. Clinical Immunology, Immunopathology 7:36.

28. Shinton R A, Jamieson D G 1989 Exercise induced diplopia as a presentation of midline cerebral tumour. Journal of Neurology, Neurosurgery, Psychiatry 52:916.

29. Dirr L Y, Donofrio P D, Patton J F, Troost B T 1989 A false-positive edrophoniumtest in a patient with a brainstem glioma. Neurology 39:865.

30. McAlpine D, Lumsden Ch E, Acheson E D 1972 Multiple Sclerosis. Churchill Livingstone, Edingburgh 135:164.

31. Keane J R 1986 Acute bilateral ophthalmoplegia: 60 cases. Neurology 36:279.

32. Mullaly W J 1982 Carbamazepine-induced ophthalmoplegia. Archives of Neurology 39:64.

33. Rosenberg M L 1986 Spasm of the near reflex mimicking myasthenia gravis. Journal of Clinical Neuro- Ophthalmology 6:106.

34. Crone R A 1973 Diplopia. Excerpta Medica Amsterdam:386.

35. Schwab R S, Perlo V P 1966 Syndromes simulating myasthenia gravis. Annals of the New York Academy of Sciences 135:350.

36. Mulder D W, Lambert E H, Eaton L M 1959 Myasthenic syndrome in patients with amyotrophic lateral sclerosis. Neurology 9:627.

37. Denijs E H, Forbes F H 1979 Amyotrophic lateral sclerosis: impairment of neuromuscular transmission. Archives of Neurology 36:202.

38. Albers J W, Zimnowodzky S, Lowrey C M, Miller B 1983 Juvenile progressive bulbar palsy. Archives of Neurology 40:351.

39. McQuillen M P 1966 Familial limb-girdle Myasthenia. Brain 89:121-132.

40. Oh S J, Kwioglu R 1992 Chronic limb-girdle myasthenia gravis. Neurology 42:1153.

41. Azulay J Ph, Pouget J, Figarella-Branger D, Colamarino R, Pellissier J F, Serratrice G 1994. Revue Neurologique (Paris) 150:377-381.

42. Susac J O, Garcia-Mullin R, Glaser J S 1973 Ophthalmoplegia in dermatomyositis. Neurology 23:305.

43. Johns T R, Crowley W J, Miller J Q, Campa J F 1971 The syndrome of myasthenia and polymyositis with comments of therapy. Annals of the New York Academy of Sciences 183:64.

44. Di Mauro S, Bonilla E, Zeviani M, Nakagawa M, De Vivo D C 1985 Mitochondrial myopathies. Annals of Neurology 17:521.

45. Eaton L M, Lambert E L 1957 Electromyography and electric stimulation of nerves in diseases of the motor unit: Observations on myasthenic syndrome associated with malignant tumors. Journal of the American Medical Association 162:1117-1124.

46. O'Neill J H, Murray N M, Newson-Davis J 1988 The Lambert-Eaton myasthenic syndrome. A review of 50 cases. Brain 111:577-96.

47. Anderson H J, Churchill-Davison H C, Richarson A T 1953 Bronchial neoplasm with myasthenia. Prolonged apnoea after administration of succinylcholine. Lancet II:1291-1293.

48. Kennedy W R, Jimenez-Pabon E 1968 The myasthenic syndrome associated with small cell carcinoma of the lung (Eaton-Lambert Syndrome). Neurology 18:757-766.

49. Lambert E H, Rooke E D, Eaton L M, Hodgson C H 1961 Myasthenic syndrome occasionally associated with bronchial neoplasm: neurophysiological studies. In: Viets H R Myasthenia gravis, Ch Thomas, Springfield:362-410.

50. Rooke E D, Mulder D W, Eaton L M, Lambert E H 1961 Studies of neuromuscular conduction in myasthenia gravis and related disorders. In: Viets H R (ed) Myasthenia gravis, 2nd International Symposium Proceedings. Charles C Thomas:435-443.

51. Wise R P, McDermot V 1962 A myasthenic syndrome associated with bronchial carcinoma. Journal of Neurology, Neurosurgery and Psychiatry 25:31-39.

52. Lennon V, Lambert E H, Whittenham S, Fairbanks V 1982 Auto immunity and the Lambert-Eaton syndrome. Muscle and Nerve 5:S21-S25.

53. Hawley R J, Cohen M H, Saini N, Armbrustmacher V W 1980 The carcinomatous neuromyopathy of oat-cell lung cancer. Annals of Neurology 7:65-72.

54. Ehrington G M, Murray N M F, Spiro S G, Newsom-Davis 1991 Neurological paraneoplastic syndromes in patients with small cell lung cancer: a prospective survey of 150 patients. Journal of Neurology, Neurosurgery and Psychiatry 54:764.

55. Taphoorn M J, Van Duijn H, Wolters E C 1988 A neuromuscular transmission disorder: combined myasthenia gravis and Lambert Eaton syndrome in one patient. Journal of Neurology, Neurosurgery and Psychiatry 51:880-2.

56. Spalek P, Orolin D, Lisy L 1989 Immuno suppressive drug treatment in overlap myasthenic syndrome: combined myasthenia gravis and Lambert-Eaton myasthenic syndrome. Neurology in Europe I, Bartko D, Gerstenbrand F, Turcani P, Eds John Libbey & Co Ldt:603.

57. Newsom-Davis J, Leys K, Vincent A, Ferguson I, Modi G, Mills K 1991 Immunological evidence for the co-existence of the Lambert-Eaton myasthenic syndrome and myasthenia gravis in two patients. Journal of Neurology, Neurosurgery and Psychiatry 54:452-543.

58. Scopetta C, Caasali C, Vaccario M L, Provenzano C 1984 Difficult diagnosis of Eaton-Lambert myasthenic syndrome. Muscle and Nerve 7:680-681.

59. Santa T, Engel A G, Lambert E G 1972 Histometric study of neuromuscular junction ultrastructure II Myasthenic syndrome. Neurology 22:370-376.

60. Fukuhara N, Tahamori M, Gutmann L, Chou S M 1972 Eaton-Lambert syndrome. Ultrastructural study of the motor end-plates. Archives of Neurology 27:67-78.

61. Fardeau M, Godet-Guillain J, Chevallay M 1974 Ultrastructural changes of the motor end-plates in myasthenia gravis and myasthenic syndrome. Neurology, Ed. A Subirana and KJ M Espadaler. Excerpia Medica International congress Series 319:427-438.

62. Hesselmans L F G M, Jennekens F G I, Kartman J, Wokke J H J, De Visser M, Klaver-Krol E G, DeBaets M, Spaans F, Veldman H 1992 Secondary Changes of the Motor Endplate in Lambert-Eaton Myasthenic Syndrome - A Quantitative Study. Acta Neuropathologica (Berl) 83:202-206.

63. Lambert E H, Elmqvist D 1971 Quantal components of end-plate potentials in the myasthenic syndrome. Annals of the New York Academy of Sciences 183:183-199.

64. Fukunaga H, Engel A G, Osame M, Lambert E H 1982 Paucity and disorganization of presynaptic membrane active t-Eaton myasthenic syndrome. Muscle and Nerve 5:686-697.

65. Lang B, Newsom-Davis J, Wray D, Vincent A, Murray N 1981 Auto immune aetiology for myasthenic (Eaton-Lambert) syndrome. Lancet II:224-226.

66. Fukuoka T, Engel A G, Lang B, Newsom-Davis J, Vincent A 1987 Lambert-Eaton myasthenic syndrome: II Immunoelectron microscopy localization of IgG at the mouse motor endplate. Annals of Neurology 22:200-211.

67. Nagel A, Engel A G, Lang B, Newsom-Davis J, Fukuoka T 1988 Lambert-Eaton myasthenic syndrome IgG depletes presynaptic membrane ective zone particles by antigenic modulation. Annals of Neurology 24:552-558.

68. Oh S J 1989 SFEMG improvement with remission in the cancer-associated Lambert-Eaton myasthenic syndrome. Muscle and Nerve 12:844-8.

69. Lundh H, Nilsson O, Rosén I, Johansson S 1993 Practical aspects of the Lambert-Eaton myasthenic syndrome. Acta Neurologica Scandinavica 88:136-140.

70. Newsom-Davis J 1982 Auto-immune diseases of neuromuscular transmission. Clinics in Immunology and Allergy 2:405-424.

71. Ueno S, Hara Y 1992 Lambert-Eaton myasthenic syndrome without anti-calcium channel antibody: adverse effect of diltiazem. Journal of Neurology, Neurosurgery and Psychiatry 55:409-410.

72. David A, Pelosi A, McDonald E, Stephens D, Ledger D, Rathbone R, Mann A 1990 Tired, weak, or in need of rest: fatigue among general practice attenders. British Medical Journal 30:1199.

73. Johns R J, McQuillen M P 1966 Syndromes simulating myasthenia gravis: asthenia with anticholinesterase tolerance. Annals of the New York Academy of Sciences 135-385.

74. Behan P O, Behan W M H, Bell E J 1985 The postviral fatigue syndrome - an analysis of findings in 50 cases. Journal Infect. 10:211.

75. Holmes G P, Kaplan J E, Gantz N M 1988 Chronic fatigue syndrome: a working case definition. Annals Intern Med 108:387.

76. Wessly S, Powell R 1989 Fatigue syndromes: a comparison of chronic 'postviral' fatigue with neuromuscular and affective disorders. Journal of Neurology, Neurosurgery and Psychiatry 52:940.

77. Landay A L, Jessop C, Lennette E T, Levy J A 1991 Chronic fatigue syndrome: clinical condition associated with immune activation. Lancet 338:707.

78. Sher E, Gotti C, Canal N, Scopetta C, Piccolo G, Evoli A, Clementi F 1989 Specificity of calcium channel auto-antibodies in Lambert-Eaton myasthenic syndrome. Lancet II:640-643.

79. Leys K, Lang B, Johnston I, Newsom-Davis J 1991 Calcium channel autoantibodies in the Lambert-Eaton myasthenic syndrome. Annals of Neurology 3:307-314.

80. Lennon V A, Lambert E H 1989 Autoantibodies bind solubilized calcium channel ω - conotoxin complexes from small cell lung carcinoma: a diagnostic aid for Lambert-Eaton myasthenic syndrome. Mayo Clinic Proceedings 64:1498-1504.

81. Motomura M, Johnston I, Lang B, Vincent A, Newsom-Davis J 1995 An improved diagnostic assay for Lambert-Eaton myasthenic syndrome. Journal of Neurology, Neurosurgery and Psychiatry 58:85-87.

82. Oosterhuis H J G H 1964 Studies in myasthenia gravis. Journal of the Neurological Sciences 1:512-546.

83. Oosterhuis H J G H 1996 Acquired blepharoptosis. Clinical Neurology and Neurosurgery 98:1-7.

Chapter 7

1. Querido A 1929 On myasthenia gravis. Journal Nervous and Mental disease 69:522-530.

2. Russell D S 1953 Histological changes in the striped muscles in myasthenia gravis. Journal of Pathology Bacteriology 65:279-289.

3. Duchenne de Boulogne G B A 1872 De l'electrisation localisée et de son application à la pathologie et à la therapeutique. Paris J.B. Balliere.

4. Singer Ch, Ashworth Underwood E 1962 The chemical transmission of nerve impulse. A short history of medicine. Oxford. At the Clarendon Press 564-577.

5. Roitt I 1956 ch 1.54.

6. Burnet MF 1959 ch 1.55.
7. Burnet MF 1962 ch 1.56.
8. Desmedt JE 1958 ch 1.49.
9. Grob D 1961 ch 1.48.
10. Bergmans J, Fannes-Breselow C, Gribomont B 1976 A reassessment of the neurophysiological evidence for presynaptic defect in myasthenia gravis. Electromyography and clinical Neurophysiology 16:337-351.
11. Famborough DM 1973 Ch 1.78.
12. Plomp J J, Van Kempen G Th, De Baets M B, Graus Y M F, Kuks J B M, Molenaar P C 1995 Acetylcholine release in myasthenia gravis: Regulation at Single Endplate level. Annals of Neurology 37:627-636.
13. Molenaar D 1993 ch 1.88.
14. Drachman D B 1994 Myasthenia gravis. New England Journal of Medicine 330:1797-1810.
15. Conti-Tronconi B 1994 ch 1.89a.
16. De Baets M H 1993 Experimental autoimmune myasthenia. In De Beats M H, Oosterhuis H J G H Ed. Myasthenia gravis CRC Press Broca Raton. 174-180.
17. Drachman DB 1978 ch 1.79.
18. Engel A G, Arahata K 1987 The membrane attack complex of complement at the endplate in myasthenia gravis. Annals of the New York Academy of Science 505:326-332.
19. Howard FM 1987 ch 3.43.
20. Vincent A, Whiting P J, Schluep M, Heidenreich F,Lang B, Roberts A, Willcox, Newsom-Davis J 1987 Antibody heterogeneity and specificity in myasthenia gravis. New York Academy of Science 505:106-120.
21. Nakano S, Engel A G 1993 Myasthenia gravis: Quantitative immunocytochemical analysis of inflammatory cells and detection of complement membrane attack complex at the endplate in 30 patients. Neurology 43:1167-1172.
22. Coërs C, Desmedt J E 1959 Mise en évidence d'une malformation caractéristique à la junction neuromusculaire dans la myasthéni. Corrélations histo- et pathophysiologiques Acta Neurologica Belgica 59:539-561.
23. Oosterhuis H J G H 1973 ch 2.45.
24. Guyon T, Levasseur P, Trouffault C, Cottin C, Gaud C, Berrih-Aknin S 1994 Regulation of acetylcholine receptor subunit variants in human myasthenia gravis: quantification of steady state levels of messenger RNA in muscle biopsy using the polymerase chain reaction. Journal of Clinical Investigation 94:16-24.
25. Theophipoulos A N 1993 Molecular pathology of Autoimmunity. In Bona C A Ed. The molecular pathology of autoimmune diseases. Harwood Academic Publishers Chur, Switserland Ch 1, 1-12.
26. Hohlfeld R, Toyka K V, Tzartos S J, Carson W, Conti-Tronconi B M 1987 Human T-helper lymphocytes in myasthenia gravis recognize the nicotinic receptor alpha subunit. Proc Natl Academy Science USA 84:5379-83.

27. Salvetti M, Jung S, Chang S F, Will H, Schalke B C, Wekerle H 1991 Acetylcholine receptor-specific T-lymphocyte clones in the normal human immune repertoire: target epitopes, HLA restriction, and membrane phenotypes. Annals of Neurology 29:508-16.

28. Sommer N, Harcourt G C, Willcox N, Beeson D, Newsom-Davis J 1991 Acetylcholine receptor-reactive T lymphocytes from healthy subjects and myasthenia gravis patients. Neurology 41:1270-6.

29. Melms A, Malcherek G, Gern U, Wiethölder H, Müller C A, Schoepfer R, Lindstrom J 1992 T cells from normal and myasthenic individuals recognize the human acetylcholine receptor: heterogeneity of antigenic sites on the -subunit. Annals of Neurology 31:311-318.

30. Pette M, Fujita, Kitze B et al 1990 Myelin basic protein-specific T lymphocyte lines from MS patients and healthy individuals. Neurology 40:1770-1776.

31. Smith C I, Aarli J A, Biberfeld P, et al 1983 Myasthenia gravis after bone-marrow transplantation. Evidence for a donor origin. The New English Journal of Medicine 309:1565-1568.

32. Lefvert A K, Bolme P, Hammerström L et al 1987 Bone marrow grafting selectively induces the production of acetylcholine receptor antibodies, immunoglobulins bearing related idiotypes, and anti idio typic bodies. Annals of the New York Academy of Science 505:825-827.

33. Nath A, Kerman R H, Novak I S, Wolinsky J S 1990 Immune studies in human immunodeficiency virus infection with myasthenia gravis: a case report. Neurology 40:581-583.

34. Vittecoq D, Morel C, Eymard B, Bach J F 1992 Recovery from myasthenia gravis of a patient infected with human immunodeficiency virus [letter]. Clinical Infectious Diseases 15:379-80.

35. Ahlberg R 1994 ch 4.162.

36. Aoki T 1985 ch 1.96.

37. Smith C I, von Sydow M, Hammerstroem L 1986 Viral etiology in myasthenia gravis? Analysis of thymic tissue. European Neurology 25:317-9.

38. Smith C I E, Hammerström L, Berg J V R 1978 Role of virus for the induction of myasthenia gravis. European Neurology 17:181-187.

39. Schwimmbeck P L, Dyrberg T, Drachman D B, Oldstone M B 1989 Molecular mimicry and myasthenia gravis. An autoantigenic site of the acetylcholine receptor alpha-subunit that has biologic activity and reacts immunochemically with herpes simplex virus. Journal Clinical Investigation 84:1174-80.

40. Seitz D, Fischer K, Hopf H Chr, Janzen R W C, Meyer W 1977 D-penicillamin-induzierte Myasthenie bei chronischer Polyarthritis. In Myasthenia Gravis. Thieme Verlag ed. G Hertel:162-165.

41. Tighe H P, Silverman G J, Carson D A 1993 Rheumatoïd arthritis. In: Bona C A Ed. The molecular pathology of autoimmune diseases, Harwood Academic Publishers. Chur. Ch. 21A, 347.

42. Oosterhuis H J G H, Willing-Versteegh E T B 1969 Human sensitivity to small doses of d-tubocurarine. Neurology (Minn) 19:760-764.

43. Wolf S M, Simmonds R L, Nastuk W L 1965 The effect of age and sex on sensitivity to d-tubocurarine in the rat. Proceedings of the Society of Experimental Biology (N.Y.) 117:1.

44. Kirchner T, Hoppe F, Schalke B, Mueller-Hermelink H K 1988 Microenvironment of thymic myoid cells in myasthenia gravis. Virchows Archives [B] 54:295-302.

45. Melm A, Schalke B C, Kirchner T, Mueller-Hermelink H K, Albert E, Wekerle H 1988 Thymus in myasthenia gravis. Isolation of T-lymphocyte lines specific for the nicotinic acetylcholine receptor from thymuses of myasthenic patients. Journal Clinical Investigation 81:902-8.

46. Sommer N, Willcox N, Harcourt G C, Newsom-Davis J 1990 Myasthenic thymus and thymoma are selectively enriched in acetylcholine receptor-reactive T cells. Annals of Neurology 28:312-9.

47. Hohlfeld R, Wekerle H 1994 The thymus in myasthenia gravis. Neurological Clinics 12:331-42.

48. Wakkach A, Guyon T, Bruand C, Tzartos S, Cohen-Kaminsky, Berrih-Aknin S 1996 Expression of acetylcholine receptor genes in human thymic epithelial cell's. Implications for myasthenia gravis. Journal of Immunology 157:3752-3760.

49. Kirschner T, Tzartos S, Hoppe F, Schalke B, Wekerle H, Mueller-Hermelink H K 1988 Pathogenesis of myasthenia gravis. Acetylcholine receptor-related antigenic determinants in tumor-free thymuses and thymic epithelial tumors. American Journal of Pathology 130:268-80.

50. Somnier F E 1994 ch 4.84.

51. Kuroda Y, Oda K, Neshige R, Shibasaki H 1984 Exacerbation of myasthenia gravis after removal of a thymoma having a membrane phenotype of suppressor T cells. Annals of Neurology 15:400-402.

52. Somnier F E, Keiding N, Paulson O B 1991 Epidemiology of myasthenia gravis in Denmark. A longitudinal and comprehensive population survey. Archives of Neurology 48:733-9.

53. Beekman R 1997 ch 2.85.

54. Feltkamp T E W 1974 ch 3.90.

55. Compston D A S 1980 ch 3.105.

56. Carlsson B, Wallin J, Pirskanen R, Matell G, Smith E I E 1990 Different HLA-DR-DQ associations in subgroups of idiopathic myasthenia gravis. Immunogenetics 31:285-290.

57. Simpson J A 1958 ch 1.43.

58. Oosterhuis H J G H 1989 ch 2.72.

59. McQuillan M P, Leone M G 1977 A treatment carol: thymectomy revisited. Neurology 27:1103-1106.

60. Rowland L P 1980 Controversies about the treatment of myasthenia gravis. Journal of Neurology, Neurosurgery, Psychiatry 43:644-659.

61. Evoli A 1996 ch 4.70.

62. Lanska D J 1990 Indications for thymectomy in myasthenia gravis. Neurology 40:1828-9.

63. Jaretzki A 1988 ch 4.66.

64. Donaldson D H, Ansher M, Horan S, Rutherford R B, Ringel S P 1990 The relationship of age to outcome in myasthenia gravis. Neurology 40:786-90.

65. Drachman D B, Mclntosh K R, Reim J, Balcer L 1993 Strategies for treatment of myasthenia gravis. Annals of the New York Academy of Science 681:515-528.

66. Strauss A 1960 ch 1.63.

67. Geld v.d. H 1963 ch 1.64.

68. Polanyi M 1969 Knowing and being. Chicago III: University of Chicago Press.

69. Simpson J A 1960 ch 1.58.

70. Myasthenia gravis 1966. Annals of the New York Academy of Science vol 135.

71. Jerne N K 1974 Towards a network theory of the immune system. Annals of Immunology (Paris) 125C:373-389.

72. Dwyer D S, Bradley R J, Urquhart C K, Kearney J F 1983 Natually occurring anti-idiotypic antibodies in myasthenia gravis patients. Nature 301:611-614.

73. Dwyer D S, Vakil M, Bradley R J, Oh S J, Kearney J F 1987 A possible cause of myasthenia gravis: idiotypic networks involving bacterial antigens. Annals of the New York Academy of Science 505:461-71.

74. Lefvert A K, Pirskanen R, Svanborg E 1985 Anti-idiotypic antibodies, acetylcholine receptor antibodies and disturbed neuromuscular function in healthy relatives to patients with myasthenia gravis. Journal of Neuroimmunology 9:41-53.

75. Vincent A C 1988 Are spontaneous anti-idiotypic antibodies against anti-acetylcholine receptor antibodies present in myasthenia gravis? Journal of Autoimmunology 1:131-42.

76. Ofosu-Appiah W, Mokhtarian F, Shirazian D, Grob D 1994 Production of anti-acetyl choline receptor -antibody in vitro by peripheral blood lymphocytes of patients with myasthenia gravis: role of immunoregulatory cells and monocytes.

77. Grob D, Arsura E L, Brunner N G, Namba T 1987 The course of myasthenia gravis and therapies affecting outcome. Annals of the New York Academy of Science 505:472-99.

LIST OF MG ORGANIZATIONS
OR NMD ASSOCIATIONS WITH MG GROUPS

AUSTRIA
Österreichische Gesellschaft
zur Bekämpfung der
Muskelkrankheiten (ÖGBM)
Postfach 23
A-1097 WIEN
Phone (43) 1 40400 3112

BELGIUM
Belgische Liga van MG
Mr Willy Thijs
Nieuwstraat 41
B-3511 KURINGEN-HASSELT
Phone (32) 11 22 75 47

BULGARIA
Bulgarian NMD Association
Mr P. Pintev
96 Pliska Street, Entr.2 App.4
ROUSSE 7004
Phone (359) 82 45 20 55

CROATIA
MG Society of Croatia
Mrs Josipa Gazibara
Kumiciceva 2
41000 ZAGREB
Phone (385) 1 440 639

DENMARK
Muskelsvindfonden
Vestervang 41
DK-8000 AARHUS-C

ESTONIA
Eesti Lihasehaigete Selts
(Estonian Ass. of Muscular Disorders)
Energia 8
EE-0013 TALLINN
Phone (372) 270 14 59 89 92

FINLAND
Suomen MG-yhdistys r.y.
PL 187
SF-00101 HELSINKI

FRANCE
Ass. Francaise contre les Myopathies
13 Place de Rungis
F-75013 PARIS
Phone (33) 1 69 47 28 28

GERMANY
Deutsche Gesellschaft
für Muskelkranke (DGM)
Im Moos 4
D-79112 FREIBURG
Tel.: (49) 7665 94470

Deutsche Myasthenie
Gesellschaft (DMG)
Langenmarckstrasse 106
D-28199 BREMEN
Phone (49) 421 59 20 60

239

GREAT BRITTAIN
Myasthenia Gravis Association
(MGA)
Keynes House, Chester Park
Alfreton Road
GB-DERBY DE21 4AS
Phone (44) 1332290219

HUNGARY
MEOSZ-MG Önsegitö
Beteg-Csoport
Özgida u. 22/a
H-1025 BUDAPEST
Phone (36) 1 325 62 87

ICELAND
MG Félag Islands
Ms O. Eysteinsdottir
Birkigrund 51
IS-200 KOPAVOGUR
Phone (345) 1 42 824

IRELAND
MGA-Ireland
Mrs Mary D. Lane
29 Chestnut Grove
NEWRY, BT 34 1JT
Northern Ireland
Phone (44) 693 684 66

ISRAEL
Ass. of MG in Israel
Mr Naftali Avital
30 Burla Street
IL-TEL-AVIV 69364
Phone (972) 3 699 18 58

ITALY
Ass. Ital. per la Lotta contra
la Miasthenia
Via Celoria 11
I-20133 MILANO
Phone (39) 2 23 60 280

LATVIA
Mrs M. Naudina
Indranu Street 11, App. 1
LV-1012 RIGA
Phone (371) 237 02 71

NETHERLANDS
Vereniging Spierziekten
Nederland (VSN)
Lt. Gen. van Heutszlaan 6
NL-3743 JN BAARN
Phone (31) 3554 18400

NORWAY
Foreningen for Muskelsyke
Post 116 Kjelsas
N-0411 OSLO 4
Phone (47) 2 23 50 50

POLAND
Polish Neuromuscular Ass.
c/o Dep. of Neurology
Ul. Banacha 1a
PL-02-097 WARSAW
Phone (48) 26 59 75 05

PORTUGAL
Ass. Portuges de MG/DNM
Centro de Estudos E. Moniz
Hospital de Santa Maria
Av. Prof. Egas Moniz
P-1699 LISBOA
Phone (351) 761 181 ext.64

SPAIN
Ass. Esp. de Enfermedades
Muskulares
Apartado de Correos 14170
ES-08080 BARCELONA
Phone (34) 3451 65 44

SWEDEN
Neurologist Handikappades
Riksforbund (NHR)
Box 3284
S-103 65 STOCKHOLM
Phone (46) 8 67 77 010

SWITZERLAND
Schweizerische Gesellschaft für
Muskelkrankheiten (SGMK)
Forchstrasse 136
CH-8032 ZÜRICH
Phone (41) 1 422 16 34

TURKEY
Association of Muscle Disorders
Hatboyu Cad., No: 12 YESILKÖY
34800 ISTANBUL
Phone (90) 1 212 573 09 75

INDEX

A

Acetazolamide 75
Acetylcholine (ACh) 6, 15, 45, 73, 98, 172, 173, 175
Acetylcholinereceptor (AChR) 9, 11, 13, 14, 73, 173
   cross-linking 174
   deficiencies 46, 149
   degradation 11
   mutations in CMS 46, 146
   subunits 46, 177
Acetylcholinesterase 15, 73
AChR-ab 11, 55-56, 73, 96, 104-105, 114-116, 175, 178
   blocking 45
   in children 47, 129, 131
   decrease after thymectomy 77, 105
   heterogeneity 14
   monoclonal 91, 176, 182
   sensitivity 50
   specificity 50
   TE 671 66
Acid maltase deficiency 166
ACTH (adreno corticotrope hormone) 10,87
Addison's disease 42, 111, 166
Adrenalitis 42, 111
Age at onset 39-40
AIDS 175
Alcohol 71,85
Aldactone A
Allopurinol 85
Alopecia totalis 111
Alpha Bungarotoxin 11
Alpha feto protein 45
AMA see antibodies, striated muscle

Ambenomium-CI 5, 6, 15, 71, 72
Amenorrhoea, secondary 111
Aminoglycosides 75, 98, 166
Aminophylline 98
ALS (amyotrophic lateral sclerosis) 54, 56, 60, 106, 159, 165
Anaemia
   haemolytic 42
   pure red cell 42, 111, 182
Anaesthesia 97-98
Animal models of myasthenia gravis 14, 173
Anorexia nervosa 103
Anovulatory drugs 69
Antiarrhytmic drugs 75
Antibiotics 74-75, 87
Antibodies
   to acetylcholinereceptor (see AChR)
   non disease specific 61-62
   end-plates 10
   to muscarine AChR 62
   to myosin 61
   to neuro blastoblastoma 61
   to nuclear factors 10, 61
   to presynaptic membrane 62
   to reticulin 61
   to rheumatoid factors 62
   to striated muscle 10, 60-61, 105-106, 116, 154
   in thymoma 60
   to thyroid globulin 10, 56, 163
   to titin 61
   to vinculin 61
   to viruses
   to Voltage Sensitive Calcium channels 168

Anticholinesterases 15, 46, 69-74, 87,
    113, 110, 125, 170, 175
    in diagnosis 54, 158
    irreversible 15
    principle of action 73
    serum measurements 98
    side effects 70
Antidepressive drugs 75
Antiepileptic drugs 75
Antihelmintic drugs 75
Antihypertensive drugs 75
Antilymphocyte globulins 91
Antimalaria drugs 75
Antirheumatic drugs 75
Antimuscle antibodies (AMA) 60-61
Anxiety attacks 112-113
Aphonia 29, 169
Apnoea, prolonged 19, 97, 149, 166
    sleep 96
Arthralgia 85, 132
Articulation 29
Arthrogryposis 46
Associations of patients 97,
Asthenic syndrome, see Chronic fatigue
    syndrome
Atrophy, see Muscle atrophy
Atropin 70, 72, 125
Atropin-neostigmine test 53, 54, 66
Auto-immune diseases, associated 41-
    43, 110, 116, 121, 137, 154, 176
Auto-immune hypothesis 9-15, 173,
    175-177
Autonomic disturbance
    in botulism 164
    in crisis 86
    in LEMS 167
Autopsy 1, 4, 110, 172
Azathioprine 10, 80-85, 110, 132, 133,
    135, 136, 182
    side effects 82, 133-135

B

Basal cell carcinoma, 86, 110, 135
Basilar artery insufficiency 160, 164
Bell's phenomenon 29, 48
Bell's palsy 27
Benzodiazepines 74-75, 97
Beta-blockers 74-75, 98
Biliary cirrhosis 56
Blalock 7
Blepharospasm 49, 112, 157, 159
B-lymphocytes 11, 174, 177, 182
Bone densimetry 84, 135, 156
Bone marrow depression 83
Bone marrow grafting 56, 175
Botulism 54, 158, 160, 164
Brain stem syndrome 54, 160
    auditory evoked potentials 96
Breast feeding 69
Brocho constriction 53, 113
Bulbäre neurose 16
Bulbar paralyse, asthenic 16
Bulbar symptoms 19, 26-30, 45
    differential diagnosis 164, 165
Bungarotoxin 11
Burnet 173
Bromide 98

C

Calcium-influx blocker 121
Cancer, see Malignancy
Carbamazepine, side effect 164
Carcinoma, basal cell 86, 110, 135
Carotid aneurysm 54
Carpal tunnel syndrome 85, 133
Cataract 81, 84, 134
Catecholamines 99, 177
Caution, drugs to be used with 74-75
Cellulair immunity 11-12
    thymectomy 77, 78
Central nervous system involvement 96
Cephalosporins 87

Chewing 26
Chinese patients 47, 62
Chlorambucil, side effects 75, 110, 112, 135
Chloroquine, side effect 75, 99, 165
Chlorpromazin, side effect 75, 99
Cholinergic crises, see Crises, cholinergic
Chronic fatigue syndrome 159, 165, 169-170
Chronic Obstructive Respiratory Disease (COPD) 68, 113
Classification of clinical state of myasthenia gravis 17, 34-36
Clinical condition, assessment of 50-53
Clonal selection theory 173
CMAP compound muscle action potential 57
CMS see congenital myasthenic syndrome
Colistin, side effect 75
Colitis ulcerosa 111
Communication, problems of 95
Complement fractions 11
  activation 11, 174
Computer tomography in diagnosis of thymoma 63-64, 78, 138
Congenital Familial MG 45-46, 144-145, 156
Congenital malformations 86
Congenital myasthenic syndrome 14, 17, 44-46, 144-151, 153
Congenital paucity of synaptics clefts (CPSC) 45, 46, 147-149
Consciousness, loss of 31, 86
Contracture, muscle 45
Contrast agents 75, 86
Convergence spasm 160, 16
Conversion 112, 114, 159, 165
Corticosteroids 73, 79-85, 81
  side effects
  see also: Prednisone
Counting test 29, 51
Course of MG 35-37

CPEO see ophthalmoplegia
Crisis 7, 35, 37, 86-88, 125, 178
  cholinergic 86-87
  incidence 35, 104, 178
  myasthenic 86-87
Crohn's disease 42, 111
Curare 5, 6, 9, 15, 86, 155, 166, 176
Curariform substance 9, 16, 172
Curare test in diagnosis of myasthenia gravis 115
Cushing's syndrome
  side effect of corticosteroids 81, 134
Cyclophosphamide 90, 135, 136
Cyclosporine 90, 121, 135

D

Deafness 28
Death, cause of, 104, 142, 154
  rate 40-41
Decrement, see Electromyography
Denervation
Depression 81
Dermatochalazis 120, 161
Diabetes mellitus 81, 85, 111, 134
Diagnosis of myasthenia gravis 49, 65-66
  delay in: 49, 102
Diaminopyridine 3, 4, 46, 168
Diary keeping 68
Diazepam, effect of, 74-75
Differential diagnosis of myasthenia gravis 155-169
Diphenylhydantion, side effects 75
Diplopia 18-25, 51, 115, 116, 118, 157, 162, 165, 166, 169
Disability Score (DS) 36, 104
Distigmin 71, 72
Diuretic drugs, side effects 73
Double vision, see diplopia
Down's syndrome 56
Drooping eyelids, see ptosis, 162

Dropping feet 106-107
  fingers 27, 106
Drugs to be used with caution 73-74
Dynamometer 32, 51-53, 66
Dysarthria 19, 26, 51, 165
Dysphagia 19, 26, 30, 51, 164, 165
Dyspnoea 32, 86
Dysthyroid ophthalmoplegia, 118, 121, 160
Dystonia focal 112

E

Early onset MG 17, 19, 121-129, 152, 178
Early treatments 5
Eaton-Lambert (myasthenic syndrome), see Lambert-Eaton syndrome
Edgeworth 5
Edrophonium 5, 6, 15, 67, 70, 164
  test 50, 54, 114, 125
  see also: Tensilon
Electrencephalography 96
Electromyography 57-60, 115, 147, 158
  convential 67
  decrement in 50, 57
  surface 48
Emotions, effect on myasthenia gravis 68, 86
Endocrinopathy 166
Endplate
  anatomy 12, 13, 14. 168
  electronmicroscopic data 12, 168
  physiology 168
Ephedrine 5, 73, 98, 125
Epidemiology 38-41, 101, 115, 121, 132, 137
Epilepsy 111, 96
Epithelial cells, thymic 76
Erb 1, 2
Eserine, see Physostigmin
Exacerbation 45, 47, 117, 123, 132, 177, 178, 182

Examination of the myasthenic patient 50-53
Exertion 32, 50-53, 170
Exhaustion 31, 48, 175
Experimental auto-immune myasthenia gravis (EAMG) 11
Experimental therapies 89, 182
Extended arm test 31, 32, 51
Extended leg test 51
External influences 38
Extra pyramidal syndrome, ptosis 159
Eye lid apraxia 112
  retraction 24, 163
  supports 119, 155
Eye muscle paresis 23
  operations 120
Eye symptoms, see Ocular symptoms

F

Facial expression 27-29
Falls, sudden 30
Familial myasthenia gravis 44
Familial infantile myasthenia gravis 45, 144-145
Familial limb girdle myasthenia 46
Fasciculations 70
Faradic stimulation 3, 172
Fatigue, see also exhaustion 30, 32, 48, 50
Female predominance 10, 40, 177
Fertility, female 129-130
  male 127
Fever, 38, 68, 86
Fisher's syndrome 163

G

Gadolinium 98
Gammaglobulin in myasthenia gravis treatment 89-90, 133
Gastritis, auto-immune 42, 111

Gastrointestinal disturbance 70, 81, 82, 83, 85, 134, 135
Genetics see heredity,
Gentamycin, side effect 75, 99
Germinal centres, in thymus 7, 8, 123, 155, 177
    in other auto-immune diseases 155
Glasses, bifocal 119
Glomerulonephritis 42
Glycolcoll 15
Goldflam 1, 2, 16
Grave's disease, see Thyroid disease
Grip strength 32, 52
Guillain-Barré syndrome 54, 160

H

Head lifting test 30
Haematological disease 56
Haemodialysis 11
Halotane 98
Hashimoto's disease, see Thyroiditis
Heart muscle, see Myocarditis
Hemicholinium 9
Hemolytic anemia 42, 111
Hepatotoxicity 83, 85, 111
Heredity of myasthenia gravis 43, 45, 62, 176
Hérard 2, 16
Hering, law of, 24
Herpes zoster 81, 83, 85, 134, 135, 176
History of myasthenia gravis 1-16, 172-173
H.I.V. 1-infection 175
HLA (human leucocyte antigen) 14, 62, 121, 123, 137, 176, 178
Hoarseness 29
Humoral immunity 14, 175
Hypalgesia 27
Hypergammaglobulinaemia 61, 111
Hyperplasia of thymus 8
Hypertension 81, 86, 134
    benign intracranial 134

Hyperthyroidism 38, 42, 86, 110, 111, 163
Hyperventilation 113
Hypogammaglobulinaemia 111
Hypokaliaemia 166
Hypothyroidism 38, 42, 110, 111

I

Idiotype antibodies 92, 184
Immunity
    cellular 11, 12, 71
    humoral 10, 71
Immunoadsorption 88
Immunofluorescence technique 10, 11
Immunoglobulins 91-92, 99
Immunomodulation 11, 62, 177
Immunoprecipation test for AChR-ab 55
Immunosuppressive drugs 47, 73, 125-129, 130, 132, 180, 182-183
Imuran, see Azathioprine
Incidence of myasthenia gravis 38-39
Incontinence, urine 33
Infantile myasthenia gravis 44, 47, 131-132, 155-156
Infections, influence on myasthenia gravis 38
    by azathioprine 83, 135
    by corticosteroids 81, 134
INH 85
Inspiratory stridor 86
Intercostal biopsy 9, 143-150
Inferon-alpha 75
Intoxication
    anticholinesterases 84
    carbamazepine 160
    clostridium botulinum 160, 164
    phenytoin 160
    snake poison 158, 164
Intracranial hypertension 81, 134
Intraspinal liposis 81
Ion conductance channel 174

Irradiation of thymoma 7, 79, 181-182
    total body - 91

J

Japanese patients 47,62
Jitter in single fibre electromyography
    58-60
Jolly 1-3, 172
Jolly, reaction of, 2, 3, 9
Juvenile myasthenia gravis 44

K

Kanamycine, side effect, 75
Keynes 7, 179
Kneebending 32

L

Lambert-Eaton myasthenic syndrome
    42, 54, 58, 159, 160, 165, 166-169
Late onset MG 17, 19, 321-136, 152,
    178
Laughing, vertical 27, 28
Levator dehiscence-disinsertion
    syndrome 159, 161
Leucopenia 81, 85
Lidocaine, side effect 73
Limb muscle symptoms 19, 30-33, 165
    examination 32
Lithium carbonate, side effect 75, 99
Local anaesthetics, side effects 75
Lundie loop in treatment of ptosis 155
Lung carcinoma, small cell 166-168
Lung function tests 32
Lupus erythematosus disseminatus 42,
    56, 111
Lymphfollicles, see Germinal centres
Lymphocytes, peripheral blood 105, 183
Lymphoproliferative diseases 110-111

Lymphorrhages in muscle 4, 172, 173,
    174

M

Macrocytosis 81, 83, 85
Main immunogenic region 13-14, 174
Major Histocompatibility Complex 176,
    184
Malignancies
    associated with myasthenia gravis
    110-111, 121
    in Lambert-Eaton syndrome 166-
    168
    thymoma and 41, 112, 137
Mary Walker effect 16
Masticatory muscles 30
Medication, see treatments
Memory function 96, 146
Menstruation, effect on myasthenia
    gravis 38, 68
Meige syndrome 159, 160, 161
Membrane attack complex 11, 174
Mercaptopurine 85, 90, 110, 112
Mestinon, see Pyridostigmine
Metabolic myopathy 166
Methotrexate 90, 135
Methylcellulose 98
Methyl prednisolone 80
Mitochondrial myopathy 54, 163, 166
Molecular mimicry 176, 184
Mood changes 81, 134
Mortality rate 39-40, 104
MRI, mediastinum 63-64, 77
Multiple sclerosis 42-43, 60, 111, 159,
    160, 164, 175
Muscle atrophy 33-34, 106-109, 154,
    158, 175
Muscle biopsy data, 109, 158, 175
    conduction velocity 48
Muscle unit potential (MUP) 67
Muscle relaxants, effect on myasthenia
    gravis 97-98

Myasthenia gravis pseudo
 paralytica 3
Myasthenia gravis in animals 9
Myasthenic myopathy 33
Myasthenischer Paralyse 15
Myocarditis 86, 109
 thymoma 86, 109, 154
Myoid cells in thymus 14, 177
Myopathy 33, 60, 81, 106
Myotonic dystrophy 58, 160, 162, 164
Mytelase, see Ambenonium-CI

N

Narcosis, see Anaesthesia
Natural course of myasthenia gravis 35,
 37, 179
Neck muscle weakness 26
Neomycine, side effect 75
Neonatal myasthenia gravis 10, 17, 43-
 45, 129-131
Neoplasms, see Malignancies
Neostigmine 5, 53, 69-72, 74, 98
 test 50
Nephrotic syndrome 111
Nerve stimulation tests, see EMG
Neuroleptic drugs, side effects 73
Neurological diseases, associated 112
Neuromuscular junction, see End-plate
Neuromuscular transmission 9, 58, 73,
 98-99, 173
 safety margin 155, 177
Neuropathy 33, 60
Neurosis 93
Non Hodgkin lymphoma 82, 110, 128
Nystagmography 24
Nystagmoid movements 24

O

Obesity 81
Ocular symptoms 18-25, 102, 155

Ocular myasthenia gravis (OMG) 17,
 114-121, 178
 diagnosis 114-115
 differential diagnosis 158-165
 examination 20-25
 incidence 47
 symptoms and signs 10, 20-25
 thymectomy 76
 treatment 118-119, 125-126
Oculopharyngeal myopathy 160, 164
Onset, age at, 39-40
 symptoms at 19
Operation 68, 73, 97
 eye muscle 120
 ptosis 120
Ophthalmoplegia 33, 45, 54, 67, 106
 chronic progressive external 60,
 160, 162, 163
 drug induced 164-165
 dysthyroid 118, 121, 163
 internuclear 164
 painful 163
 pseudo internuclear 23, 164
Oppenheim 1, 2, 20
Orbicularis oculi weakness 22, 27, 67
Orbicularis oris weakness 27, 29
Osserman's categories 34
Osteoporosis 81, 84, 134, 156
Overdosage anti AChE 72, 86, 118

P

Palatal weakness 30
Palpebral fissure widening 22, 24
Pancreatitis 81, 83, 85
Pancytopenia 83, 111, 182
Paraesthesias 27, 158, 168
Paralysie glosso-labiolaryngée 16
Paraneoplastic syndrome 14, 177
Patient's Associations 97,
Pathophysiology 174
Peak flow measurements 30, 32
Peek sign 22

Pemphigus 42
Penicillamin 56, 61, 74, 116, 121, 133, 176, 184
    inducing myasthenia gravis 14, 116, 159, 164
Periodic paralysis 164
Pernicious anaemia 42, 111
Pharyngeal muscle insufficiency 30
Phenytoin, side effect 75, 99, 164
Phrenicus nerve, lesion 125
Physiotherapy 92-93
Physostigmin 5, 6, 15, 172
Piperazine, side effect 75
Plasma-pheresis (exchange) 14, 84, 88-89, 99, 133, 180
    in myasthenic crises 86, 87
Pneumomediastinography 63, 137
Polioencephalitis 16
Polymyalgia rheumatica 111
Polymyositis 33, 42, 54, 109, 111, 165-166
Polymixin B, side effect 75, 99
Postsynaptic membrane 14, 174
Posttetanic exhaustion 58
Potassium 85
Prednisone 11, 79-85, 107, 109, 119, 120, 123, 181-182
    alternate day 83
    in crises 87
    exacerbation at onset 83, 84
    examination before starting 84
    side effects 81, 133-134
    thymoma 63
Pregnancy 38, 129-131
Prevalence rate 38-39, 101
Primary ovarian failure 42
Prism, press-on 118
Probanthine 70
Procainamide, side effect 75,99
Prognosis 35, 97
Prolonged eye lid closure 112
Propranolol, side effect 75
Prostigmin 5, 6, 15
Pseudo-internuclear ophthalmoplegia 23

Pseudo myasthenia 56, 157-158
Pseudo ptosis 159-162
Psoriasis 111
Psychiatric disease 103, 112
Psychological aspects 93-97, 125-128, 177
    premorbid personality 93
Psychotic periods 81, 95, 134
Ptosis 18-25, 45, 51, 115, 116, 157-163, 166
    fluctuating 20
    at awakening 20
    shift 20
    slowly progressive 160, 163
    therapeutic advise 118
Puerperium, effect on myasthenia gravis 38, 130
Pupil areflexia 24, 48
Pymantel palmoate 75, 99
Pyridostigmine 5, 6, 69-74, 98, 168
    plasma measurements 97
    side effects 70

Q

Qualification systems 34-35
Quinidine 38, 74-75, 147
Quinine 38, 74-75, 147
Quiver movements 23

R

Radiation therapy
    in treatment of thymoma 78, 138-139
    side effects 138
Reaction centres, see Germinal centres
Reaction to muscle relaxants 9, 97-98
Receptors of acetylcholine see Acetylcholinereceptor
Red-green glass test 23
Regurgitation of fluids 26

Reinnervation in muscle 175
Relatives of MG patients 61, 60
Remission rate of myasthenia gravis 35,
    132, 179
    after thymectomy 74-76, 122-124
Repetitive nerve stimulation, see
    Electromyography
Resochine, side effect 75
Respiration, symptoms at onset 19, 31
Rest: 73
Restlessness 87
Rethymectomy 64, 123, 124, 180
Retro-orbital tumour 160, 164
Rheumatoid arthritis 42, 56, 61, 74, 110,
    111, 137, 176
Rire verticale 28
Rubinstein-Taybi syndrome 131

S

Saccadic eye movements 24
Sarcoidosis 42, 111
Scleroderma 42
Scoring system 34, 36
Seronegative myasthenia gravis 56, 67,
    147, 158
Severity, maximum clinical 39-40, 104
Simpson 10, 173, 184
Single fibre electromyography 58-60,
    67, 164, 165
Sinus caroticus denervation 5
Sjögren's disease 42, 111
Sleep, apnoea 96
Skin changes 81, 134
    infections 85
Slow channel syndrome 45, 58, 144-148,
    159
Snake venoms 10, 158
Snarl, myasthenic 27
Somatization disorder 49, 112, 114, 159
Speech therapy 92
Splenectomy 99
Spironolacton 136

Stapedius reflexometry 28
Streptomycin, side effect 75
Strabismus, latent 162
Stress 38, 86
Succinylcholine 6, 15
Sunglasses 20
Surgery 68, 86, 97-98
Suxamethonium 97
Swallowing 30, 51
Synaps, see End-plate
Systemic lupus erythematodes 42, 56

T

Tardive dyskinesia 56
Tensilon test 53, 54, 87
Temperature 38, 68, 86
Test, diagnostic 50
    sensitivity 67
    specificity 67
Tetracycline, side effect 74-75, 99
T helper cells 11, 13, 73, 77, 174, 175,
    177, 182
Therapies of myasthenia gravis, early 5
Thoracic duct lymph drainage 11
Thrombopenia, A-1, 111
Thrombosis 81, 134
Thymectomy 7-9, 47, 75-77, 122-125,
    131, 179-182
    cervical 64, 76, 124, 180
    complications 124-125
    indications 76, 122-123
    reoperation 77, 123, 124, 132
    results 7-9, 47, 75-77, 121-122
    surgical approach 76
    thoracoscopic 64
Thymoma 4, 19, 137-143, 153, 177, 178
    associated diseases 79, 137
    chemotherapy 78, 181-182
    classification 78
    diagnosis 63-64, 132, 137-139
    incidence 41
    invasiviness 78, 139-140, 181-182

metastases 79, 181
    prognosis 79, 143, 182
    radiological examination 63-64
    radiotherapy 78, 139, 182
    recurrence 78, 138, 141
    without MG 56, 65
Thymomectomy 7, 8, 78-79, 139-143
    effect on myasthenia gravis 142
Thymus 176-178
    anatomy 74
    extracts 5
    function 177
    histology 123, 132, 143, 155
    hyperplasia 8
Thyroid diseases 42, 87, 111, 163
Thyrotoxicosis 87
Titin antibodies to, 61
Tobramycin, side effect 75
Tolosa-Hunt syndrome 163
Tongue
    atrophy 34, 107
    protrusion of 109
    thick 27
    weakness 30
Torticollis 112
Tracheostomy 87, 124-125, 179
Treatment of myasthenia gravis 68-97,
    139-141, 178-182
    plan 69, 73
Trials, controlled 99, 180
Tricho epithelioma 42
Trihexyphenidyl 75
Trimethadione, side effect 75
Trunk symptoms 30-33
    examination 32, 51
T suppressor cells 77
Tubocurarine see curare
Tumour of the thymus, see Thymoma
Twin studies in Myasthenia gravis 43,
    176

U

Ulcerative colitis, 42
Unconciousness 31, 86
Urine incontinence 33, 70

V

Vaccinations 86
Vasculitis 111, 161
Vena cava syndrome 139, 181
Vencuronium 97
Ventilation, artifical, 86-87, 124
Ventilatory insufficiency, 71 see also
    crisis
Verapamil 75, 99
Vertebral collapse 134
Vinculin, antibody to 61
Viruses, role in auto-immunity 15, 176
Vital capacity measurements 32, 51, 86
Vitiligo 111
Voice, nasality 26, 29
Voltage Stimulated Calcium Channels
    (VSCS) 168

W

Walker, Mary 5, 172
    effect 16
Weigert 4
Weight loss 26
Wernicke-Korsakow, syndrome 160
Willis, Thomas 16

For Product Safety Concerns and Information please contact our EU representative GPSR@taylorandfrancis.com Taylor & Francis Verlag GmbH, Kaufingerstraße 24, 80331 München, Germany

T - #0105 - 160425 - C0 - 234/156/14 - PB - 9789090106007 - Gloss Lamination